Jan 9/86

S0-BXG-607

STRESS FOR SUCCESS

A Holistic Approach to Stress
and Its Management

STRESS FOR SUCCESS

A Holistic Approach to Stress
and Its Management

Donald Roy Morse, D.D.S., M.A.
Associate Professor
Department of Endodontology
Temple University School of Dentistry
Philadelphia, Pennsylvania

M. Lawrence Furst, Ph. D., M.P.H.
Associate Professor
Division of Behavioral Sciences
Temple University Health Sciences Center
Philadelphia, Pennsylvania

With a Foreword by
Patricia Carrington, Ph.D.
Department of Psychology, Princeton University, Princeton, New Jersey

VAN NOSTRAND REINHOLD COMPANY
NEW YORK   CINCINNATI   TORONTO   LONDON   MELBOURNE
LONDON   TORONTO   MELBOURNE

Van Nostrand Reinhold Company Regional Offices:
New York   Cincinnati   Atlanta   Dallas   San Francisco

Van Nostrand Reinhold Company International Offices:
London   Toronto   Melbourne

Copyright © 1979 by Litton Educational Publishing, Inc.

Library of Congress Catalog Card Number: 79-15002
ISBN: 0-442-26646-4
ISBN: 0-442-26228-0 pbk.

All rights reserved. No part of this work covered by the copyright hereon may
be reproduced or used in any form or by any means—graphic, electronic, or
mechanical, including photocopying, recording, taping, or information storage
and retrieval systems—without permission of the publisher.

Manufactured in the United States of America

Published by Van Nostrand Reinhold Company
135 West 50th Street, New York, N.Y. 10020

Published simultaneously in Canada by Van Nostrand Reinhold Ltd.

15 14 13 12 11 10 9 8 7 6 5 4 3 2 1

Library of Congress Cataloging in Publication Data

Morse, Donald R
    Stress for success

    Bibliography: p. 359
    Includes indexes.
    1. Stress (Psychology) 2. Psychology,
Pathological. 3. Medicine, Psychosomatic.
I. Furst, Merrick L., joint author. II. Title.
[DNLM: 1. Stress. 2. Stress, Psychological.
WM172 M884s]
BF575.S75M67   616'.001'9   79-15002
ISBN: 0-442-26646-4
ISBN: 0-442-26228-0 pbk.

Foreword

Until very recently, people suffering from illnesses were viewed as relatively helpless victims of invading forces (microbes, viruses, and so on), and the effective treatment was thought to be an attack on these biological invaders by chemical or mechanical means. Such a counterattack is an external one—by drugs or surgery—and is usually launched *after the fact,* i.e., when the individual is already showing signs of being ill.

Obviously this "invader-invaded" view of illness is the appropriate one in a number of circumstances—in fact it is the cornerstone of modern medicine. But today it is no longer the *sole* approach.

Nonpharmaceutical preventive measures are rapidly gaining momentum and are leading us to a new view of each person's responsibility for his or her own state of health. The individual is increasingly considered to play a major role in creating his or her own good or ill health. This is a fundamental shift in perspective. It implies that we can alter the odds in our favor.

That we very much need to alter them becomes apparent when we view the rapidly accumulating data on the toll that stress takes in terms of our national health. An example of this is the fact that for executives alone, American industry loses between $10 billion and $20 billion annually through lost work days, hospitalization and early death caused by stress.* With society's stress index spiraling and strategies to combat it proliferating, some 6,000 research reports a year are now generated on this crucial subject.

Prescribing tranquilizers is still the most popular approach to controlling stress, with their manufacture a multi-billion-dollar industry, but the use of nonchemical means of lowering stress is increasing as growing numbers of people seek natural means of stress reduction such as relaxation and exercise techniques. One reason for this is that there is no danger of becoming addicted to these approaches. In addition, rather than furthering a reliance on chemical aids (which ultimately brings about a feeling of dependence and futility), these new stress-reducing techniques increase personal autonomy and self-pride and add to the basic enjoyment of life.

Reporting on stress and these new means of managing it, Donald Morse and Larry Furst have taken a significant step. They have assembled nuggets of information from many diverse fields to forge a multifaceted approach to stress management that can easily be understood by the untrained person as well as the health professional. Their statement is remarkably unbiased, with no single technique emphasized at the expense of other equally useful ones. The result is an impressive survey of stress factors in our lives today and a wealth of usable information on how to combat them.

The work done by Morse and Furst is particularly interesting to me because their research studies are so relevant to my own field. I am engaged in research on the westernized meditative-relaxation techniques, and in this area the authors have had the courage to try some exciting things. They were the first researchers to combine meditation with hypnosis, and the first to study the use of meditation for pain control (either meditation used by itself, or as a form of hypnotic induction); and they have conducted a pioneering study on the differential effects of internally repeated sounds (mantras) with varying types of personalities. In their approach to stress control,

* The New York Times Magazine, November 20, 1977, p. 49.

they have also made imaginative use of what I have termed the "meditative mood."

Meditation, conceived of in its broadest sense, has been with us, in one form or the other, through all of recorded history. It appears to be rooted in the predilection of human beings to retreat periodically from the pressures and cares of the external world and turn inward to experience a mentally "idling" state, which possesses distinct therapeutic qualities, of both a stabilizing and a pain-mitigating nature.

The meditative mood is characterized by a dreamy, drifting state of consciousness that is often accompanied by an unusual openness to experiences ordinarily obscured by active, goal-directed awareness, and by a sense of harmony with our own inner rhythms and the greater rhythms of the universe. It is an antianxiety state, a time when we are in control of ourselves and can establish an inner balance.

What is particularly important is that *all* of us have experienced this meditative mood at times—perhaps when we were close to nature; perhaps when we were lying in the darkness just before going to sleep; or at any other moment when a sense of tranquility and inner stillness was deeply felt. It is therefore readily available for therapeutic purposes.

Some people require little assistance in entering such a mood. They are fortunate enough to experience a sense of inner silence frequently enough in the course of everyday life that it is second nature to them. This ability to establish a meditative mood at will may have a profound effect upon their lives—bring them back periodically to an inner "center" of themselves, as though a psychological gyroscope were working to right a balance. For such people, too much outwardly focused stimulation tends automatically to be followed by a period during which the motor seems to idle as the person regains a balance between his or her inner and outer self, between the experiencing of activity and the experience of being. Perhaps such people as these do not need *formal* meditation for purposes of maintaining an optimal adjustment to life, and they may well be more stress-resistant than others.

For most of those living in modern, industrialized society, however, the pace of life is determined largely by economic considerations rather than by the rhythms of human life or natural growing things, and there is a dearth of spontaneously occurring quiet inner space into which the individual can retreat for refurbishing. Therefore the authors supply those of us faced with these modern high-pressure lifestyles with numerous ways of reducing tension by returning to satisfying inner rhythms of rest, exercise and relaxation. Among the methods they advocate is one I know particularly well because it relates to my special area of research—the eliciting of the "relaxation response."

Beyond the immediate tension-reducing effects of the meditative mood, there is another benefit that comes to us when we systematically schedule-in deeply quiet moments in our lives. A leisurely stroll, a prayer or listening to the gentle patter of rain as "change of pace" are not possible for most of us in today's world, especially during working hours. Even in our leisure time we may subject ourselves to prolonged sensory bombardment from a television set rather than seek quietude. Within this context of haste and perpetual stimulation, the average human being moves from task to task with almost no time to sense his or her own self and to reaffirm the basic tenet "I exist."

It is scarcely surprising, therefore, that the conflicts engendered by our uncertain and stressful environment are often left unresolved and that their effects upon the human organism may accumulate until a variety of psychosomatic illnesses or behavioral disturbances emerge and a stress-prone individual is created. Although the more fortunate may not become ill from such conflicts, they will in all likelihood experience a sense of meaninglessness or unease about their lives—they will have lost touch with the core of their beings.

It is within this vacuum within our society that the new meditative techniques have gained their popularity. The widespread use of commercially available forms of meditation (and more recently of clinically based forms such as CSM or Benson's Technique*) undoubtedly reflects a hunger on the part of Westerners for the meditative mood. Not being supplied this kind of inner refurbishing by other modalities in our society, many people are now turning to formal meditation as a means for attaining it.

This has resulted in enough solid research on the meditative-

---

* CSM (Clinically Standardized Meditation) is a modern form of mantra meditation taught by the use of tapes and a programmed instruction text; Benson's Technique is a modern form of breathing meditation.

relaxation techniques that the question to be answered is no longer whether meditative relaxation works to relieve stress (it very often does), but rather for *whom* and under what circumstances. We must also ask *which* meditative-relaxation technique is most beneficial for a particular individual. It is to these questions that those conducting research on the meditative-relaxation techniques are now addressing themselves.

Within this important area of inquiry, the present book assumes a unique place. Morse and Furst have drawn together a mass of data and related it to a goal that has meaning for all of us—the introduction of a more truly human perspective into our lives. The authors do not see people as present or future "patients" to be "managed." Nor do they see them as dependent upon outside assistance to meet *all* health needs. Instead they clearly view the individual as being in charge of his or her own destiny, as free to choose a rewarding lifestyle and in so doing to reduce excess stress and the likelihood of premature unnecessary illness. The emphasis in this book is upon the positive aspects of life. The authors ask us to increase our enjoyment and self-confidence; we are not asked to concentrate upon disease and distress per se—a true shift of emphasis.

We can all benefit by heeding the authors' well-stated message. By so doing we will be partaking of a new era in health care—an era in which the "humanistic" management of stress may well be the most satisfying as well as one of the most effective of all preventive medicine strategies.

PATRICIA CARRINGTON, PH.D.
Department of Psychology
Princeton University
Author of *Freedom in Meditation*

Preface

Stress has been defined as a "mentally or emotionally disruptive or disquieting influence; distress;" whereas one definition of success is "the achievement of something desired; planned or attempted; the gaining of fame or prosperity."* A logical question you might ask is: How can stress, which is negative lead to success, which is positive? Let's investigate.

The dictionary definition of stress is similar to the one that most people hold; stress = distress. Yet as is emphasized later, distress is only one type of stress. Another type of stress is actually beneficial. It is known as positive stress or eustress. It can occur in many day-to-day activities including working, gardening, running, dancing and lovemaking. And recent findings have shown that physiological and psychological benefits can accrue from positive stress. Even negative stress or distress is necessary at times for survival. For example, suddenly swerving your car away from an oncoming car to avoid a fatal

* Morris, W., ed. The American Heritage Dictionary of the English Language. New York: American Heritage Publishing Co. Inc., 1969.

collision creates a lot of temporary distress, but it is a life-saving move.

All right! you may add, stress may help someone to survive at times and there may be some healthful benefits from it, but how can stress lead to success? The answer lies in emphasis. As the familiar song states, "you've got to accentuate the positive" and at the same time cut down on the negative. By managing stress positively, one can achieve health, happiness, prosperity and longevity, all aspects of success. The overriding theme of "Stress for Success" is that stress can be used to allow an individual to reach his full potential in life without being burdened by physical, mental and social problems.

This book is a textbook on stress. The many reference sources are keyed to the text and are listed at the end of each chapter. Also included is a list of suggested supplementary readings at the back of the book. Although it is a textbook, it is written in a flowing style where each chapter leads into the next. This should make it easy to read for anyone with at least a minimal scientific background. It is not our purpose to give the reader a simplistic panacea for overcoming stress. Rather we present an up-to-date, scientifically based, holistic* approach, which can help each reader cope with the stress of daily living. This format also allows the use of the text for assignment in psychology and behavioral science courses.

The book is divided into four parts. Part I is the "Stress Story," in which stress is thoroughly examined. In Part II, the consequences of distress are covered, including diseases, disorders and premature aging. Dealing with stress is the concern of Part III, and topics include diet, psychological coping methods, diversion, drugs, exercise, meditation, hypnosis and biofeedback. Because of our belief in their importance and effectiveness, meditation and hypnosis are considered in detail. In Part IV, all the coping methods are packaged in an integrated whole. Throughout the book are interspersed various stress-assessment methods, which give the reader a way of evaluating himself** and rating his progress. A final stress-assessment system is given in Chapter 20.

---

* Holistic means a complete, integrated, mind-body orientation toward prevention, diagnosis and treatment of symptoms, diseases and disorders. It is opposed to the specialized approach where only one area (e.g., the eyes) is thoroughly examined, but the interrelationship with the rest of the body and the mind is ignored. Holistic also emphasizes a many-faceted approach toward the achievement of optimum health.

** In accord with popular usage, the male gender is employed throughout the book, there being no simple way to cover both male and female in one word.

Some of the concepts discussed are relatively simple but are often ignored by the public (e.g., the ill effects of smoking). Therefore, they have been included for reinforcement. Other concepts, of necessity, are quite technical, but we have tried to simplify the scientific aspects and amplify them with frequent research findings, anecdotes and illustrations. We have also included a touch of humor. This helps lighten the load for those who might be taxed by reading about stress.

We would like to thank Mr. Alex V. Mucha, Director of Visual Education, Temple University School of Dentistry, and both Andrew and Brian Morse for the photography. Thanks are also extended to Dr. Norma Furst, Dean of Student Affairs, Temple University for editorial advice, and Mr. Ashak M. Rawji, Senior Editor of the Van Nostrand Reinhold Company for his sincere cooperation in the publication of this book.

Donald Roy Morse
M. Lawrence Furst

Contents

Part I
The Stress Story

What is stress? The answer seems to come easily enough through personal experiences. But we may be confused about cause and effect. And what about individual differences? The answers to these and other questions about stress are contained in Part I.

Chapter 1 is concerned with the causes of stress—those physical, social and emotional factors that can upset one's equilibrium. In Chapter 2, the ways people differ in the perception and management of stress are covered. In Chapter 3, the mechanisms of the stress response are considered.

1

From Adam to Stressors

And when the woman saw that the tree was good for food, and that it was pleasant to the eyes, and a tree to be desired to make one wise, she took of the fruit thereof, and did eat, and gave also unto her husband with her; and he did eat.*

IN THE BEGINNING

The Garden of Eden began as a tranquil, stressless environment. But when Adam was given the tantalizing chance to eat of the forbidden fruit, he was thrust into mankind's first stressful situation. Adam was offered a choice, and as we now know, decision making is the breeding ground for conflict, frustration and distress. Biblical scholars may argue over whether Adam made the correct choice, but whatever path he chose would have been beset with potential stress.

If we turn from the biblical interpretation of mankind to the anthropological description of ancient man, it appears that the cavemen fared somewhat better than Adam. They led active lives in

*Genesis 3:6.

3

which they had to cope effectively or die. In their quest for food, shelter and survival, they had to fight against, run away from or avoid potential predators and enemies. They did not have the time for worry or anxiety or the luxury of lawsuits. And as a result, our cave-dwelling ancestors were not prone to incapacitating stress-related diseases such as bleeding ulcers and coronaries—that is, if they escaped a wild boar's tusks or a native's club.

Along with the great scientific advances mankind has made since the caveman era, there have come a whole host of stress-induced diseases and disorders. It is unrealistic to believe that we can return to the tranquility of the Garden of Eden or the caveman's methods of physically coping. In fact, even if we tried to emulate the caveman, we'd be in a lot of trouble. With our current sugar- and cholesterol-rich diets and automatized devices, we have grown into a race of inactive, overweight, flabby-muscled individuals. Moreover, we no longer have the sharp, strong teeth of our ancestors, and even our fingernails have become brittle. No doubt, there are still some of us who might be able to compete with our ancient forebears, but as a race we're simply in bad shape.

Yet, there is much that we can do—we can make stress work for us in a positive way. It is true that stress has a great potentiality for destruction, but it can also be constructive. If stress is perceived and managed poorly, it can lead to grief, disease and premature death. On the other hand, the correct use and management of stress can actually lead to a longer, healthier and happier life. In the remainder of this book, we try to show how each of us—regardless of age, sex, occupation or position in life—can achieve that tripartite goal of health, happiness and longevity.

The two possible paths are now presented, and they serve as an introduction to all that follows. It is sincerely hoped that the reader will not find himself confined to the negative stress path, shown in Path 1. We certainly hope to guide the reader in following the positive stress path, shown in Path 2. (See Figs. 1.1 and 1.2.)

In order to follow the positive path, it is necessary to change one's orientation. One cannot sit back, wait for the arrival of distress symptoms and then run to his doctor for a cure. He must—himself— be actively concerned with prevention of distress and disease. Whether one is religious or not, the saying, "God helps those who help themselves" is completely applicable. With this in mind, let us

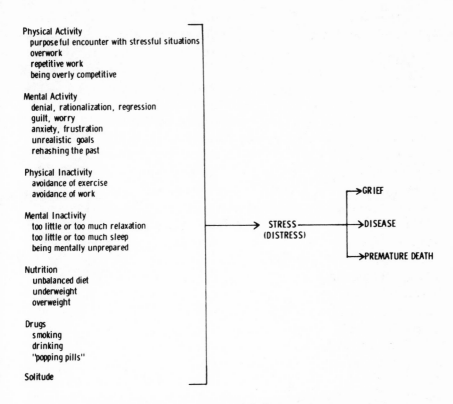

Fig. 1.1 Path 1: The stress path to grief, disease and premature death.

begin by trying to understand what is meant by stress, distress and eustress.

DEFINITIONS

Stress

Over 40 years ago, Hans Selye—the "father" of stress—wrote his first article on the subject.[1] Since then, there have been over 110,000 scientific publications related to stress. Yet, the meaning of stress is still elusive, partly because of the confusion engendered by the incorrect adaptation of terms drawn from the discipline of physics. One definition of stress in physics is, "an applied force or system of forces that tends to strain or deform a body." The resultant deformation of the body (or object) is called "strain."

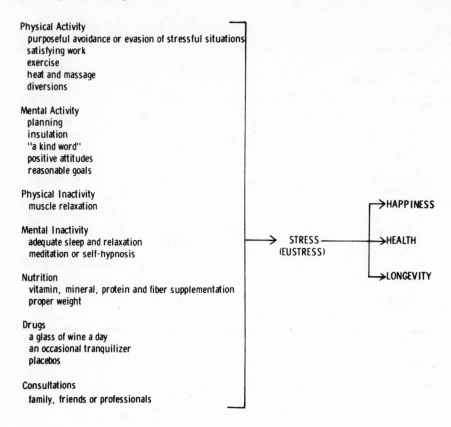

Fig. 1.2 Path 2: The stress path to happiness, health and longevity.

When Selye first used the term stress biologically, he inadvertently applied it to the reaction of the body.[2] As he later admitted, he should have called the reaction "strain," so that it would agree with the physics use.[3] In order to differentiate the causative factors from the body's reactions, Selye coined the term "stressors" for the causative factors. Hence, Selye's "stressor" is the equivalent of the "stress" of physics. This compromise would have been fine except that the majority of researchers and writers decided *not* to follow Selye's lead. They used biologic stress for the causative factors without choosing a separate term for the stress response.[3-8] Selye and many of his followers did not accept this viewpoint.[9-12] So, we now have the current situation where the cause and the result are both called "stress" by different investigators.

There is a second problem with the usual definition of stress. Consider this version: "Stress is a mental or emotional disruptive or disquieting influence; distress." This definition and most people's concept is that stress is a negative or disruptive outcome. Yet, as Selye has pointed out, there are positive as well as negative aspects to stress.

Pressure

To add to the confusion, the physics terms of "pressure" and "tension" have also been used as synonyms for biologic stress. In physics, pressure has been defined as, "a force applied over a surface, measured as force per unit of area." One commonplace, biologic definition of pressure is, "a burdensome, *distressing* (authors' italics) or weighty condition." This definition of biologic pressure is similar to the negative, external-force concept of biologic stress.

Tension

One physics definition of tension is, "a force tending to produce elongation or extension." To give an example of twisted logic, when "tension" was incorporated as a biologic term, it reverted to the Selye "stress" meaning. Consider this definition of biologic tension: "a mental, emotional or nervous *strain* (authors' italics)." In other words, in physics tension is the external force, but in biology it is the reaction of the body. As if that's not enough, there are three types of biologic tension.

Mental Tension. First of all, there is "mental," "nervous" or "emotional tension." A person in this state is "keyed-up" and has feelings of uneasiness and anxiety.

Muscle Tension. The second type of tension is "muscle tension." The "tense" individual is also described as being "tensed-up" or "up-tight." The body's muscles are presumed to be in an extreme state of contraction and are "coiled or bracing for action," but no action takes place to relieve the stress. The late comedian Fred Allen gave a vivid description of such an individual: "He was so high-strung that he could have gone to a masquerade as a tennis racket."*

However, this popular version of muscle tension is in error. The correct meaning of muscle tension refers to the partial contraction of the supporting muscles of the body that maintain a state of muscle tone. This partial contraction is important for body stability and posture. Under stressful conditions, the entire body's muscles are *not* overcontracted, but certain muscle groups can show *partial* contraction. This often occurs along with strong emotions such as anger, frustration, hate, worry, fear and anxiety. The partial contraction closes down blood vessels and causes nerves to be overreactive. The end result is muscular pain. Most commonly affected sites are the scalp ("tension" headache), the jaws (myofascial pain), the neck and shoulders ("a pain in the neck" or shoulder ache) and the lower back (backache).

Visceral Tension. The third kind of tension is "visceral tension." Although its meaning is not clear, this term apparently relates to the reaction of viscera (e.g., the heart, the lungs, the blood vessels, the kidneys) to stressful stimuli. The result of "visceral tension" tends to be marked increases in blood pressure,** heart and breathing rates.

Let us now review some of these terms and their definitions and see if we can develop some semblance of order out of them.

> Stress: for Selye, it is the body's reaction and can be positive as well as negative; for most others, it is the physical and mental factors that cause the body to react, and it is generally considered to be negative.
> Pressure: the mental negative factors.
> Tension: the body's negative reactions; emotional for nervous tension, muscular for muscle tension and physiological for visceral tension.

In our opinion, pressure and tension are incorrectly used as biologic terms; therefore, we shall not consider them further. Although

---

* From Allen, Fred, *Treadmill to Oblivion,* Boston: Little, Brown and Co., 1954.
** Increased blood pressure is known as high blood pressure or hypertension. The latter could be considered another kind of biologic tension.

it would be more correct to use the terms stress and strain as they are used in physics, "strain" has other meanings, and its use here would only complicate matters. Hence, we will use the term "stressor— as Selye does—for the causative factors and "stress" or the "stress response" for the body's reactions.

Now let us look at the stress concept as it is shown in the following equation:

STRESSORS + INDIVIDUAL "MAKEUP" = STRESS

Stressors, Individual "Makeup" and the Stress Response

There are three kinds of stressors: physical, social and psychological. The "makeup" of the individual is determined by hereditary and environmental factors. Stress (or the "stress response") results from the interaction between the stressor and the individual, modified by the person's state at the time. Therefore, to expect that stress takes only one form is unreasonable. We consider that there are three types of stress.

The Stress Response. If the stress response is necessary for the day-to-day adaptability of man to his environment and results in the maintenance of an internal steady state (homeostasis), it is designated *neustress* (prefix neu = neutral). For example, one produces neustress in order to breathe, walk and perform the bodily functions.

If the stress response is unfavorable and potentially disease-producing, it is labeled *distress* (prefix dis = bad or negative). For example, constant worry in a susceptible individual can lead to ulcers.

If the stress response is favorable and results in improvement in physical and/or mental functioning, it is called *eustress* (prefix eu = good or healthy, as in the word eugenics). For example, vigorous exercise can improve the functioning of the heart and lungs and could result in a decreased chance of getting a heart attack (Selye coined the term "eustress," but he only used it for positive mental responses).[10,13]

The details of this discussion are illustrated in Figs. 1.3 and 1.4.

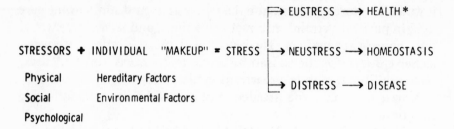

Fig. 1.3 The stress path.

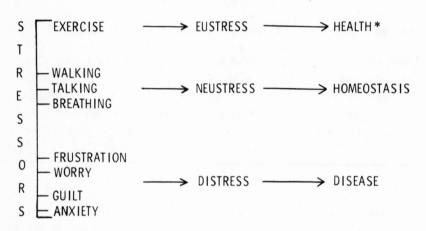

Fig. 1.4 Kinds of stress.

STRESSORS

As mentioned, there are three kinds of stressors: physical, social and psychological, to be considered here in that order.

Physical Stressors

Physical stressors are external factors, including chemicals, pollutants, drugs, foods, infectious microbes, shock therapy, radiation (e.g., light, X-rays, laser beams), noise, temperature (hot, cold),

---

* Health is not just the absence of disease. It is a positive condition in which an individual has no untoward symptoms (e.g., headache, backache, cough) and is in a state of physical and mental well-being. For example, a middle-aged man can have a blood pressure reading of 145/90 and have no clinical manifestations of disease and medically would be considered "normal." Yet, another similar-aged man with a blood pressure reading of 115/60 and a pulse rate of 60 and all other considerations similar to the first man should be considered to be in a state of health rather than just "normal."

humidity, exercise and trauma. The resistance of the individual will modify the stress response, but if the agents are sufficiently intense and enduring, then distress will result in any person. For example, atomic radiation plays no favorites, and if the dose is strong enough, then third-degree burns, leukemia and finally death can result. Physical stressors are often related to a person's occupation, and with certain jobs the stressors are intense. Consider the high noise exposure of pneumatic drill operators, dentists, airline personnel, riflemen, artillerymen and rock musicians.

In our first study at Temple University,* we compared the physiological responses of 48 subjects while they were in a state of hypnosis or meditation.[14] As part of the study, blood pressure was taken using a sphygmomanometer. The taking of the blood pressure acted as a physical stressor. The subjects were monitored for pulse rate, breathing rate and skin resistance. It was found that people varied greatly in their responses to the blood pressure detection. For some individuals, even their hypnotic or meditative state was not disturbed; others were brought out into a state of agitation. A polygraph record of a representative subject is shown in Fig. 1.5.

Social Stressors

Social stressors** are externally induced and result from the interaction of the individual with his environment. Many social stressors are unavoidable and traumatic. They include occurrences such as the death of a loved one, forced relocation of one's home, loss of a job, retirement, divorce and financial reversal. Apparently, pleasant events such as engagement announcements, marriage ceremonies and financial windfalls can also be social stressors. The unforeseen social stressors are the most difficult to cope with. Even the most stable individual will react with distress to an event such as the death of a spouse.

Psychological Stressors

Psychological stressors, because of their recurrent nature, are often the most damaging kind. They may be brought on by physical or

* Discussed in detail in Chapter 15.
** Also known as life-change events or life-stress events; covered more thoroughly in Chapter 4.

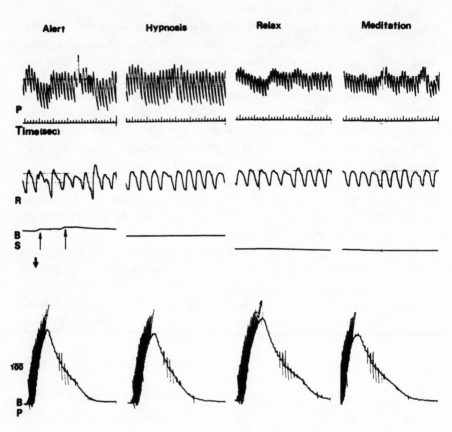

Fig. 1.5 Blood pressure detection as a physical stressor. P = pulse rate; R = respiratory rate; BS = skin resistance level; ↑ = skin resistance, nonspecific fluctuations (indicative of a stressful reaction); ↓ = direction of increased skin resistance (less stress); BP = blood pressure; and subject's blood pressure was approximately 107/87. For this subject, the taking of blood pressure acted as physical stressor only in the alert state, as shown by the decreased skin resistance level and increased nonspecific fluctuations. During hypnosis, relaxation and meditation no significant changes occurred in pulse rate, respiratory rate or skin resistance.

social stressors, or they may be self-induced. The psychological stressors are intense emotions and include frustration, guilt, worry, anger, resentment, hate, love, disgust, jealousy, happiness, sadness, grief, self-pity, fear, anxiety and inferiority feelings. The more one harbors these feelings or emotions, the greater and more cumulative is the resultant distress. Two particularly severe and repetitive psychological stressors are frustration and anxiety.

Frustration. Frustration occurs when a person is blocked from achieving a goal and feels confused, annoyed or angry as a result. The closer a person is to reaching his goal when the blockage occurs, the greater is the ultimate frustration. Frustration often comes not only from failure to achieve a single goal, but from a conflict of two important goals or needs in which choosing either alternative means frustration with regard to the other.

Neal Miller—the "father" of biofeedback*—has classified frustration and conflict into the following three kinds: approach-avoidance, double-approach and double-avoidant.[15] With *approach-avoidance* conflicts, a person simultaneously wants to approach and to avoid the same goal. Consider the married executive who has strong sexual desires toward his receptionist and simultaneously experiences anxiety about being caught. With *double-approach* conflicts, a person must choose between two desirable goals. For instance, the women's liberation movement may have intensified for many women the conflict between pursuing a satisfying career and maintaining a happy home. With *double-avoidant* conflicts, a person wants to avoid both goals. Consider the plight of the individual short of funds who has a conflict over cheating on his income tax return and worrying about whether or not he would be caught.

People often become frustrated when they must choose between their personal goals and pleasing other people. There are five basic ways to react in this situation, and each can be a source of frustration. Let us consider these five ways (labeled A–E for later reference purposes).

(A) First of all, a person may pursue his personal desires and forget about interpersonal relationships. The individual so described would be the egoist who cares little about stepping on others as long as he gets to the top of the ladder. His frustration results from the displeasure of others. The others may outwardly smile at him because of his power, but they secretly would like to "stab him in the back."

(B) Second, a person may try to please everyone by setting aside his own aspirations. This is the person who can't say no. His frustration results from lack of personal achievement and the realization that complete altruism is not self-satisfying.

* Discussed in Chapter 16.

(C) Third, a person may try to achieve all his ambitions and simultaneously please everyone. This person is the typical "wheeler and dealer." He is maximally frustrated, since it is virtually an impossible task to be all things to all people, including one's self.

(D) Fourth, a person may decide to be an ostrich and bury his head in the sand. This describes the hermit. He also becomes very frustrated because he achieves nothing and pleases no one, not even himself.

(E) Fifth and finally, one may choose to go halfway. Such a person is the compromiser or the person who can't seem to make up his mind. But even he is frustrated because he may sacrifice worthwhile personal goals or fail really to please some important people, since he has decided on a middle course.

A graphical representation of these five choice points (A–E) is displayed in Fig. 1.6. From the wide range covered, it would appear that frustration is a way of life in today's society. In Chapter 8, methods of dealing with frustration are covered.

After examining this figure, which one are you? That is, A(10,0), B(0,10), C(10,10), D(0,0), or E(5,5)? Or are you somewhere in be-

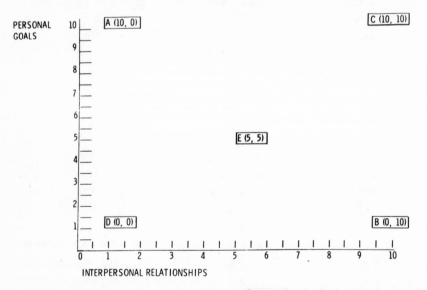

Fig. 1.6 The paths to frustration. (Adapted from a presentation by Rodney Napier at the Philadelphia Society of Periodontists in Philadelphia, 1977.) A(10,0) = the "egoist;" B(0,10) = the "altruist;" C(10,10) = the "wheeler-dealer;" D(0,0) = the "hermit;" E(5,5) = the "compromiser."

tween? Do you change with different goals and different people, or is your behavior consistent with everyone? In short, understanding yourself is the first step in the management of stress.

Fear and its Close Relatives. Fear, anxiety, panic and phobia are somewhat similar psychological stressors. Their important differences are now examined. Fear is derived from the old English word, "faer," which means a sudden calamity or danger. Fear is a normal response that engenders feelings of alarm or disquiet brought on by the realistic expectation of pain, danger or disaster. For instance, many patients in the office of a physician or dentist are frightened at the sight of a hypodermic needle.

Anxiety. [16-18] Anxiety is derived from a Greek word that means, "to press tight" or "to strangle." Anxiety is a response that brings forth feelings that are indistinguishable from fear. The difference is that anxiety is an irrational fear. Anxiety may be brought on by some external happening, but it is more often based on an individual's subjective, distorted view of the situation. The anxious individual has intense fear or dread, but there is usually no realistic object or situation that engenders the fear. As Mark Twain put it, "I'm an old man and have known a great many troubles, but most of them never happened."*

There are two kinds of anxiety. The first type is "generalized trait anxiety," in which the person experiences anxiety as a personality characteristic or as a stable aspect of his life. This individual would be anxious about every new situation. The second type of anxiety is "transitional situational anxiety," in which a person who is usually not anxious could temporarily become anxious because of a specific event or stressful occurrence. Again referring to the dental situation, dental anxiety is the illogical fear of having dental treatment. It can occur with either of the two types of anxiety. It is generally brought on by hearing "horror stories" or "tales of woe."

For most people, forewarning them about the stressful situation to come greatly diminishes their anxiety; but this is not true for everyone. This was borne out in the second study the authors performed at Temple University, in which 48 subjects were meditating while

---

* Quoted in *The Home Book of Humorous Quotations,* A. K. Adams (ed.), New York: Dodd Mead and Co., 1969.

heart rate, breathing rate and skin resistance responses were monitored.[19] As part of the study, a stressful verbal phrase was spoken in the presence of the meditating subjects. The phrase was: "John, may I please have the needle." In the beginning, the subjects were not told about the impending verbal stressor and, as might be expected, the "needle" phrase caused a significant alerting reaction for most of these subjects. In the second phase of the experiment, the subjects were forewarned about the forthcoming "needle" phrase. For most of these subjects, forewarning was effective in reducing the stress response (37 of 48, or 77%). A polygraph record from one of the subjects showing this effect is presented in Fig. 1.7.

To use this information in a clinical situation, it would appear that advance knowledge would help reduce anxiety of most patients. On the other hand, some of the subjects (11 of 48, or 23%) actually became more alarmed when they were forewarned. This was probably the result of anticipation.

Hence, for people falling into this category, advance information about subsequent medical or dental procedures would increase anxiety. Thus, we should each consider how we react to advance information before we ask for a detailed explanation of upcoming surgical procedures. To help the reader assess his anxiety level, a simple anxiety level test is presented in Table 1.1.

The reader should take a sheet of paper and number it from 1 to 33. Then he should read the following 33 statements, after which he should mark a "yes" or "no" next to the appropriate place on the paper. A "yes" response to 0–8 statements indicates low anxiety; 9–16 indicates moderate anxiety; 17–24 indicates high anxiety; and 25–33 suggests an extreme anxiety level. If one has a score of 8 or more "yes" responses, he should make every effort to decrease his anxiety level. (See Chapter 8 for methods on how this may be accomplished.)

Panic. Panic is derived from the Greek word "Pan." Pan was a Greek god who was the originator of sudden and unexplainable terror. Panic means a sudden surge of intense terror that can be brought on by any condition that causes severe anxiety. Some people panic in the hospital "O.R." or dental waiting room. The panic in these situations is usually related to fear of the unknown.

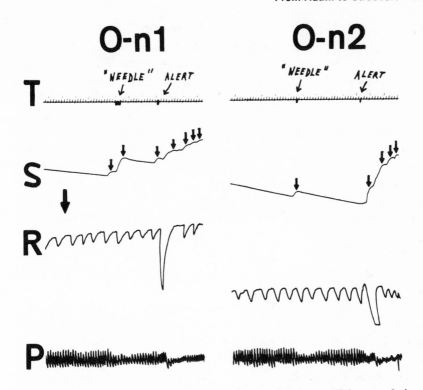

Fig. 1.7 Forewarning decreases anxiety. O-n1 = the stressful phrase, "John, may I please have the needle," was stated while the subject was meditating with the word, "one." The subject was not forewarned. O-n2 = same as for O-n1 except that this time the subject was forewarned about the impending stressful phrase. T = time in seconds; S = skin resistance; ↓ = skin resistance nonspecific fluctuations (indicative of a stressful reaction; ⬆ = direction of increased skin resistance (less stress); R = respiratory rate; P = pulse rate. For this subject, the "needle" phrase was stressful, as shown by the decreased skin resistance level, increased fluctuations, irregular breathing and increased pulse rate (O-n1). Forewarning (O-n2) decreased the stressful effects of the "needle" phrase. (From Morse, D. R. et al., 1979, A physiological and subjective evaluation of neutral and emotionally-charged words for meditation. Reprinted from *The Journal of the American Society of Psychosomatic Dentistry and Medicine,* Volume 26, 1979.)

Phobia. Phobia is another Greek-derived word, originating from the word "Phobos." Phobos was also a Greek god, who provoked panic and flight in his enemies. A phobia is a persistent, abnormal and usually illogical fear, which is out of all proportion to the object or situation that engenders it. The phobia results in avoidance of the feared situation or object. There are all sorts of phobias, including

TABLE 1.1 Rate Your Anxiety Level

MENTAL SIGNS

_____ I frequently worry.

_____ Many times I feel nervous.

_____ Bothersome thoughts run through my mind.

_____ I often imagine frightening scenes.

_____ I can't concentrate well.

_____ I often belittle myself.

_____ It takes me a long time to make a decision.

_____ I find it difficult to stick to a job.

_____ I don't feel happy.

SOMATIC SIGNS

_____ My heart frequently races.

_____ I get chest pains (my doctor says my heart is fine).

_____ I have a tense stomach.

_____ I vomit for no apparent reason.

_____ I often get diarrhea.

_____ I often lose my breath.

_____ Sometimes I feel as if I'm being smothered.

_____ I have a habit of sighing.

_____ I get dizzy for no apparent reason.

_____ When upset, I sometimes feel like fainting.

_____ I frequently have headaches.

_____ I perspire a lot.

_____ I get frequent chills.

_____ I frequently blush.

_____ I cry a lot over minor things.

_____ My body often becomes immobilized (I find it difficult to react).

_____ I fidget around a lot.

_____ Frequently, my whole body feels jittery.

_____ I often pace around.

_____ I often have no energy.

_____ I tire easily.

_____ I have trouble sleeping.

_____ I don't have a good appetite.

_____ I frequently stammer or have difficulty with my speech.

such common ones as claustrophobia (a pathological fear of being confined), acrophobia (an intense fear of heights) and hydrophobia (an exaggerated fear of water).

Inferiority Feelings. Feelings of inferiority are another major psychological stressor, at least according to Alfred Adler (one of the early psychoanalysts who broke away from Freud).[20] If a person can overcompensate for a weakness, he can, in effect, deny its existence. For example, Napoleon, being of short stature, may have suffered a sense of powerlessness. He effectively overcompensated for his lack of height by becoming politically strong. Thus, if an individual can use an energetic and effective—though not necessarily admirable— way of combatting a particular weakness, his stress response could be considered as eustress. On the other hand, if the person continually reflects on his particular weakness, he can develop an inferiority complex, and his stress response would be considered distress.

Mental Condition. The effects of physical and social stressors are primarily based on the strength and duration of the involved stressor. However, with psychological stressors, the individual's mental condition can seriously affect the outcome. Mental replay, such as in rehashing past events, intensifies the stress response. In contradistinction, mental preparation, such as being prepared to deliver a lecture, greatly diminishes the stress response. Knowing one's material often overcomes the fear of talking to an audience of strangers. Sometimes the situation is so intense that the psychological stressors induce distress for almost everyone. A good example is battle fatigue. The combination of fighting an unseen enemy for days and weeks on end without rest and the intense anxiety experienced from not knowing whether death or serious injury will occur, leads to the mental breakdown known as "shell shock" (a term used in World War I) or battle fatigue. Many individuals who cope well with severe stressors in civilian life suffer battle fatigue under the trying combat situation.

Now that the three types of stressors have been considered, we shall next focus on the individual's makeup.

REFERENCES

1. Selye, H. A syndrome produced by diverse nocuous agents. *Nature* 138:32, 1936.
2. Selye, H. *The Stress of Life*. New York: McGraw-Hill Book Co., 1956.
3. Rees, W. L. Stress, distress and disease. *Br. J. Psychiat*. 128:3–18, 1976.
4. Wolff, H. G. *Life Stress and Bodily Disease*. Springfield, Ill.: Charles C. Thomas Publ., 1950.
5. Becker, B. J. A holistic approach to anxiety and stress. *Am. J. Psychoanal*. 36: 139–146, 1976.
6. Kopin, I. J. Catecholamines, adrenal hormones, and stress. *Hosp. Pract*. 11(3):49–55, 1976.
7. Hurst, M. W., Jenkins, C. D. and Rose, R. M. The relationship of psychological stress to onset of medical illness. *In* Creger, W. P., Coggins, C. H. and Hancock, E. W. (eds.), *Ann. Rev. Med*. 27: 301–312, 1976.
8. Glass, D. C. Stress, behavioral patterns and coronary disease. *Am. Sci*. 65:177–187, 1977.

9. Selye, H. *The Stress of Life,* Second Ed. New York: McGraw-Hill Book Co., 1976.
10. Selye, H. *Stress Without Distress.* Philadelphia: J. B. Lippincott Co., 1974.
11. Rabkin, J. G. and Struening, E. L. Life events, stress, and illness. *Science* 194: 1013–1020, 1976.
12. Monjan, A. A. and Collector, M. I. Stress-induced modulation of the immune response. *Science* 196:307–308, 1977.
13. Selye, H. Further thoughts on "stress without distress." *Med. Times* 104(11):125–144, 1976.
14. Morse, D. R., Martin, J. M., Furst, M. L., and Dubin, L. L. A physiological and subjective evaluation of meditation, hypnosis and relaxation. *Psychosom. Med.* 39:304–324, 1977.
15. Miller, N. E. Liberalization of basic S-R concept: Extensions to conflict behavior, motivation, and social learning. *In* Koch, S. (ed.), *Psychology: A Study of a Science,* Vol. 2. New York: McGraw-Hill Book Co., 1959, pp. 196–292.
16. Leder, M. and Marks, I. *Clinical Anxiety.* New York: Grune & Stratton, 1971.
17. Evans, F. J. The placebo response in pain reduction. *Adv. Neurolol.* 4:289–296, 1974.
18. Crosby, J. F. Theories of anxiety: A theoretical perspective. *Am. J. Psychoanal.* 36:237–248, 1976.
19. Morse, D. R., Martin, J. M., Furst, M. L. and Dubin, L. L. A physiological and subjective evaluation of neutral and emotionally-charged words for meditation. *J. Am. Soc. Psychosom. Dent. Med.* 26(1–4): (1979), in press.
20. Adler, A. *Study of Organ Inferiority and its Physical Compensation.* Washington, D.C.: Nervous and Mental Disease Publishing Co., 1917.

2

Individual Makeup

In moments of crisis my nerves act in the most extraordinary way. When utter disaster seems imminent my whole being is instantaneously braced to avoid it. I size up the situation in a flash, set my teeth, contract my muscles, take a firm grip on myself, and without a tremor, always do the wrong thing.*

ON HEARING THE FIRST NEEDLE IN TEMPLE**

Many of us do the "wrong" thing in a stress situation, but few are as candid about it as was Shaw. However, whether our responses are "right" or "wrong" depends upon many factors, including the specific circumstances and our individual makeup. In that previously mentioned study at Temple University, we observed how people vary in their responses to a psychological stressor.[1] While the subjects were deep in meditation, they were suddenly confronted with a voice asking about a "needle" ("John, may I please have the needle?").

* George Bernard Shaw; quoted by Hesbeth Pearson in *Lives of the Wits*.
** No relation to Delius's *On Hearing the First Cuckoo in the Spring*.

In the subsequent alert state, the subjects were questioned about their impressions upon hearing the "needle" phrase. Some were indifferent; they said they heard nothing, and perhaps for them the stimulus was not functional—the physiological responses showed absolutely no change. Others were so frightened that they literally jumped out of the chair; they really expected to get an injection—and their physiological responses showed it.

A few acknowledged hearing what was said but believed that the needle was for the machine and so they ignored it. Their physiological changes were minimal. Some clever individuals realized that it was just to test their response to a stressor, so they were not afraid. A few of them had slight physiological changes, but others showed moderate changes. The remaining subjects heard the phrase and were alerted, but they were uncertain: "Was he really going to give me a 'shot' or was it just a test?" Some opened their eyes to peek. Physiologically, their changes varied from slight to those indicative of a marked stress response. (For a typical response, refer back to Fig. 1.3 in Chapter 1.) This experiment seems to show that people vary greatly in their responses to a stress situation.

Let us now consider how different individuals react to stressors. We begin with personalities, traits and attitudes, follow with genetic factors and conclude with environmental factors.

PERSONALITIES, TRAITS AND ATTITUDES

Personality Types and Typology

Many so-called personality types have been classified by various investigators. It is presumed that people of a particular type tend to react in certain patterned ways to particular stressors. Although personality types are described as having certain characteristic ways of functioning, there is considerable overlap between types. And some theorists dismiss the whole concept of personality, stating that instead of having unique personalities people have certain characteristic traits or methods of functioning.[2] Nevertheless, let us consider some of the classic personality types and describe how each might react to stressors. But, as with stress definitions covered earlier, there are many different definitions of personality. Hence, let us first attempt to define personality.

We consider personality to be specific behavioral patterns of an individual which reflect thoughts, attitudes and emotions as he adapts to his life situations.

The Humors.   The first recorded attempt at categorizing individuals into personality types was by the ancient Greek physician Hippocrates (circa 400 B.C.). He assigned people to one of four temperaments that were attributable to the predominance of the four bodily humors. Thus, choleric individuals were irritable and presumbly had an excess of yellow bile. Melancholic individuals were depressed and presumably had too much black bile. Sanguine individuals were optimistic, which supposedly reflected a predominance of blood. Finally, phlegmatic individuals were calm and listless and presumably had an overabundance of phlegm. At the present time, this concept is not scientifically supported, but we may hypothesize how people with these supposed characteristics might react to stressors. Thus, the choleric person should react with anger—which is usually a self-defeating response. The melancholic individual would tend to give up when faced with stressful situations. A sanguine person should react well, as his mental outlook would be positive. Finally, the phlegmatic individual would have an ineffectual response or might try to avoid or evade the situation.

Introverts and Extroverts.   The first modern attempt at personality typing was by Carl Jung, another early psychoanalyst who broke away from Freud.[3] Jung categorized people as either "introverts" or "extroverts." Introverts tend to react to stressors by withdrawing into themselves and "seething" internally. At the other extreme, extroverts tend to lose themselves among others and "blow off steam" as a stress-release mechanism. At the present time, most psychologists do not go along with this strict categorization, but believe that people have varying degrees of introversion and extroversion (i.e., are ambiverts).[2]

Body Type.   William Sheldon tried to correlate physique type with temperament.[4] In his classification, the "endomorphic" individual is overweight, tends to be relaxed and sociable and should react well to stressors (i.e., he tends to let things "roll off"). It is as if his excess layer of fat acts as a cushion to protect him from the outside world.

The "mesomorphic" person is strong and muscular. He is inclined to be energetic, assertive and courageous. The mesomorph has a tendency to "grab the bull by the horns" and as a result should react relatively well to stressors. The "ectomorphic" individual has a long thin body and is supposed to have a large brain and a sensitive nervous system. He is considered to be restrained, fearful and introvertive. As such, he would tend to manage stressors poorly.

Most current investigators have failed to replicate Sheldon's findings.[2] Therefore, it is probable that there is no significant link between physique and personality.

"Internals" and Externals": Locus of Control. Julian Rotter categorized people as either "internals" or "externals."[5] Internals believe that they have control over their environment and what happens to them. Their self-confidence tends to ensure that they react well to most stressors. At the other extreme, externals believe that whatever happens to them is the result of luck, fate or "superior beings." Thus, they would tend to react poorly to stressors. This is an example of another "black-or-white" classification where most people fall somewhere between the extremes.

"Uppers-and-Downers" and "Inners-and-Outers." We are not talking here about drugs, but in simple terms we have classified people into "uppers-and-downers" as well as "inners-and-outers." Uppers-and-downers are described as having mood swings that go from excitement or elation to flatness, sadness or despondency. During the "up" phase, stressful situations tend to be fairly well managed. During the "down" phase, stress tends to be poorly handled. In its pathologic form, uppers-and-downers may be classified as manic-depressives (i.e., a psychiatric classification). Finally, inners-and-outers may be regarded as a popularized version of introverts and extroverts.

Various Typologies. * Various investigators have proposed a variety of other personality types.[2,6] Although we do not support these

---

* Notions of personality types stem from a few dramatic instances of somebody's behavior, from contact with relatively rare personalities or from exposure to fictional characters who have purposely been overdrawn to make them interesting. Thus, characterization of people by type tends to be oversimplified and, therefore, incorrect in current psychological thinking.

conceptions, it is of interest to consider how people with these presumed characteristics might react under stress. Hence, let us now consider them in turn.

The "aggressive" or "explosive" individual is a common personality typing. The so-called aggressive person tends to lose control when he is confronted with minor stressors. He often becomes frustrated when he fails to achieve his goals.

The "obsessive-compulsive" person tends to be a perfectionist who pays strict attention to minor details. The obsessive-compulsive tries to avoid conflicts by adhering rigidly to all rules and regulations. Any change or deviation from the accustomed routine tends to be upsetting and distressful. In brief, it seems that the obsessive-compulsive has a lack of tolerence for stressors.

The "hysterical" personality tends to seek out physical stressors that cause pain and suffering. This individual may have an unconscious need to be hurt (i.e., psychiatrically speaking: masochism).

The "negativistic" or "passive-aggressive" individuals do not express open aggression. They try to avoid or ignore stressors whenever possible.

The "passive-dependent" person is sad, shy and submissive. Such an individual usually offers no opinion, is afraid to offend, rarely exercises independent judgment, and holds in his emotions. As a result, the passive-dependent person copes poorly with stressors and suffers from many physical and psychosomatic ailments.

The "sociopathic" or "antisocial" personality gratifies egocentric desires and impulses. These people tend to lie, blame others and are inclined to use defense mechanisms such as denial and rationalization. They easily become frustrated and often harm others as a stress-release mechanism (i.e., psychiatrically speaking: sadism).

The "asthenic" or "detached-passive-asocial" individual has a low energy level. He is easily fatigued by physical stressors and lacks a zest for living.

The "dependent-passive," "submissive" or "inadequate" personality does not appear to do anything correctly. He is inept, gives poor responses to stressors and is continually frustrated.

The "narcissistic" individual is the perpetual "spoiled-child." He tends to be egocentric, boastful, disdainful of others and acts self-assured. The narcissistic person expects others to subordinate their desires for his comfort so that he is always "No. 1." When left to himself, he handles stressors poorly.

The "noncompetitive" individual continually avoids competition or other potentially stressful encounters. When forced into a stress-inducing situation, he tends not to manage adequately.

Stress Seekers. There are people who actively seek certain stressors which are not immediately pleasurable in order to experience the exhilaration following the relief of the stress. Let us consider some examples. According to R. L. Solomon, many parachutists engage in that dangerous activity for the "rush" experienced upon landing safely.[7] The jump is life-threatening and the relief is in averting death. Similarly, many soldiers seek the stress of battle not for the pleasure of fighting, but because of the stress release that follows from the realization that they survived the engagement. Then there is the person who beats himself or allows himself to get beaten (i.e., a form of masochism). He may tolerate it for the same stress-release reason ("Oh! It feels so good when you stop!").

Some people take pills, alcohol or tobacco in increasing amounts (i.e., adjusting to body tolerance) for the subsequent "high," even though they know that they are causing damage and that it is a slow form of suicide (i.e., psychologically speaking: cognitive dissonance). These individuals may initially detest the taste of the drug (e.g., scotch), but persist for the subsequent pleasure. There are even some patients who go to the dentist expecting to be hurt and feel pain. Again, it may be the pleasure of the relief that they seek. Loren Borland observed dental patients who reported enjoying painful dental treatment. "One of these was a woman who insisted upon having her teeth removed without anesthesia, and gave every indication of a kind of detached ecstasy in the face of what must have been excruciating pain."*

Accident-Prone Personality. Flanders Dunbar has described an accident-prone personality.[8] The individuals are described as aggressive, angry and hostile, harboring self-punishment impulses (see Chapter 5).

---

* Borland, L. R., Odontophobia—Inordinate fear of dental treatment, *Dent. Clin. North Am.* 6:683, 1962.

Type A and Type B Personalities. Friedman and Rosenman have categorized people into Type A and Type B personalities.[9] The Type B personality is described as passive, restrained, not overly ambitious and not prone to develop stress-related diseases such as coronary artery disease. On the other hand, the Type A individual is seen as a competitive achiever who is constantly striving. He has feelings of time urgency, hostility and aggressiveness. The Type A person is a compulsive, hard-driving individual who often sets deadlines and quotas. He is impatient with delay; he suppresses fatigue and tries to control his environment. When he is unsuccessful, he tends to become helpless. The Type A individual is prone to develop high blood pressure and coronary artery disease. (See Chapter 4 for amplification of this and the following personalities.)

Cancer Personality. Beyond the classification of Type A and Type B personalities according to heart attack potentiality, people have also been classified according to whether or not they are prone to develop certain other stress-related diseases. For instance, there is a "cancer personality."[10] These individuals are generally "low-geared," have few outbursts of emotion and have a history of feelings of isolation from their parents that began in childhood. They are described as being depressed prior to the onset of their disease.

Ulcer Personality. The "ulcer personality" is considered to be an oral individual. Some of his characteristics are: the desire to be fed; continually leaning on others; seeking close body contact with people; tendency to repress anger; and being prim, tidy, mild-mannered, conscientious, inhibited and punctual.[11,12]

Rheumatoid Arthritis Personality. Another stress-disease-related type is the "rheumatoid arthritis personality."[13] Most cases of rheumatoid arthritis occur in women who are described as being unhappy in the traditional female sex role. These individuals are considered to be perfectionists who are easily frustrated, self-sacrificing, punctual, tidy and orderly.

Ulcerative Colitis Personality. Still another stress-disease-related type is the "ulcerative colitis personality."[14] These individuals supposedly have problems both at home and at work. They are considered to be mild, restrained, well-mannered, prim, conscientious and dependent upon others.

Depression-Prone Personality. Recently, the "depression-prone personality" has been described.[15] Although outwardly happy, hardworking and conscientious, inwardly these people are tormented individuals.

Migraine Headache Personality. A final disease-personality type we shall mention is the one associated with migraine headaches.[16,17] These individuals tend to be hypersensitive to stressors, possessing obsessional-perfectionist traits, repressed hostility and a great amount of bottled-up resentment.

A summary of personalities and associated stress responses is presented in Table 2.1. For later use, the reader should note which personality types seem to "fit" him personally, keeping in mind their speculative nature.

Traits and Attitudes

Not only do personality types differ in management of stressors, but specific traits and attitudes of people can influence their reactions to stressors and their susceptibility to stress-induced diseases. Strong positive attitudes enable people to cope better with stressors (e.g., think positively; be optimistic; see the bright side of things; have the "will to live"), whereas negative attitudes can lead to distress and disease.

Attitudes and Heart Surgery. A landmark study with respect to attitude and recovery from heart surgery was conducted by Chase Kimball at the University of Rochester.[18] Four groups of patients were interviewed prior to open-heart surgery. Group 1 individuals were categorized as "adjusted" and tended to cope well with stressors; they were optimistic about the forthcoming surgery. Group 2 individuals were considered to be "symbiotic"; they adapted well to their disease and approached the impending surgery with mixed feelings, hoping at least to maintain the status quo.

TABLE 2.1   Personality and Stress

PERSONALITY	CHARACTERISTICS	STRESS RESPONSE
Hippocrates		
choleric	irritable	reacts with anger
melancholic	depressed	"gives up"
sanguine	optimistic	reacts positively
phlegmatic	calm and listless	reacts ineffectively
Jung		
introvert	withdrawn	internalizes
extrovert	outgoing	"blows off steam"
Sheldon		
endomorph	overweight	lets things "roll off"
mesomorph	muscular	"grabs the bull by the horns"
ectomorph	underweight	reacts poorly
Rotter		
internals	control their own lives	react well
externals	"others" control their lives	react poorly
(simple labels)		
"uppers and downers"	mood swings from elation to depression	reacts well when "up"; poorly when "down"
"inners and outers"	mood swings from withdrawn to outgoing	goes from internalizing to externalizing
Kraepelin		
aggressive	explosive	loses control
obsessive-compulsive	attends to details	reacts poorly, avoids stressors
hysterical	masochistic	reacts with pain and suffering
negativistic	nonaggressive	internalizes, avoids stressors
passive-dependent	sad, shy and submissive	reacts poorly
sociopathic	sadistic	reacts with frustration
asthenic	low energy level	reacts with fatigue
dependent-passive	inept	reacts with frustration
narcissistic	egocentric	reacts poorly
noncompetitive	avoids choices	reacts inadequately
Solomon		
stress-seekers	masochistic	tolerate stress so that they can enjoy relief
Dunbar		
accident-prone	aggressive, self-punishing, angry and hostile	reacts poorly, prone to accidents

TABLE 2.1 Personality and Stress (*cont.*)

PERSONALITY	CHARACTERISTICS	STRESS RESPONSE
Friedman and Rosenman		
Type A	competitive achiever, compulsive, hard-driving	suppresses fatigue, reacts poorly, prone to cardiac diseases
Type B	passive, restrained, not overly ambitious	reacts well, not prone to cardiac diseases
Weiner		
"ulcer type"	prim, tidy, mild-mannered, conscientious	reacts poorly, suppresses anger, prone to ulcers
Le Shan		
"cancer type"	low-geared, depressed	reacts poorly, suppresses emotions, prone to cancer
Moos and Solomon		
"rheumatoid arthritis"	punctual, tidy, orderly, perfectionist	reacts poorly, easily frustrated, prone to rheumatoid arthritis
Grace, Wolf and Wolff		
"ulcerative colitis"	mild, well-mannered, conscientious, overdependent	reacts poorly, prone to ulcerative colitis
Sword		
"depression-prone"	hard-working, conscientious, inwardly tormented	reacts poorly, prone to depression
Pelletier		
"migraine type"	obsessional-perfectionist, repressed hostility and "bottled-up" resentment	overreacts to stressors, prone to migraine headaches

Group 3 individuals were considered to be unrealistic and were described as "denying anxiety." They coped poorly with the upcoming surgery, and were suspicious, hyperalert and rigid. Group 4 individuals were categorized as "depressed"; they were not enthusiastic about their chances, and just went along with their doctors' advice. Persons in the four groups did not differ significantly with respect to age, disease entities and duration of surgery. After surgery, the results were as follows:

Group 1: Thirteen patients were in this group; one died, nine improved, and three remained unchanged.

Group 2: Fifteen patients were in this group; one died, one imimproved, eight remained unchanged, and five deteriorated.

Group 3: Twelve patients were in this group; four died, three improved, three remained unchanged, and two got worse.

Group 4: Fourteen patients were in this group; eleven died, one improved, one remained unchanged, and one became worse.

Thus, it is apparent from this study that if you go into surgery with a negative or uncaring attitude, your chances of survival greatly decrease.

Changing Attitudes. There is also some evidence that attitudes of people can change during surgery, and this change can affect their chances of survival. David Cheek hypnotized patients who had recently had surgery performed.[19] He regressed the patients back to the time of the operation. (See Chapter 14 for details about hypnosis.) Surprisingly, the patients were able to recollect details of the conversation carried on by the surgeons and their aides. Even though the patients were under general anesthesia at the time and "out," they apparently could still hear while in that state. Cheek found that when negative comments were passed (e.g., "The poor guy hasn't got a chance!"), the patients did poorly and often succumbed. When positive statements were spoken, under similar conditions, the patients did better. These findings seem to show two things: the first is that even under general anesthesia people can hear; and the second is that negative comments can affect the patients in a detrimental way.

Attitudes and Diseases. The investigations of Grace, Holmes and their associates have shown that the attitude of an individual influences his susceptibility to a particular stress-related disease.[20-22] Some examples cited are the following: A person who feels deprived and wants to get even with someone tends to develop ulcers; an individual who is threatened with bodily harm and must be constantly prepared is prone to get hypertension (high blood pressure); someone who feels that he is being neglected counters by trying to shut out others from himself and winds up becoming an asthmatic; a person who believes that everyone is trying to injure or degrade him tries to get rid of the causative agents and often comes down with ulcerative colitis; an individual who feels restrained, confined and restricted in his movements but wants to get free has a tendency towards rheumatoid arthritis. A more complete list of attitudes and stress-related diseases is given in Table 2.2. For later use, the reader should note whether any of the given attitudes are personally appropriate—keeping in mind that they may be speculative although based on the findings of Graham and others.

Despite the foreboding connections between all these attitudes and diseases, there are four mitigating points to bear in mind. One is that many people who seem to have these attitudes do not come down with these diseases. Second is that people with specific attitudes associated with one disease can still come down with a different disease. The third is that individuals with certain attitudes can get the

TABLE 2.2   Attitudes and Diseases

ATTITUDES	SYMPTOMS AND DISEASES
_____feels nagged at	acne
_____feels neglected	asthma
_____wants to escape	backache
_____sticks to unliked situations	constipation
_____feels as if he is starving in the midst of plenty	diabetes
_____wants impending tasks to be done with quickly	diarrhea
_____feels continually frustrated	eczema (skin rash)
_____feels as if he has too much responsibility	edema
_____feels he has been tampered with or poisoned	enteritis (intestinal disease)
_____feels that he is getting what he wants	heartburn
_____feels that he must control his anger	hernia
_____feels that he is being mistreated	hives
_____tries to hold on to someone he loves	hyperthyroidism
_____feels threatened by bodily harm	hypertension (high blood pressure)
_____feels he must reach goals and then relax	migraine headaches
_____feels he must work without help	multiple sclerosis
_____feels responsible for some wrongdoing	nausea and vomiting
_____needs close physical contact	neurodermatitis (skin disease)
_____feels nagged at constantly	psoriasis (skin disease)
_____feels restrained	rheumatoid arthritis
_____feels conditions are too slow and must be speeded up	tachycardia (irregular, rapid heart beat)
_____feels overwhelmed by circumstances	tuberculosis
_____feels as if everyone is "out to get him" and tries to free himself	ulcerative colitis
_____feels deprived and wants to get even	ulcers

generally associated disease and also other nonrelated diseases. And finally, most of these associations were arrived at by retrospection, which means that the people had to recall their attitude prior to the onset of the disease. It is quite possible that the attitudes could have followed or merely accompanied the disease.

GENETIC FACTORS

Personality, traits and attitudes have a genetic basis, but they are primarily influenced by the environment. However, certain individuals are genetically programmed with specific ways of reacting to stressors. Let us consider some of these factors.

Congenital Dysautonomia

Rarely people are born without the ability to perceive pain and other external stimuli. This condition is called congenital dysautonomia.[23] Such people can receive severe physical stressors such as burns, cuts and trauma and yet not react or report pain. At first glance this might seem to be an advantage, but it is not, since these people may suffer severe inflammatory and degenerative diseases without the warning benefit of pain.

Sympathicotonics and Vagotonics

When we consider the stress response in Chapter 3, the autonomic nervous system (ANS) is described. The ANS has two components: the sympathetic (SNS) and the parasympathetic (PNS) divisions. For normal individuals, the SNS is the primary system activated during stress. Associated with ANS activation are two rare types of people.[24] One type—the "sympathicotonic"—reacts to stressors by developing severe stress responses as a result of extreme SNS activation and the outpouring of catecholamines (adrenaline and noradrenaline). These individuals—about 8% of the population—can easily develop high blood pressure and suffer heart attacks. The other rare type is the "vagotonic" (also about 8% of the population). He responds to stressors by activation of the PNS with a corresponding release of acetylcholine. The vagotonic is prone to develop low blood pressure, fainting reactions and asthma.

Other primarily genetic characteristics of the individual's makeup that can affect how he reacts to stressors are age, sex, ethnic origin or background, brain laterality and biorhythms.

Age

With age, during normal development certain periods have more stress potentiality than others. The ages from seven to ten are less stressful than the teen-age years. For instance, young children often react well to the potential stressors of the medical or dental office if they have not been "brainwashed" by their parents. Gail Sheehy (author of *Passages*[25]) and R. Gould (author of *Transformations*[26]) have described stages in adult development during which distress can result. Sheehy's stages include: "pulling up roots," the division between self and parents; "the trying twenties," the first stand as adults; "the catch-thirties," potential disharmony; and the "mid-life crisis of the forties," the dangerous years. Older individuals have a poorer reaction to physical stressors, such as infectious microbes and trauma. This vulnerability is related to their diminished immune responses, generally weaker bones and muscles and greater tendency to be out of condition.

The Sexes

With respect to the sexes, women react better than men to many stressors, including infection and frustration. The female hormones may help decrease the incidence of serious infections and heart attacks in women.

Two recent studies seem to show that the female hormone estrogen may help protect women against heart disease. In the first study—using female rats—it was found the estrogen "binds" in certain select parts of the heart (atria and auricles; see Fig. 2.1).[27] To quote: "This suggests that estrogen has a direct effect on atrial myocytes through which its 'protective' action may be mediated."*

In the second study, a tissue-culture experiment,** it was found

* Stumpf, W. E., Sar, M. and Aumüller, G., The heart: A target organ for estradiol, *Science* 196:319–320, 1977.
** A "tissue culture" is a growth of live cells taken from a part of an individual's body. The cells are grown in a nutritive medium inside a plate. Various materials can then be tested against the cells.

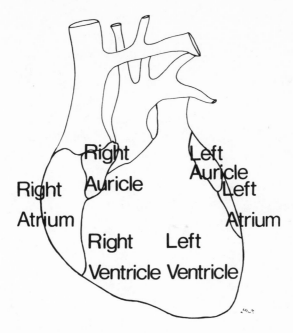

Fig. 2.1 The chambers of the heart. The auricles are appendages on the outside of the heart above the atria. The blood is pumped from the atria to the ventricles. (See Fig. 3.5 for greater detail.)

that estrogen also binds on the endothelial lining of blood vessels (innermost lining; see Fig. 2.2).[28] It is hypothesized that it may exert a protective shield against the development of the cholesterol-rich atherosclerotic patch that can occlude the coronary arteries and cause a heart attack. From the time of menopause onward when these hormonal levels greatly decrease, women become just as susceptible as men to heart disease.

Recent studies have shown that during the reproductive years women produce less adrenaline, noradrenaline and cortisone (i.e., three of the stress hormones discussed in Chapter 3) than men when exposed to various challenging and demanding influences in the psychological and social environment.[29-31] However, the sex differences in stress responses may not be solely genetic. Other recent findings seem to show that when women adopt male work roles, their stress responses and tendencies toward the development of stress-related diseases is similar to that of men.[32] Women may ex-

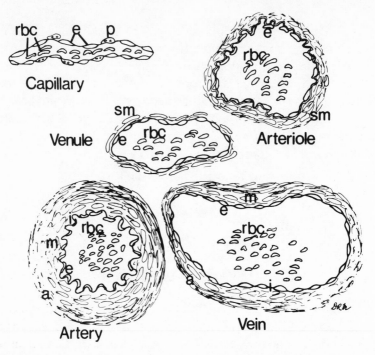

Fig. 2.2 Blood vessels. Cross section of five types of blood vessels beginning with the smallest (capillaries) and ending with the largest and thickest (arteries). rbc = red blood cells (erythrocytes); e = endothelial cells (the innermost lining cells); p = pericyte; sm = smooth muscle cells; i = intima, innermost layer of veins and arteries; m = media, middle muscular layer of arteries and veins (it is thickest in arteries); a = adventitia, outermost layer of arteries and veins (it is thickest in veins). Atherosclerotic plaque can attach to the intima of coronary arteries and can lead to a heart attack. Oxygen (O_2)-rich blood goes from the arteries to the arterioles, then to the capillaries and finally into the tissues. Carbon dioxide (CO_2), the waste gas, goes from the tissues to the capillaries and then to the venules and veins. (See Figs. 3.5 and 3.6 for further amplification.)

perience even greater stress because of job-related sexual discrimination.

Notwithstanding the gay rights movement, homosexuals still have many personal and socially related stressors. Employment opportunities are limited, and there may be anxieties about finances, family and personal health.

When confronted with stressful situations, men are prone to become angry, since society dictates that they are not supposed to show fear. In contrast, women are more likely to become anxious and cry. Crying is a beneficial stress-releasing mechanism, whereas anger is often only an illusion of strength. That is, the beneficial eustress role of fight is substituted for by the harmful distress role of anger. Of course, women don't always have the better of it. For instance, during the few days before and after the menses, women often react worse to stressors than during the remainder of the month (a condition known as premenstrual tensional syndrome; see Chapter 4).

Ethnic Origin and Background

Ethnic origin and background are also related to stress. People of different races, nationalities and religions may show different ways of reacting to stressors. For instance, studies have shown that when painful stimuli were presented to different ethnic groups, reactions were quicker among Jews, Italians and Frenchmen as compared to Orientals, "Yankees," and Scandinavians.[23,33] Certain primarily genetic diseases that may be precipitated by stressful incidents occur in different ethnic groups. These include diabetes and Gaucher's disease in Jews, sickle cell anemia in blacks and Cooley's anemia in Italians and Greeks.[34] Blacks also have a higher incidence than Caucasians of hypertension and coronary artery disease.[35]

People belonging to the so-called repressed minorities in the United States (e.g., black Americans, Hispanics, American Indians and Oriental Americans) may experience strong social stressors. In some areas of the country, Jews, Catholics and Moslems are discriminated against and may also experience similar social stressors. All of these individuals, at some time or other in their life, may experience school- and job-related stressors.

Brain Laterality

There is some recent evidence that the hemispheres of the brain are specialized with respect to how they process information (see Fig. 2.3).[36,37] In a right-handed person, the associated left hemisphere is considered to be responsible for processing analytical, logical and verbal information (i.e., rational type). The right hemisphere purportedly controls gestalt, holistic and spacial information (i.e., emotional type). In Western societies such as the United States emphasis is placed on left brain activity. In Eastern cultures such as India right

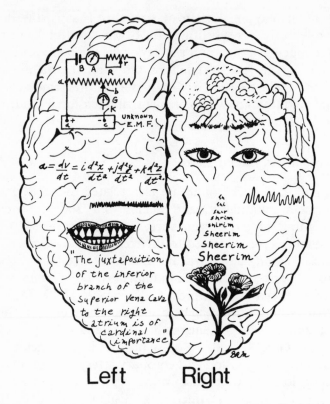

Left   Right

Fig. 2.3 The two hemispheres of the brain: functional representation. The left hemisphere is basically concerned with logic, analysis and speech. The right hemisphere is considered to be the seat of holistic, spacial and emotional-type thinking.

brain activity is emphasized. Apparently, as a result, Yogis and Zen meditators handle stressors well; hence it may be important for people of the Western countries to train themselves to increase right brain activity. This reorientation may permit all of us to cope better in this "age of anxiety."

Cyclic Changes

People appear to experience cyclic changes related to genetic background, emotional state, hormonal and enzymatic activity, weather, time of day, season, geographic location, atmospheric ions and astrological signs (according to some believers). Some of these changing cycles have been called "biorhythms." [38,39] At present, the scientific basis of biorhythms has been called in question. During so-called bad periods, people are presumably more inclined to react negatively to stressors, and vice versa during "good" periods.

Although many people blame their vicissitudes and moods "on the stars" and the weather, part of their changing attitudes may be related to nothing more than atmospheric ions! Atmospheric ions are small, charged (positive or negative) particles that are found in the air as a result of radioactivity, cosmic rays, movement of hot, dry winds and waterfall activity. Some studies have shown that negative ions reduce anxiety when mice and rats are exposed to stressful situations.[38] The opposite effect seems to have been found during certain severe weather fronts—meteorologists have named them, for example, the foehn and the sharav—that cause high concentrations of positive ions, and it has resulted in many people becoming ill.[38] Hence, people should be legitimately wary of "winds of ill repute" such as the foehn, the sharav, the zonda of Argentina and the chinook of the Rocky Mountain states.

A summary of the important genetic factors is given in Table 2.3. For later use, the reader should note any of the given conditions that seem to "fit."

Now that we have examined the primarily genetic factors of an individual's makeup, it is time to turn our attention to the environmental factors.

ENVIRONMENTAL FACTORS

A number of factors in the environment interact with individual makeup. The important environmental factors that help determine

TABLE 2.3   Genetic Factors and Stress

CONDITION OR FACTOR	STRESS PROFILE
Congenital dysautonomia	No pain perception.
Sympathicotony	Proneness to high blood pressure and heart attacks.
Vagotony	Proneness to low blood pressure and fainting.
Age	Poorer responses in old age.
Sex	Females react better than men.
Ethnic origin or background	Blacks tend toward high blood pressure; Jews and Italians more susceptible to pain.
Brain laterality	Left hemisphere: rational reaction; right hemisphere: emotional reaction.
Biorhythms	Poor reaction during down cycles.

how a person will react to stressors include disease, fatigue, diet, drugs, occupation, location, family and social structure, physical and mental fitness, emotional stability and the ability to relax.

Disease

If a person is sick, that will affect how he responds to stressors. Let us look at some examples. People with immunological diseases (e.g., Addison's disease, decreased cortisone production; Cushing's disease, increased cortisone production) or people who are taking immuno-suppressant drugs such as cortisone (i.e., to fight cancer, leukemia, arthritis, asthma and other diseases) often have poor ability to cope with stressors. In addition, people with diabetes mellitus have a poor capacity to fight infection and for repair following surgery. Also, people with mental diseases such as schizophrenia or individuals who have had treatment for mental diseases (e.g., drugs, shock treatment, pre-frontal lobotomy) have impaired ability in stressful situations.[34] Moreover, when a person is either physically or mentally fatigued, his ability to cope with stressors is greatly diminished. In Chapter 17, the specific problems in stress management by individuals with various diseases are considered.

Diet

Although the evidence is inconclusive, it does appear that inadequate diets can contribute to poor resistance to stressors. The malnourished individual is prone to vitamin-deficiency diseases such as pellagra, beri-beri and scurvy. The overweight person is a prime candidate for a "coronary." Vitamin, mineral, and fiber supplementation can enhance one's ability to counteract stressors. (The subject is discussed more fully in Chapter 10.)

Drugs

Many drugs can affect resistance to stressors. For example, excessive alcohol consumption decreases the body's immune mechanisms. This effect, in turn, can produce inadequate responses to microbial and viral stressors, which may result in severe disease.[34]

Occupation

Undoubtedly, a person is subjected to a number of different stressors depending upon his occupation. Let us consider a few examples. Studies showed that blood cholesterol levels rose by as much as 100 mg% for accountants during tax collection time (usually right before April 15). Furthermore, the accountants' blood pressure and blood clotting time increased significantly during the same time period.[40] In other studies air traffic controllers have developed high blood pressure four times as frequently as second-class licensee controllers (i.e., the occupation of the former demands more responsibility than that of the latter). Also high blood pressure was shown to occur sooner in controllers working in towers with high volume control than in controllers working in towers with low volume control.[41]

Decision-making business executives are prone to develop ulcers, heart attacks and nervous breakdowns. Decision-making and frustration have repeatedly been shown to induce ulcers in animals. Joseph Brady's work with "executive" monkeys is classic.[42] In this study, "executive" and control monkeys were both subjected to electric shocks. However, only the "executive" monkey could push a lever that would prevent *both* monkeys from receiving the shocks. Which monkey would you think developed the ulcers? If you said the "executive," you are correct—apparently you have a pretty good idea of what goes on in the upper echelons of the business world. Thus, the monkey with responsibility suffered the decision-making aftermath.

Neal Miller compared two groups of rats in an ulcer study.[43] The A group regularly received electric shocks, and developed "some" ulcers. On the other hand, the B group was constantly in conflict because those rats were forced to take shocks in order to avoid getting considerably more shocks. That is, the rats in the B group were continually frustrated,* and as a result developed a much higher incidence of ulcers than was found in rats of the A group. If we recognize that business executives are constantly making decisions and oftentimes are frustrated in achieving their objectives, then we

---

* When investigators speak of animals being frustrated or showing emotions such as anger and fear, it is understood that it is by inference. Actually, the animal's behavior is observed and measured, and then an interpretation follows.

can see why they are so prone to stress-related disorders such as ulcers.

That stressors can be compounded for business executives is pointed up in a news release. A California cardiologist, Martin Krauthamer, discussed extramarital sex and sudden death.[44] According to his findings, it is not a question of retribution, but simply a matter of cause and effect. Krauthamer found that heart stoppage occurred more often with extramarital sex than when sexual involvement was with one's legal spouse. He recited the following compounding stressors: a strange partner; a heavy meal mixed with alcohol; intense guilt feelings; and a fear of detection. The prime candidate for a heart attack under these circumstances is the 40-plus male business executive (or other individual in a stressful occupation) who eats poorly, doesn't exercise and, of course, is unfaithful. It may be a poor play on words, but "if one has a mistress, it is difficult to miss stress."

Medicine and dentistry are also stressful occupations. In fact, psychiatrists and dentists have been vying for the honor of being at the head of the professional suicide parade. Physicians and dentists also have a higher than average incidence of drug addiction, alcoholism, divorce, depression and other mental disorders.[45]

One special stress-filled occupation is that of concert musician. A study by a team of University of Vienna investigators came up with some interesting findings.[46] Aside from the physical stressor of the loud music, the musicians have many psychological stressors. Bear this in mind: In general, the average span of comfortable concentrated attention is about 30 minutes; within one hour, heavy fatigue sets in. As a rule, symphony concerts generally last about two hours, with a 15-minute break. Hence, since concert musicians have prolonged periods of concentrated attention, considerable stress is experienced—with soloists undergoing the greatest amount. Moreover, members of the orchestra are required to exhibit perfect teamwork; their timing can be off by no more than one hundredth of a second. When the concert is going well, each player's performance is taken for granted. But if one wrong note is played, "all hell breaks loose."

It follows that concert musicians must experience constant fear of failure. Severe periods of anxiety can occur beginning two weeks before a concert. During the performance, the musicians may worry about missing cues and thus suffer bouts of perspiration, giddiness and trembling. After the concert, many musicians experience total exhaustion and are beset with insomnia. Conductors must have it well though—consider how many of them live and practice into their eighties!

The various occupations may be stressful, but being unemployed can be even more so. H. and M. Lewis reported that when Olin Chemical Works closed down its Saltville, Virginia, plant many of the newly unemployed came down with cases of hypertension, stomach distress and alcoholism.[47] I. Barmash described a steel and aluminum company where executives were forced to retire.[48] Within a few months, one individual developed a stroke, a second had a heart attack, and a third came down with a bleeding ulcer.

Business and Home Location

Stress levels are affected by where one works and lives. Undoubtedly, there are more stressors associated with city living than with living in the suburbs or rural areas. For instance, consider the noise, unsanitary conditions, cramped living quarters and lack of sunshine of the typical slums of a center city.

Infectious microbes are more easily transmitted in a crowded environment. One example is that tuberculosis occurs much more frequently with the poor in crowded cities. Rickets, which is related to lack of sunshine, is also more prevalent in such an environment. A recent study showed that overcrowding, as might be found on subways, causes such stress-induced changes as increases in heart rate, blood pressure, breathing rate and sweating of the palms.[49]

Also, the part of the country where one lives and works can be related to stress. One study showed that major illnesses and depression had a much lower incidence in the traditionally relaxed South as compared to the "hustle-bustle" East.[50]

Not only can location cause stress, but it has been repeatedly shown that change in location can be very stressful. One interesting example involving the Navajo Indian tribe was reported by Moorman.[51] It was found that when the Navajos were forced from their homes and put onto reservations a few miles away, they became severely stressed, and many came down with fatal tuberculosis. This occurred even though the new location had generally improved food, clothing and hygiene (and, of course, was similar to the old location in other respects).

Family and Social Situation

The family and the social situation affect stress levels. Single (never married) people have a higher incidence of stress-related diseases and disorders such as cancer and suicide than married persons. Those who have been divorced or widowed also have increased risks for these conditions.[35] People who have few social contacts have an increased mortality rate as compared to those with many social relationships. In a recently concluded nine-year study, Lisa Berkman found that the socially-isolated were 2 to 4½ times more likely to die of any disease as compared to their gregarious counterparts.[52]

Another consideration is the particular religious and cultural mores of the society in which the individual grows up. For example, certain deeply religious people consider death as a way to attain a "oneness with God" and thus to "live" in heavenly bliss. For them, the death of a loved one would not have the same stress-inducing potential it would for someone else without those beliefs. In biblical times and in some primitive cultures, human sacrifice was an important means of appeasing the gods; again this view would lessen the stress impact on the "honored" families of those sacrificed.

Physical and Mental Fitness

Physical and mental preparation are very important in the management of stressors. For example, a well-trained weightlifter might easily lift 200 pounds overhead with a consequent beneficial eustress response. An overweight, sedentary business executive attempting that same feat would probably have a severe stress reaction that might precipitate a hernia or a heart attack.

Trained perception can change potential distress into eustress. Let us look at a hypothetical situation. An average American is relaxing outdoors, and suddenly a harmless water snake crosses his field of vision. The usual startle reaction of such an individual would be based on fear, and panic might ensue. In contrast, a typical Yogi in that same situation would continue to meditate even if the snake slithered across his feet.

Emotional Stability

Emotional stability is a key element in the management of stressors. A positive outlook can change negative into positive stress. All of these factors can promote psychological health: being calm in the face of adversity; smiling instead of frowning; giving praise instead of negative criticism; and thinking before acting.

Part of this philosophy is found in the Bible: "A soft answer turneth away wrath."* An old epigram emphasizes another part: "Think and you won't sink."** And Hans Selye says it all when he advises that one act so as to "Earn one's neighbor's love."***

Being just a bit apprehensive, without panicking, can also be effective. Before a speech or an athletic contest, "psyching oneself up" promotes the "flow of adrenaline" and often makes for a better performance. The mental methods of coping with stress are covered more fully in Chapter 8.

Relaxation

Finally, the ability to relax plays a major role in how one reacts to stressors. Fortunately, one can learn to relax, and detailed discussion of this topic may be found in Chapters 12 and 13. The environmental factors are summarized in Table 2.4. For later use, the reader should consider which of the given conditions are personally appropriate.

SUMMARY

It can be seen that the individual's makeup is of great importance in how he will react to a particular stressor to produce stress. There are many personality types, traits and attitudes along with genetic and environmental factors that come together in a particular individual. It is recommended that the reader carefully review this past section and judge which of the various characteristics "fit" him. Then, when methods of coping are described in the later chapters, he will be better able to consider how he could effectively allow stress to work for his benefit.

Now that stressors and the individual's makeup have been covered

* Proverbs 15:1.
** Forbes, *Epigrams.*
*** Selye, H. *Stress Without Distress,* Philadelphia: J. B. Lippincott Co., 1974.

TABLE 2.4   Environmental Factors and Stress

FACTOR OR CONDITION	STRESS RESPONSE
Disease	Immune response is decreased in many chronic diseases.
Diet	Poor diets mean poor resistance to stressors; obesity inclines one toward heart attacks.
Drugs	Alcoholism means impaired immune response.
Occupation	Accountants get high blood pressure during tax time; business executives are prone to ulcers.
Location	City living is most stressful.
Family situation	Single people have higher incidence of stress-related diseases and disorders.
Social situation	Socially isolated persons are more prone to disease and tend to die prematurely.
Religious affiliation	Deeply religious persons seem to manage severe stressors well.
Physical and mental preparation	Well-conditioned athletes respond well to physical stressors; mental preparation permits someone to handle assignments well.
Emotional stability	Stable people react well to stressors.
Ability to relax	Negative effects of stress may be overcome by those who can relax.

in detail, we turn in the next chapter to consideration of the actual physiological and psychological changes that make up the entity known as stress.

REFERENCES

1. Morse, D. R., Martin, J. M., Furst, M. L. and Dubin, L. L. A physiological and subjective evaluation of neutral and emotionally-charged words for meditation. *J. Am. Soc. Psychosom. Dent. Med.* 26(1-4): (1979), in press.
2. Mischel, W. *Introduction to Personality,* Second Ed. New York: Holt, Rinehart and Winston, 1976.
3. Jung, C. G. *Psychological Types.* New York: Harcourt, Brace and World, 1923.
4. Sheldon, W. H. *Atlas of Men: A Guide for Somatotyping the Adult Male at All Ages.* New York: Harper, 1954.
5. Rotter, J. B. Generalized expectancies for internal versus external control of reinforcement. *Psychol. Monogr.* 80:1-28, 1966.
6. Kraepelin, E. *Clinical Psychiatry.* New York: Macmillan, 1907.
7. Solomon, R. L. and Brush, E. S. Experimentally derived conceptions of anxiety and aversion. *In* Jones, M. R. (ed.), *Nebraska Sympostium on Motivation.* Lincoln: University of Nebraska Press, 1956.
8. Dunbar, F. *Psychosomatic Diagnosis.* New York: Harper, 1943.

9. Friedman, M. and Rosenman, R. H. *Type A Behavior and Your Heart.* New York: Knopf, 1974.

10. Le Shan, L. An emotional life-history pattern associated with neoplastic disease. *Ann. N.Y. Acad. Sci.* 125(3):780–793, 1966.

11. Wolff, H. G., Wolf, S. and Goodell, H. *Stress and Disease,* Second Ed. Springfield, Ill.: Charles C. Thomas Publ., 1968.

12. Arehart-Treichel, J. Can your personality kill you? *New York Magazine* 10:62–67, Nov. 28, 1977.

13. Moos, R. H. and Solomon, G. F. Psychologic comparisons between women with rheumatoid arthritis and their non-arthritic sisters. *Psychosom. Med.* 27:150–164, 1965.

14. Grace, W. J., Wolf, S. and Wolff, H. G. *The Human Colon.* New York: Paul B. Hoeber, 1951.

15. Sword, R. O. The depression-prone personality: Almost "too good" to be true. *Dent. Surv.* 53(3):12–18, 1977.

16. Pelletier, K. R. *Mind As Healer Mind As Slayer. A Holistic Approach to Preventing Stress Disorders.* New York: Dell Publ. Co. Inc., 1977, pp. 151–153.

17. Cohen, M. J., Rickles, W. H. and McArthur, D. L. Evidence for physiological response stereotyping in migraine headaches. *Psychosom. Med.* 40:344–354, 1978.

18. Kimball, C. P. A predictive study of adjustment to cardiac surgery. *J. Thorac. Cardiovasc. Surg.* 58:891–896, 1969.

19. Cheek, D. B. Unconscious perception of meaningful sounds during surgical anesthesia as revealed under hypnosis. *Am. J. Clin. Hypn.* 1:101–113, 1959.

20. Grace, W. J. and Graham, D. T. Relationship of specific attitudes and emotions to certain bodily diseases. *Psychosom. Med.* 14:243–251, 1952.

21. Graham, D. T., Lundy, R. M., Benjamin, L. S., Kabler, J. D., Lewis, W. C., Kunich, N. O. and Graham, F. K. Specific attitudes in initial interviews with patients having different psychosomatic diseases. *Psychosom. Med.* 24:257–266, 1962.

22. Holmes, T. H., Jaffe, J. R., Ketcham, J. W. and Sheehy, T. F. Experimental study of prognosis. *J. Psychosom. Res.* 5:235–252, 1961.

23. Hilgard, E. R. and Hilgard, J. A. *Hypnosis in the Relief of Pain.* Los Altos, Calif.: William Kaufman, 1975, pp. 32–33.

24. Schlesinger, Z., Barzilay, J., Stryjer, D., and Almog, C. H. Life-threatening "vagal reaction" to emotional stimuli. *Israel J. Med. Sci.* 13:59–61, 1977.

25. Sheehy, G. *Passages: Predictable Crises of Adult Life.* New York: Dutton, 1976.

26. Gould, R. *Transformations.* New York: Simon and Schuster, 1978.

27. Stumpf, W. E., Sar, M. and Aumüller, G. The heart: A target organ for estradiol. *Science* 196:319–320, 1977.

28. Colburn, P. and Buonassisi, V. Estrogen-binding sites in endothelial cell cultures. *Science* 201:817–819, 1978.

29. Johansson, G., Frankenhaeuser, M. and Magnusson, D. Catecholamine output in school children as related to performance and adjustment. *Scand. J. Psychol.* 14:20–28, 1973.

30. Johansson, G. and Post, B. Catecholamine output of males and females over a one-year period. *Acta Physiol. Scand.* 92:557–565, 1974.
31. Frankenhaeuser, M., von Wright, M. R., Collins, A., von Wright, J., Sedvall, G. and Swahn, C. G. Sex differences in psychoneuroendocrine reactions to examination stress. *Psychosom. Med.* 40:334–343, 1978.
32. Collins, A. and Frankenhaeuser, M. Stress responses in male and female engineering students. *J. Human Stress* 4(2):43–48, 1978.
33. Seltzer, S. *Endodontology: Biologic Considerations in Endodontic Procedures.* New York: McGraw-Hill Book Co., 1971, p. 408.
34. Morse, D. R. *Clinical Endodontology: A Comprehensive Guide to Diagnosis, Treatment and Prevention.* Springfield, Ill.: Charles C. Thomas Publ., 1974.
35. Editorial. Hypertension more likely among less educated and blacks. *Med. World News* 19(2):13, Jan. 23, 1978.
36. Samples, R. E. Learning with the whole brain. *Hum. Behav.* 4(2):16–23, 1975.
37. Galaburda, A. M., LeMay, M., Kemper, T. L. and Geschwind, N. Right-left asymmetries in the brain. *Science* 199:852–856, 1978.
38. Krueger, A. P. and Read, E. J. Biological impact of small air ions. *Science* 193:1209–1213, 1976.
39. Gittelson, B. *Biorhythm: A Personal Science,* Third Ed. New York: Arco Publ. Co., 1977.
40. Friedman, M., Rosenman, R. H. and Carrol, V. Changes in the serum cholesterol and blood clotting time in men subjected to cyclic variation of occupational stress. *Circulation* 18:852–861, 1958.
41. Leff, D. R. Stress-triggered organic disease in this year of economic anxiety. *Med. World News.* 16:74–92, Mar. 24, 1975.
42. Brady, J. V. Ulcers in "executive monkeys." *Sci. Am.* 199(4):95–100, 1958.
43. Miller, N. E. and Dworkin, B. R. Effects of learning on visceral functions—Biofeedback. *N. Engl. J. Med.* 296:1274–1278, 1977.
44. Editorial. The penalty of sin. *Exec. Fitness Newsletter.* Sample Issue 1, 1977.
45. Morse, D. R. and Furst, M. L. *Stress and Relaxation: Application to Dentistry.* Springfield, Ill.: Charles C. Thomas Publ., 1978.
46. Editorial. Musicians' stress likened to pilots'. *The New York Times*:34, Feb. 24, 1970.
47. Lewis, H. R. and Lewis, M. E. *Psychosomatics: How Your Emotions Can Damage Your Health.* New York: The Viking Press, 1972.
48. Barmash, I. *Welcome to Our Conglomerate—You're Fired!* New York: Delacorte, 1971.
49. Editorial. Feeling tense on subway? Leave. *Philadelphia Eve. Bull.:*10, Nov. 8, 1977.
50. Redmond, P. What your questionnaire told us about your health. *Dent. Econ.* 67(3):28–33, 1977.
51. Moorman, L. T. Tuberculosis on the Navajo reservation. *Am. Review of Tuberculosis* 61:586–591, 1950.
52. Editorial. Loneliness really can kill you. *Philadelphia Eve. Bull.:*23, Dec. 15, 1977.

3

The Stress Response

The pulse is altered by quarrels and alarms which suddenly disturb the mind.*

A HOUSE IS NOT A HOME

You turn the knob, and the door squeaks open. Your eyes peer into utter darkness. Suddenly, you hear a loud, reverberating sound, almost like the roar of a kettledrum. Just when you're about to dash out the door, the realization dawns, "Hey! That's *my* thump—that's my heart." Temporarily reassured, you re-enter the house cautiously—and just then a gust of wind slams the door shut. The crash of the door startles you; you leap into the air, and as you return to Earth, you get a sinking feeling in the pit of your stomach. You freeze—being unsure of who or what closed the door—trying not to make a sound.

Now trickles of sweat begin their journey across the bridge of your

* From a letter by the Greek physician Galen (A.D. 130–201) in his book *On Prognosis,* translated by A. J. Brock, *Greek Medicine,* London: J. M. Dent and Sons, Ltd., 1929.

nose; and try as you may, you can't stop the sound of your breathing or the pounding of your heart. Although the room seemed pitch black a few minutes ago, you now can make out several objects. You listen intently—and, aside from your own internal sounds, all you hear is the clamor of the chirping crickets penetrating from the outside: "I *knew* the house wasn't haunted."

With faltering courage, you head for the shadowy stairs, but you can't stop your body from trembling. "Gee! There are *two* staircases." At the same time, you realize that you have an overwhelming need to find a bathroom. So you reverse your steps, waver nervously out the door and . . .

"Hi, Jim! How are you feeling now?"

You look up and there's your buddy Jack—and you wonder what you're doing lying in the grass with a wet towel on your head.

Postscript

Needless to say, you, Jim, were in a stressful situation, and your various reactions were components of the stress response. You experienced both physiological and psychological stress reactions, including a culminating fainting episode. Let us now examine these responses more thoroughly, beginning with the physiological responses.

THE PHYSIOLOGICAL RESPONSES

The key to learning about stress is to understand how the body reacts under stress—to become aware of the mechanics of the stress response. When certain components of the stress response get out of hand, disease generally results. Hence, we feel it is important for the reader to understand the stress response, and we give a thorough description of it in the following pages, moving slowly and giving simplified explanations along the way. In reading the later chapters, the reader may want to return to these pages for review and clarification.

Before turning our attention to the actual changes that are characteristic of the stress response, we cover the general involvement of the systems of the body. Simple diagrams to help in the discussion are shown in Figs. 3.1 to 3.6.

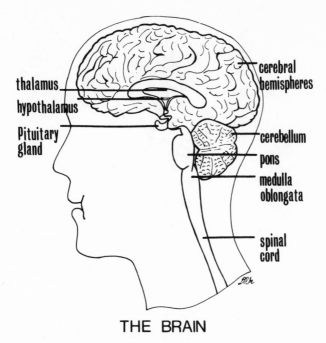

THE BRAIN

Fig. 3.1 The brain. The cerebral hemispheres are the presumed seat of consciousness, thinking and muscle activity initiation; the cerebellum is concerned with muscle coordination, equilibrium and balance; the pons is involved with autonomic nervous system functions; the medulla oblongata contains the centers for breathing, heart beat and blood flow control; the spinal cord is important in reflex activity; the thalamus is a pain center; and the hypothalamus and the pituitary gland (hypophysis) are involved in the stress response in addition to other autonomic functions.

Whether a stressor is local (e.g., a burned hand) or general (e.g., falling into an ice-cold pool), there is a rather specific stress response generated. Aside from the stress response, other changes occur that are caused by the specific stressor. For example, with the burned hand an inflammatory response is generated. Given this response, various substances are released at the local site, including histamine, plasma kinins and lysosomal enzymes. At the same time that the inflammatory substances are released, an internal message from the burned hand initiates the stress response. This reaction is illustrated in Fig. 3.7.

There is some evidence that the first stress mediator is one of the prostaglandins (i.e., small chemical substances involved in inflammation).[1-3] The message is carried to the hypothalamus in the brain stem. Once the hypothalamus is alerted, two primary systems

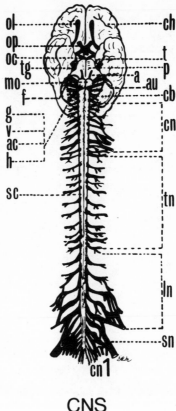

CNS

Fig. 3.2 The central nervous system (CNS) and associated cranial and spinal nerves. The CNS consists of the brain and the spinal cord. The brain parts are: ch = cerebral hemispheres; p = pons; cb = cerebellum; mo = medulla oblongata; and sc = spinal cord. The cranial nerves are ol = olfactory (1, smell); op = optic (2, sight); oc = oculomotor (3, eye movement); t = trochlear (4, eye movement); tg = trigeminal (5, chewing, teeth sensation); a = abducens (6, eye movement); f = facial (7, facial expression, salivation); au = auditory (8, hearing, equilibrium); g = glossopharyngeal (9, swallowing, salivation); v = vagus (10, swallowing, speech; stimulates digestion, slows the heart); ac = spinal accessory (11, neck muscles and palate); and h = hypoglossal (12, moves tongue). The spinal nerves are: cn = cervical (neck) nerves; tn = thoracic (chest) nerves; ln = lumbar (upper back) nerves; sn = sacral (lower back) nerves; and cn1 = coccygeal (tail) nerves.

become activated.[4] The first is the hypothalamus–anterior pituitary (adenohypophysis)-adrenal cortex (H–AP–AC) axis, with the primary release of corticosteroids (e.g., cortisone). The second system activated is the autonomic nervous system (ANS), with the principal release of epinephrine (adrenaline) and norepinephrine (noradrenaline).[5] Collectively, epinephrine and norepinephrine are known as catecholamines. A preliminary view of the stress response is illustrated in Fig. 3.8.

The Cortisone Story

Once the hypothalamus is activated, the H–AP–AC axis releases into the blood stream a corticotropic-releasing factor (CRF), which induces the anterior pituitary (also located in the brain stem) to produce adrenocorticotropic hormone (ACTH). ACTH then travels in the blood stream to the adrenal cortex (located above the kidneys) which responds by releasing the syntoxic steroids (anti-inflammatory hormones; e.g., cortisone). There is another hormone released by the anterior pituitary called somatotropin (STH or growth hormone).[6–8] It also travels to the adrenal cortex and apparently causes the release of the catatoxic steroids (pro-inflammatory hormones; e.g., aldosterone).[4]

These two groups of steroid hormones work in harmony to regulate the body's reactions during the neutral and beneficial stress responses (i.e., neustress and eustress). However, with distress, there appears to be an excessive build-up of corticosteroids (e.g., cortisone). The aspects of the stress response discussed to this point are shown in Fig. 3.9.

Since cortisone is so important in the stress response, we now consider its major actions in the body.[4,9–11] Cortisone shuts down inflammation, whereas aldosterone increases inflammation. The result of cortisone's action is to gear the body to take care of any major danger. Hence, it causes the temporary suppression of local reactions, such as the inflammatory response, so that the body is better prepared to deal with any stressor in a rapid and integrated manner. In order to slow down inflammation, cortisone reduces the action of the thymus gland and the lymph nodes, which are important in immunological responses (i.e., responses that fight infection and cancer cells). Cortisone also paralyzes the defensive cells of the body such as lymphocytes, polymorphonuclear leucocytes and macrophages (i.e., scavenger cells). A bad side effect of cortisone's action is that infections and tumor cells could spread. Hence, it can be seen that if cortisone were continually being produced, as with chronic stress reactions, there is a good chance that a person could come down with serious infections and/or cancer (although the latter is conjecture).

Cortisone stimulates glucose production (gluconeogenesis) in the liver. This reaction is important during the normal stress response, since glucose (i.e., a type of sugar) supplies energy needed for muscular work (e.g., fighting a foe or fleeing a fire). However, with chronic stress, an excessive production of glucose in a susceptible individual could lead to diabetes. Also, for the glucose to be used it

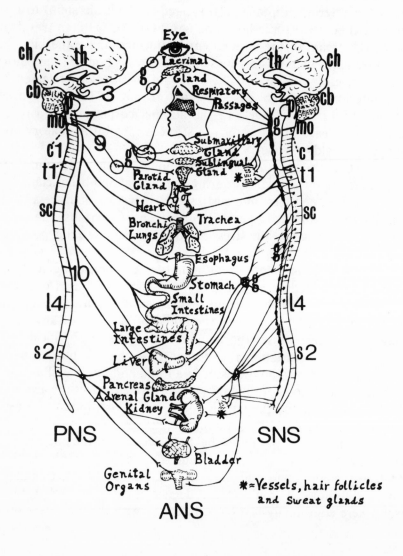

must pass from the blood into the cells, an action that requires insulin from the pancreas. But one of the side effects of cortisone production is to inhibit insulin. With chronic stress this depletion of insulin could further increase the chance of diabetes.

One breakdown product of glucose metabolism is lactic acid (lactate). Studies by Ferris Pitts, Jr. have shown that individuals who suffer severe anxiety and who are under chronic stress produce large amounts of blood lactate.[12]

Cortisone acts on the lungs to cause dilation of the bronchi. This action apparently aids in the stress response by allowing for increased intake of oxygen (also needed for energy) and elimination of carbon dioxide (i.e., waste gas). This broncho-dilatory action of cor-

---

Fig. 3.3 The autonomic nervous system (ANS). The ANS is divided into the parasympathetic nervous system (PNS; cranial-sacral) and the sympathetic nervous system (SNS; thoracolumbar). The SNS is activated during stress and the PNS during relaxation; and their reactions are generally opposite in effect. Both systems are integrated with the CNS (brain and spinal cord). Brain parts are: ch = cerebral hemispheres; th = thalamus; cb = cerebellum; p = pons; mo = medulla oblongata. The spinal cord (sc) divisions are: c = cervical; t = thoracic; l = lumbar; and s = sacral. The cranial nerves involved with the PNS are: 3 (oculomotor); 7 facial); 9 (glossopharyngeal); and 10 (vagus). Nerve cell bodies and connections between nerves are found in structures called ganglia (g).

PNS	STRUCTURE	SNS
constricts	pupil of eye	dilates
contracts	eye muscle (ciliary)	relaxes
stimulates	lacrimal (tear) gland	inhibits
stimulates	respiratory passages	inhibits
large amount of watery saliva	salivary glands: submaxillary sublingual parotid	small amount of thick saliva
contracts muscles	trachea, bronchi and lungs	relaxes muscles
inhibits	heart	accelerates
	blood vessels of skin	constricts
	sweat glands	secretion
	hair follicles	contraction
activates	esophagus, stomach and intestines	inhibits
	liver and pancreas	increases activity
	adrenal medulla	secretion of adrenaline primarily
constricts muscles	kidneys and bladder	relaxes muscles
increases activity	genital organs	inhibits activity

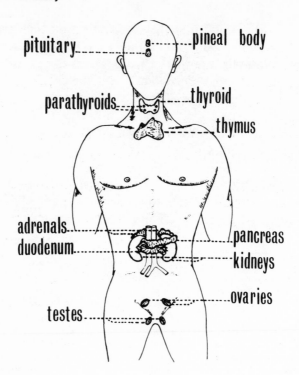

Fig. 3.4 The endocrine system. Major endocrine glands are shown and their principal hormones (chemical messengers) are given below. Pineal body → melatonin (regulates pigmentation); anterior pituitary (adenohypophysis) → adrenocorticotropin (ACTH), somatotropin (STH or growth hormone), thyrotropin (TSH), melanocyte stimulating hormone (MSH, concerned with pigment formation), gonadotropins (stimulate reproductive functional activity); posterior pituitary (neurohypophysis) → oxytocin (contracts uterus, activates milk secretion from mammary glands), antidiuretic hormone (ADH or vasopressin; facilitates water retention and salt balance and raises blood pressure); parathyroids → parathormone (bone metabolism); thyroid → thyroxine (energy metabolism) and calcitonin (bone metabolism); thymus → thymic hormone (?) (thymus is primarily concerned with cellular immunity); adrenal cortex → cortisone, aldosterone and related compounds; adrenal medulla → adrenaline (epinephrine) and noradrenaline (norepinephrine); pancreas (islets of Langerhans are the site) → insulin (brings glucose out of the blood and into cells) and glucagon (reverses actions of insulin); duodenum (a part of the small intestines) → secretin (stimulates the pancreas to secrete; aids in digestion) and cholecystokinin (stimulates the gall bladder to discharge bile; aids in fat digestion); kidneys → renin and angiotensin (concerned with regulation of body fluids and raises blood pressure); ovaries → estrogen and progesterone (important female hormones); and testes → androgens (important male hormones).

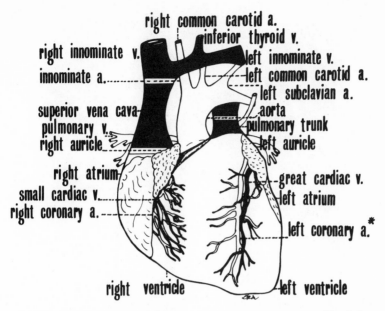

Fig. 3.5 The heart and associated blood vessels. v = vein; and a = artery. Blood that comes from the rest of the body (i.e., blood is filled with the waste gas CO_2 and deficient in O_2) enters the right side of the heart through the superior vena cava (shown in black). The blood goes from the right atrium to the right ventricle. It is then pumped out through the pulmonary trunk to the lungs. In the lungs, the CO_2 is given off and is removed with the expired air. With the inspired air, O_2 goes into the lungs. Oxygenated blood from the lungs passes into the left side of the heart via the pulmonary veins. The O_2-rich blood goes from the left atrium to the left ventricles. The oxygenated blood is pumped through the aorta and then throughout the body. O_2-rich blood is carried to the heart muscle itself via the coronary arteries, and CO_2 leaves the heart muscle via the cardiac veins (shown in black). Coronary artery thrombosis (clot formation) occurs primarily in the left coronary artery* causing severe damage to the left ventricle (called myocardial infarction). Together, the thrombosis and infarction are known as a heart attack.

tisone is effectively used for the treatment of asthma. The cortisone helps open the previously collapsed and constricted lung bronchi. Chronic stress could conceivably cause the lung tissues to lose their flexibility, which would decrease the individual's breathing effectiveness.

Another site of action of cortisone is the gut (i.e., gastrointestinal tract). Again in order to shut off unneeded activity so as to have a coordinated stress response, the action of cortisone closes down the

* Anderson, W. A. D. and Kissane, J. M. Pathology, Seventh Ed. St. Louis: C. V. Mosby, 1977, p. 761.

ARTERIAL SYSTEM

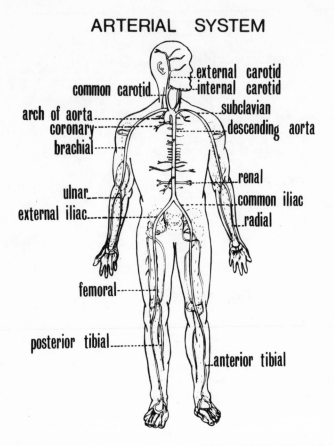

external carotid
internal carotid
common carotid
subclavian
arch of aorta
coronary
descending aorta
brachial
renal
ulnar
common iliac
external iliac
radial
femoral
posterior tibial
anterior tibial

Fig. 3.6 The circulatory system. The arterial system is shown. Oxygenated blood from the left ventricle of the heart is pumped out through the arch of the aorta to the systemic circulation where eventually all the body's tissues are supplied with oxygen. Carbon dioxide gas from the tissues returns to the right side of the heart via the venous system. The venous system is not shown, but the vessels generally parallel those of the arterial system. (For a complete picture of the circulatory system, see also Figs. 2.2 and 3.5.)

gut's digestive activity. However, in this action, an unwanted side effect can be irritation of the lining of the digestive tract. If this action becomes repetitive, then duodenal (i.e., a part of the small intestine) or peptic (i.e., stomach) ulcers can result.

A further result of cortisone's action on the gut is to inhibit the activity of vitamin D. Vitamin D is needed to bring calcium into the blood stream in a usable form. Chronic production of cortisone may lead to brittle bones (osteoporosis).[13]

Cortisone also travels to the kidney. At this organ site, it

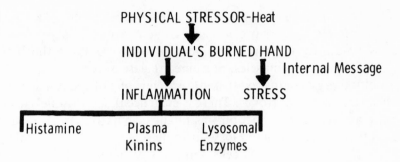

Fig. 3.7 The local response.

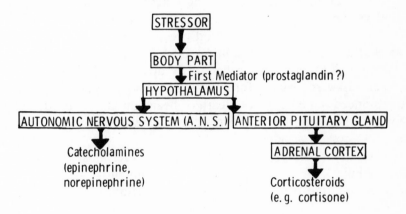

Fig. 3.8 A preliminary view of the stress response.

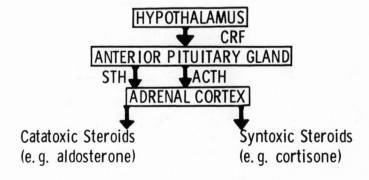

Fig. 3.9 A further stage in the stress response. CRF = corticotropic factor; STH = somatotropin hormone; ACTH = adrenocorticotropic hormone.

stimulates the release of renin,[8] a substance that causes a rise in blood pressure (i.e., a pressor agent). A rise in blood pressure is necessary during the stress response in order to force the blood quickly to the active muscles. Sustained release of renin could lead to high blood pressure (hypertension), which is one of the prime causes of heart attacks and strokes. There is evidence that cortisone's action during a severe stress reaction—as might occur from an accident in which there is major blood loss—is to help restore the blood volume by withdrawing fluid from cells and transferring it to the interstitial (tissue) spaces. Donald Gann, at Johns Hopkins, has presented some preliminary findings indicating that during severe stress reactions even without blood loss, cortisone's activity results in increased blood volume.[14] A series of such reactions, as in chronic stress, is believed to lead to increased blood pressure. Hence, this is another way that cortisone's action could raise blood pressure.

In animal experiments, when high doses of sodium and corticosteroids were given before physical stressors such as experimentally induced bone fractures, death of heart muscle occurred.[15] Conceivably, this might also happen to humans who become involved in severely stressful accidents.

These major roles of cortisone in the stress response are summarized in Fig. 3.10. In Fig. 3.11 are shown potential symptoms and diseases resulting from cortisone overproduction.

The Thyroxine Story

If we now return to the anterior pituitary gland, we find that another hormone is released during stress. This chemical messenger is known

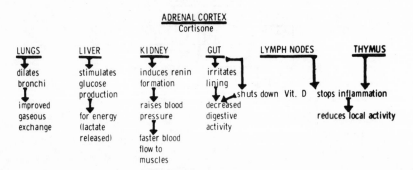

Fig. 3.10 The major roles of cortisone in the stress response.

ACTION	POTENTIAL SYMPTOM OR DISEASE
inhibits inflammation	infections or cancer
produces glucose ⟶ yields lactate ⟶	diabetes / anxiety neurosis
causes excessive dilation	impaired breathing
irritates lining	ulcers
shuts down Vitamin D	osteoporosis
releases renin	hypertension

Fig. 3.11 Potential symptoms and diseases from cortisone overproduction.

as thyrotropic hormone (TTH).[4,7] It goes to the thyroid gland and causes the release of thyroxine and other thyroid hormones, which act to increase the body's metabolism. This action is important for normal stress responses in which an active, alert body is essential (as in fighting and running). But with chronic stress responses, excessive thyroid activity in a susceptible individual could lead to the development of hyperthyroidism (Grave's disease).[16] This stress pathway is shown in Fig. 3.12.

Returning to the hypothalamus for a moment, in addition to activating the anterior pituitary gland, the hypothalamus activates the posterior pituitary gland, resulting in the release of the hormone vasopressin.[17] Vasopressin acts on arteries causing them to contract, which is still another way that blood pressure is raised. This reaction is shown in Fig. 3.13.

Now that we have examined the first component of the stress response (i.e., the H-AP-AC axis), let us consider the other component: the autonomic nervous system (ANS) response.

The Adrenaline Story

The first mediator that alerts the H-AP-AC axis also activates the ANS and principally the sympathetic division (SNS).[9,18] This causes the release of epinephrine (adrenaline) and norepinephrine

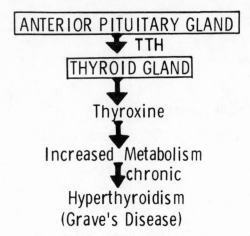

Fig. 3.12 The thyroid pathway. TTH = thyrotropic hormone.

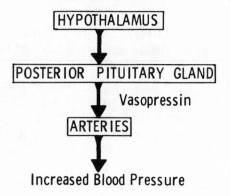

Fig. 3.13 Vasopressin's role in the stress response.

(noradrenaline) from the endings of sympathetic nerves and epinephrine (principally) from the adrenal medulla.*

The adrenal cortex which produces cortisone is on the outside of the adrenal gland. The adrenal medulla which produces epinephrine is on the inside of the adrenal gland (see Fig. 3.14). ACTH from the

---

* In humans, both of these hormones are produced during the stress response. In animals, there is some evidence that these are hormones related to different functions. "Fighting" animals such as lions, tigers and bears produce much norepinephrine. As a result, it has received the pseudonym "the aggression hormone." "Frightened" animals like rabbits and deer "pump out" large amounts of epinephrine. Hence, it has been called "the fear hormone." It is not definitely known whether humans selectively produce these hormones under the differing conditions of aggression and fear. A number of years ago, D. H. Funkenstein experimentally showed that noradrenaline is produced under the condition of anger, and adrenaline is produced during depression and anxiety.[19]

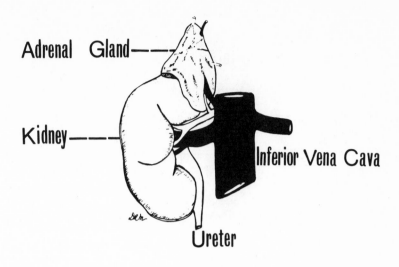

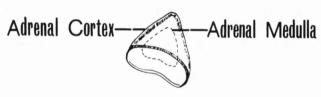

Fig. 3.14 The adrenal gland. The adrenal (suprarenal) glands lie above the kidneys. The outer surface is called the adrenal cortex. Hormones released include cortisone and aldosterone. Within the gland is found the adrenal medulla. Hormones released include adrenaline (epinephrine) and noradrenaline (norepinephrine).

anterior pituitary also appears to signal the adrenal medulla (as well as the adrenal cortex) to produce epinephrine.[9] This aspect of the sympathetic nervous system response is shown in Fig. 3.15.

The action of epinephrine and norepinephrine (i.e., the catecholamines) is the other major activity in the stress response. The catecholamines act on the heart and blood vessels to cause an increase in blood pressure. Remember that cortisone and vasopressin also cause an increase in blood pressure, but with cortisone the action is on the kidney (i.e., renin production), while with vasopressin the action is only on the arteries. Similarly to the action of cortisone, the catecholamines cause increases in blood glucose and dilation of the bronchi. The catecholamines are also used to control acute attacks of asthma. Also, as is the case with cortisone, the catecholamines act on the gut to irritate the lining.

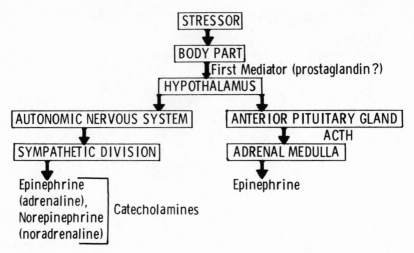

Fig. 3.15 Activation of the sympathetic response. ACTH = adrenocorticotropic hormone.

Hydrochloric acid (HCl) is present in the stomach. Its primary purpose appears to be to destroy bacteria and any other microbes that might get into the stomach. However, if there is too much HCl produced, then the stomach's lining could become eroded. Animal experiments have shown that chronic psychological stressors such as fear can cause an increased release of HCl.[20] This could further increase the chance of development of peptic ulcers.[21]

The reactions described so far are added to the similar ones produced by cortisone. These catecholamine reactions are shown in Fig. 3.16.

In addition to these responses, there are a series of reactions triggered solely by the catecholamines. Together these constitute the "fight or flight" response (first described by Walter Cannon).[5,9] This response enables a person to react to a stressor by mobilizing all of his resources so that he may either fight or run (i.e., take some definitive action). Let us consider the various components of the "fight or flight" response. The catecholamines' effect on the heart is such as to cause an increase in heart activity (i.e., gets the blood to the muscles for action). If this response were to become chronic, then it could lead to irregular heart sounds (arrhythmias).[22] Another action on the heart is to cause an increase in heart rate. If this were repeated regularly, it could develop into very rapid heart beats (tachycardia). Sudden release of large amounts of catecholamines

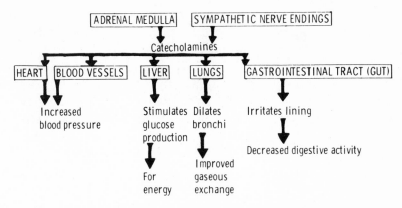

Fig. 3.16 Some stress responses from the catecholamines.

has been shown experimentally to cause severe damage to the heart muscle.[23]

The catecholamines travel to the motor nerves (those that "fire off" the muscles) and make them more excitable. In turn, the major muscles of the body "tense" (partial contraction) as the person is prepared to fight, flee or "freeze" (i.e., bracing for action). If stress becomes chronic, then spasms or "knots" can develop in muscle groups, and pain can occur. This can result in tension headaches, jaw aches (myofascial pain-dysfunction syndrome), backaches and neck and shoulder pain.[24]

If muscles become too active during the stress response, then trembling or "nervousness" can result. If this reaction were to become chronic, it could lead to muscle tremors.

Another reaction seen is sweating of the palms and soles (i.e., getting rid of waste products resulting from increased bodily activity). This can be measured—well before the actual sweating is seen visually—by using small electrodes attached to the palms of the hands. The response is called the galvanic skin response (GSR) and is one of the key features of the "lie detector test."[25] When a person lies, he is generally stressed, a fact that can be detected by increased sweating.[26] Excessive sweating can lead to malodor.

Epinephrine and norepinephrine affect the breathing centers to cause increases in breathing rate, oxygen intake and carbon dioxide removal. The chest also expands more, and the throat relaxes. All of these responses allow for a better exchange of gases so that the active muscles will have enough oxygen for energy and the means for rapid removal of waste products. If these breathing reactions were prolonged, hyperventilation could occur, which might cause a person to lose consciousness.

When a person is under stress, he must be able to see as clearly as possible (in order to fight or flee). Increased visual perception occurs as a result of catecholamine action on the eyes, causing dilation of the pupils. Of course, adequate light must be available for him to see optimally. It is possible that continual pupillary dilation could interfere with proper accommodation of eye muscles (i.e., one might develop a "beady-eye" look). E. H. Hess found that strong emotional reactions, including extreme pleasure, cause dilation.[27] After the initial shock, distasteful stimuli cause pupil constriction. This is an instance of an initial sympathetic response followed by a parasympathetic response.

In addition to seeing well, it is also essential to have the other senses operate at an optimum level. Although it is not known whether catecholamines are involved, it does appear that hearing, smell and touch receptors become hypersensitive during stress. For example, during a stressful encounter, a dog's ears point toward the source of stress, and the nostrils flare. Although most humans' external ears no longer are able to adjust, people do tend to turn toward the stress source, and the nostrils of many people do dilate. (Have you ever noticed an angry man's flaring nostrils?)

Although not related to the catecholamines, another bodily sensation is altered under stress, namely, the perception of pain. It is well known that under war combat conditions and during physical activity, people can suffer severe injuries and yet not report pain.[28] Recent findings give a clue as to how this might occur.[29] During stress, the anterior pituitary gland releases a large protein, called pro-opiocortin. This protein soon breaks up into smaller proteins including the previously mentioned ACTH (which then activates cortisone) and morphine-like substances called endorphins and enkephalins. The latter substances apparently can block the perception of and/or reaction to pain. There is also some evidence that endorphins are produced as a result of acupuncture, and that could explain—especially for the benefit of skeptics—how pain blockage is effected when that technique is employed.[30]

The catecholamines also work in the mouth, causing a decrease in the flow of saliva. Although saliva is necessary for digestion, it is temporarily inhibited so that the body can be mobilized to deal with the emergency situation. If the decrease in saliva persisted, it could lead to a perpetual dry mouth (xerostomia). There are some interesting applications based on the connection between stress and the dry mouth. Let us look at a few.[26,31] The Bedouins of the Middle East formerly required witnesses who gave conflicting evidence about a crime to lick a hot iron. The witness whose tongue was burned was considered to be the liar. In ancient China, an individual being interrogated about a reported crime was given rice powder to chew and then spit out. If the expectorated powder came out dry, then the suspect was considered to be guilty. Many years ago in England, a criminal suspect was given a "trial" slice of bread and cheese. If he could not swallow that combination, he was judged to be guilty. In all of these cases, the guilt of the suspect was based on the common observation that when a person is under stress, his salivation diminishes until his mouth becomes dry. Did you ever notice what happens when you go to the dentist—especially if you are anxious? Your saliva changes; it decreases in amount and tends to become thick and "ropy" and sticks to everything when you try to spit out. Another effect associated with a dry mouth is the loss of one's voice under stress.

Again in order to shut down the food digestion process, the catecholamines cause the transfer of blood from the intestines to the heart and skeletal muscles. This is important for muscular work.

Epinephrine acts on the skin to cause vasoconstriction of the blood vessels.[32] This shutting down causes the skin to blanch. Notice how pale some people become under stress. It has been hypothesized that closing down the skin circulation is to prevent excessive blood loss. For example, if you should get cut during a struggle, since you are under stress you'll probably not bleed too much; if you get bitten, you may still have to worry about rabies and tetanus. Another related reaction under stress is an increased tendency for the blood to clot (i.e., increased blood platelet aggregation),[33] which would also help reduce blood loss. However, if stress becomes chronic, this reaction might lead to the development of internal blood clots which could result in a thrombosis that might precipitate a heart attack or a stroke. All of the changes of the "fight or flight" response are shown in Fig. 3.17. Potential symptoms and diseases from catecholamine overproduction are shown in Fig. 3.18.

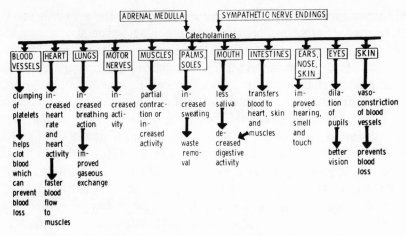

Fig. 3.17 Physiological changes of the "fight or flight" response.

SITE	ACTION	POTENTIAL SYMPTOM OR DISEASE
Skin	vasoconstriction	pallor
Liver	excess glucose	diabetes
Lungs	excessive dilation	impaired breathing
Lungs	increased breathing rate	hyperventilation
Gut	irritates lining	ulcers
Blood Vessels	increased tendency to clot	heart attack or stroke
Blood Vessels ⎤ Heart ⎦	increased blood pressure	hypertension
Heart	muscle damage	heart damage or death
Motor Nerves	increased excitability	muscle tremors
Muscles	partial contraction	headache, backache, jaw ache, shoulder pain, neck pain
Palms and Soles	increased sweating	malodor
Eyes	increased visual perception	"beady" eyes
Mouth	decreased saliva	xerostomia (dry mouth)
Blood Lactate	waste product	acid-base imbalance
Uric Acid	waste product	gout
Cholesterol and Fatty Acids	energy	heart attack or stroke

Fig. 3.18 Potential symptoms and diseases from catecholamine overproduction.

In addition to the previously mentioned blood lactate (breakdown product of glucose), other blood changes found are increases in blood cholesterol and fatty acids.[34] (These substances are probably used for energy.) If this reaction were to become chronic, it could irritate coronary and cerebral (brain) blood vessels and lead to heart attacks and strokes. A final blood change that may be observed is an increase in uric acid (i.e., another waste product).[34] Under certain chronic conditions, accumulations of uric acid could lead to gout.

During stress, the brain is active. This is reflected in fast beta wave activity in the electroencephalogram (EEG). As part of the first study reported at Temple University comparing meditation with hypnosis, the subjects' reactions were also monitored during the hyperactive condition (a stress state).[35] Using the EEG, it was found that during this state subjects showed pronounced beta wave activity (see Fig. 13.1 in Chapter 13 for an example).

Various Responses

Not everyone shows all of the previous reactions: Some people respond primarily by breathing faster; others principally show a rise in blood pressure; still others have a faster heart beat; and there are some who react with sweating palms. One reason that the "lie detector" is not universally applicable is that not everyone sweats profusely under the stress of lying. In our experiments at Temple University, it was found that certain individuals showed practically no change in skin resistance (i.e., sweat gland activity) regardless of the stressful stimuli.[35,36]

There is also evidence that under different kinds of stressors there are slightly different responses. For example, the physical stressor of exercise shows different responses depending upon a person's emotions while he is exercising. One study showed that the responses varied during exercise depending upon whether the people had feelings of anger, fear, happiness, jubilation or sadness.[37] A recent study by Benson's group showed that oxygen consumption was less for subjects when they meditated while they were engaged in stationary bicycle riding as compared to the same exercise without meditation.[38] This process may account for the apparently better physiological responses during eustress as compared to distress. Hence, the next time you jog, try meditating as well; and the next time you lift weights, think positively.

Even animals react better to stressors if they are content. It was experimentally observed that petting a dog while it was simultaneously being shocked caused less severe stress responses than if the dog was just shocked.[39] Apparently the petting made the dog tranquil or happy, which in turn positively affected the stress response. The results also seem to show that the dog's "subjective" responses were altered favorably. This is inferred from the fact that the petted-shocked dogs showed no outward signs of being shocked. There is a lesson to be learned from this experiment. If you must mete out punishment, try tempering it with some praise ("honey counteracts vinegar").

Chronic Stress

There are also different responses when the stress becomes chronic. Hans Selye points up the differences in his description of the stages of the General Adaptation Syndrome (GAS).[4] In the first stage—acute stress (the "alarm" reaction)—the previously described reactions occur (i.e., the H-AP-AC axis and the sympathetic nervous system responses). In the second stage—resistance to stress—the body adapts to the chronic stressors, and there are decreased cortisone and catecholamine levels. In the third stage—exhaustion (fatigue)—the body's reactions are no longer sufficient to respond to the stressors. At this final stage, there are the highest levels of cortisone and catecholamines, and the body is most likely to succumb to serious disease and death.

The Parasympathetic Role

Although we have emphasized the sympathetic nervous system response (the "adrenaline story"), the parasympathetic division of the autonomic nervous system is also activated during stress. The parasympathetic's role—with the release of acetylcholine—is to "dampen down" the sympathetic response (e.g., lower blood pressure) so that things don't become unstable. As mentioned in Chapter 2, there are certain individuals who are genetically programmed to have a predominant parasympathetic response during stress (i.e., the "vagotonics").[40] Stress reactions seen in these people include cold-sweating, a slow heart beat, low blood pressure, shallow and irregular breathing, low blood sugar, nausea, dizziness and fainting. In certain instances, serious or even fatal reactions can occur. This may be why some people without any evidence of heart disease react to a severe stressor by a complete slowing up—simply dropping dead.

Summary

Let us now review what has been discussed up to this point about stress. The two major pathways of the stress response have been considered. The first is the H-AP-AC axis with the release of cortisone and related hormones. The second is the autonomic nervous system with predominant activation of the sympathetic nervous system and the release of epinephrine and norepinephrine. Together these two systems mobilize the body's resources so that it can cope with an emergency situation. Although these two systems have been described separately, there are important interactions between the two. First, ACTH from the anterior pituitary gland activates the release of cortisone from the adrenal cortex, and it may also be partly responsible for the release of epinephrine from the adrenal medulla. Next, it has been shown that ACTH and cortisone are both involved in the formation of epinephrine (see Fig. 3.19). And, finally, recent evidence indicates that precursors of epinephrine and norepinephrine in the brain may be involved in activating the entire stress response.

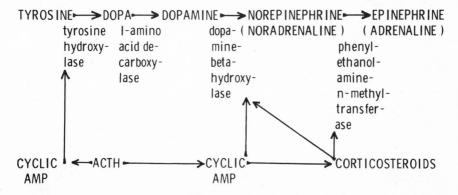

Fig. 3.19 Pathways of epinephrine biosynthesis showing the interrelationship of the two stress systems. AMP = adeno-mono-phosphate; ACTH = adrenocorticotropic hormone. (From Morse, D. R. and Furst, M. L., *Stress and Relaxation: Application to Dentistry,* 1978. Courtesy of Charles C Thomas, Publisher, Springfield, Illinois.)

A general summary of the major physiological changes involved in the stress response is shown in Fig. 3.20.

THE PSYCHOLOGICAL AND ASSOCIATED RESPONSES[4,17]

When people are under stress, they experience strong emotions, which are often accompanied by clearly observable signs. For example, people under stress often feel "nervous." They may be seen to shake, tremble or fidget (i.e., displaying excessive muscle activity). Other observable manifestations are squinting the eyes, pursing the

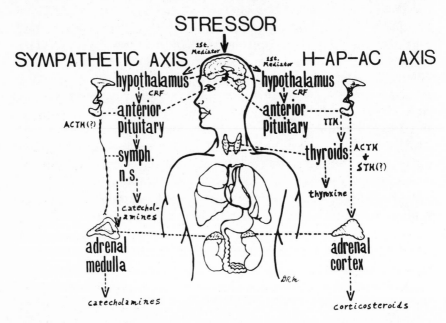

Fig. 3.20 Major physiological changes of the stress response. CRF = corticotropin releasing factor; ACTH = adrenocorticotropic hormone; TTH = thyrotropic hormone; STH = somatotropin; and symph. n. s. = sympathetic nervous system. The stressor activates the 1st mediator which turns on both the sympathetic axis and the H-AP-AC (hypothalamus–anterior pituitary–adrenal cortex) axis. CRF is released and activates the anterior pituitary, which in turn releases ACTH, STH and TTH. ACTH activates the adrenal cortex to release the syntoxic steroids (anti-inflammatory; e.g., cortisone) and possibly the adrenal medulla to release the catecholamines. STH apparently activates the adrenal cortex to release the catatoxic steroids (pro-inflammatory; e.g., aldosterone). TTH induces the thyroid to release thyroxine. The sympathetic nervous system and the adrenal medulla are also activated to release the catecholamines (epinephrine [adrenaline] and norepinephrine [noradrenaline]). (See text for details of the actions resulting from the release of these various stress hormones.)

lips and clenching the hands and jaws. Stress can cause a person to feel giddy, "high," confused—giving the observer the impression that the person is drunk—or experience mood changes. He may report having "chills running up and down my spine." These signs are all related to the release of cortisone and the catecholamines.

The increased heart rate during stress can make a person have heart palpitations (one feels as if his heart will leap out of his chest). The digestive changes associated with stress cause a "sinking feeling in the gut." The sweat gland activity may cause excessive perspiration. The catecholamine action on the skin can cause the following: a ghostlike appearance; cold, clammy hands; cold feet (the literal expression of the "coward's" response to stress); or even the opposite rebound effect—blushing. Blushing is an interesting phenomenon. It indicates embarrassment or perhaps guilt, or as Mark Twain so aptly said: "Man is the only animal that blushes. Or needs to."* With anger a person can appear extremely pale ("white with anger") or flushed ("red with rage").** The resultant reactions are related to vasoconstriction (pale reaction, primarily adrenaline) and vasodilation (flushed reaction, primarily noradrenaline).

Under stress, speech may be speeded up, show hesitation, quiver or stop altogether. The speech reactions are also related to catecholamine action.

Other subjective feelings with visible signs of their presence are as follows: feelings of restlessness (i.e., can't sit still); weakness (i.e., may be forced to sit or lie down); chills (i.e., shivering when the ambient temperature is quite high); malaise (feeling "spent," having no energy); and inability to work or concentrate. The more the stress response goes toward distress, the more severe are the manifestations. Thus, if a person is distressed greatly, he may vomit, urinate, defecate, become dizzy or faint. With severe distress, the stress response begins as a predominantly sympathetic response and then changes to a predominantly parasympathetic response. Hence, it can go from high blood pressure and rapid heart beat (tachycardia) to a slow, feeble heart beat, low blood pressure and loss of consciousness.

* From *Pudd'nhead Wilson's New Calendar.*
** *"As the blood vessels of the face flush, the skin reddens, the angular vein which runs upward from the bridge of the nose is especially distended and has been referred to as the temper or anger vein." (From Guthrie, R. D., Body Hot Spots,* New York: Van Reinhold Co., 1976. Reprinted with permission.)

POPULAR TECHNOLOGY

Both the physiological and the psychological changes of the stress response have been used in popular technology to determine when a person may be under stress. Let us look at some examples. The "lie detector" (polygraph? is a well-known instrument employed to detect characteristic stress responses that occur when a person presumably is not telling the truth.[26] The usual polygraph records heart rate, blood pressure, the rate and depth of breathing and skin resistance (to detect sweating). (In our studies at Temple University, polygraphs were used; see Fig. 3.21.)

The rationale for the "lie detector" is based on the assumption that when a person lies, his effort at deception triggers emotional responses such as anxiety, fear and guilt. These psychological stressors, in turn, set off typical stress reactions such as increased heart and breathing rate and decreased skin resistance. However, some people can "trick" the "lie detector" when they are being questioned by surreptitiously contracting or relaxing appropriate muscles or by concentrating on distracting mental pictures. And there are people who naturally show only slight physiological changes even when under severe distress. These things were found to be true in the previously mentioned study conducted at Temple University.[35] To refresh the reader's memory, 48 subjects were meditating when the stressful verbal phrase was uttered: "John, may I please have the needle." The subjects, who were hooked up to a polygraph at the time, were monitored for heart rate, breathing rate and skin resistance. Later, in the debriefing session, the subjects were asked whether or not they found the intruding phrase to be stressful.

Of the 48 subjects, 38 (79%) found the phrase to be stressful, and 10 did not. With 30 of the 38 who reported finding it to be stressful, there was correspondence with the physiological measures, indicating that they actually were stressed; the other 8 subjects (21%) who said they were stressed evidenced no stress in terms of the physiological measures. Thus, those 8 subjects could conceivably take a "lie detector" test and feel stressed, yet there would be no discernible physiological changes.

However, it is not that easy to pass a lie detector test. Competent polygraph operators can readily detect accompanying stressful signs

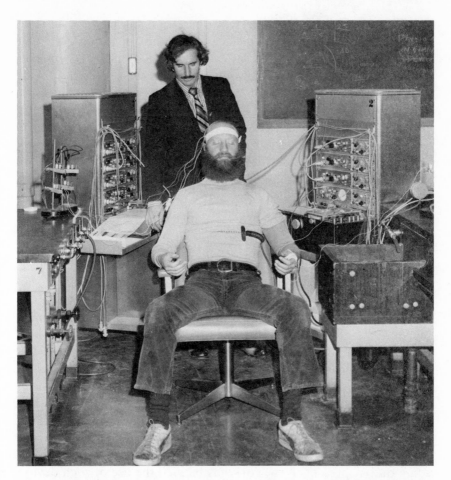

Fig. 3.21 The polygraph. While he is meditating, a subject is being monitored by the author (DM) for alpha wave rhythms (viz., white band on forehead), respiratory rate (viz., bellows around chest), pulse rate (viz., small clamp around finger of left hand) and skin resistance levels and nonspecific fluctuations (viz., attached to palm of left hand). The various leads are connected to two polygraphs comprising attached pens and recording devices. (From Morse, D. R., Overcoming "practice stress" via meditation and hypnosis, *Dental Survey,* 53 (7):33, 1977. Copyright© 1977 by Harcourt Brace Jovanovich, Inc.)

and responses of the subject such as stammering, hesitation, fidgeting and blushing. Also, a "trick" question may be employed: "Do you ever take things?" Since just about everyone takes things not belonging to them, the operator of the equipment is in a position to determine the "baseline" of the individual undergoing the test.

On the other hand, less competent operators may miss the obvious stress-related clues and rely too heavily on the apparatus. For these several reasons, the "lie detector" test is not universally accepted or indicated. Finally, the cooperation of the subject is required (i.e., the subject cannot be other than a "volunteer" who is willing to sit quietly).

With respect to the last point, a popular version of the "lie detector" has emerged recently. For example, a Radio Shack catalogue advertises its "pocket lie detector kit" at only $11.95.[41] The ad states: "Test your family, friends, party-goers! Fingertip sensors reveal body changes due to nervousness!" Undoubtedly, this is a miniature skin resistance device designed to analyze palmar sweating.

Another recent development is the Hagoth.[31,42] This hand-held voice analyzer is a cut-down version of either the Psychological Stress Evaluator (PSE) or the Mark II Voice Stress Analyzer (the latter two sell for about $4,000 each). All three machines attempt to determine when an individual is not telling the truth by measuring the amount of stress manifested in his speech. The hand-held Hagoth is not as inexpensive as the pocket lie detector, but it is less expensive than the more elaborate PSE and Mark II analyzers—it sells for $1,500.

The Hagoth is being used by some business executives. One is told that with the Hagoth, it is possible to monitor friend and foe alike during routine telephone conversations. And, of course, the person being monitored is completely unaware of anything unusual going on. At present, New York has banned the use of such devices for job interviews, and Pennsylvania and California legislatures are in the process of banning the covert use of voice stress analyzers.

There is also controversy over whether these machines really measure what they are supposed to. At the very least, most experts do consider them less reliable than a polygraph.[31]

The State of Israel has purportedly developed an instrument that it uses to screen people crossing the border.[31] From a short distance, the gadget takes measurements focusing on a person's chest cavity. Apparently, it is sensitive enough to detect variations from normal in blood pressure and breathing rate—giving an indication of stress reactions.

In the mid-1970s, stress was measured for still another purpose, employing a rather unusual method. During that period, the "mood" ring came into vogue. The changing colors of the stone were supposed to indicate an individual's physiological and psychological state. For instance, when the color of the stone changed to dark blue or black, this was interpreted as meaning that the ring wearer was sad, depressed or dejected. On the other hand, if the ring shone with a yellow glow, this was viewed as signaling a calm, relaxed and happy person.

Actually, there was a scientific basis for these implausible determinations. Within the stone were cholesteric crystals which changed colors with variations in skin temperature.[13] Thus, the mood ring was based on blood flow changes that occur during stress and relaxation. Since with stress there is a closing down of skin blood vessels (peripheral vasconstriction), there is a resultant decrease in skin temperature and cold extremities. On the other hand, with relaxation there is an opening up of skin blood vessels (peripheral vasodilation), with a resultant increase in skin temperature and warm extremities.

There are two negative aspects of the mood ring that probably led to its rapid demise. First, external temperatures affected the ring so that it was not reliable out-of-doors and hence, made the interpretations seem arbitrary. Second, the enclosed crystals were quite fragile and many a "bad" mood was triggered by a ring's cracking. There is a third possible reason why this ring went out of existence. It simply may be that people do not want or need verification that they are in a bad mood, especially if they are unable to do anything about it.

SUMMARY

Let us review what we have discussed in Part I. There are three kinds of stressors: physical, social and psychological. Physical stressors are the least damaging kind unless they are severe (e.g., an overwhelming infection) or great and repetitive (e.g., noise of a pneumatic drill). Social stressors, such as the death of a family member, can cause the most severe single stressful response. Psychological stressors are generally the most destructive, since they can be self-induced and self-perpetuated (e.g., anxiety, guilt, frustration).

The reaction to the stressors is modified by the makeup of the particular individual. The individual's makeup includes personality factors (e.g., the introvert tends to withhold anger), genetic factors (e.g., the coronary-resistant female) and environmental factors (e.g., the accountant's soaring blood pressure at tax time). As a result of the interaction between the stressor and the individual, a rather specific stress response occurs. The stress response is comprised of physiological and psychological changes. These changes generally result from the release of cortisone, adrenaline and related hormones. But there are individual variations depending upon the type and frequency of the stressor as well as the condition of the individual.

If the stress changes are neutral but necessary for normal body functioning, the stress is designated neustress. If the stress changes are destructive to the individual, the response is known as distress. And finally, if the stress response promotes improved physical and/or psychological functioning, it is called eustress.

In Part II, consideration is given to the consequences of distress. In Part III, the management of distress and methods of promoting eustress are covered.

REFERENCES

1. Hanukoglu, I. Prostaglandins as first mediator of stress. *Lancet* 1:193, 1977.
2. Hedge, G. A. Roles for prostaglandin in the regulation of anterior pituitary secretion. *Life Sci.* 20:17, 1977.
3. Kehlet, H., Brandt, M., Enguist, A. and Medsen, S. N. Prostaglandins as mediators of stress reaction. *N. Engl. J. Med.* 297:672, 1977.
4. Selye, H. *The Stress of Life,* Second Ed. New York: McGraw-Hill Book Co., 1976.
5. Cannon, W. B. The emergency function of the adrenal medulla in pain and the major emotions. *Am. J. Physiol.* 33:356-372, 1914.
6. Brown, W. A. and Heninger, G. Stress-induced growth hormone release: Psychologic and physiologic correlates. *Psychosom. Med.* 38:145-147, 1976.
7. Noel, G. R., Diamond, R. C., Earll, J. M. and Frantz, A. G. Prolactin, thyrotropin, and growth hormone release during stress associated with parachute jumping. *Aviat. Space Environ. Med.* 47:543-547, 1976.
8. Syvälahti, E., Lammintausta, R. and Pekkarinen, A. Effect of psychic stress of examination on serum growth hormone, serum insulin, and plasma renin activity. *Acta Pharmacol. Toxicol. (Kbh.)* 38:344-352, 1976.
9. Kopin, I. J. Catecholamines, adrenal hormones and stress. *Hosp. Pract.* 11:49-55, 1976.
10. Monjan, A. A. and Collector, M. I. Stress-induced modulation of the immune response. *Science* 196:307-308, 1977.

11. Perchellet, J. P., Shanker, G. and Sharma, R. K. Regulatory role of guanosine 3′5′ monophosphate in adrenocorticotropin hormone induced steroidogenesis. *Science* 199:311–312, 1978.
12. Pitts, F. N., Jr. The biochemistry of anxiety. *Sci. Am.* 220(2):69–75, 1969.
13. Morse, D. R. *Clinical Endodontology. A Comprehensive Guide to Diagnosis, Treatment and Prevention.* Springfield, Ill.: Charles C. Thomas Publ., 1974.
14. Shore, D. Research news: it's happening at Hopkins. *Johns Hopkins Mag.*:35–39, Mar. 1977.
15. Editorial. Before they ski, stress cardiography. *Phys. Sports med.* 2(1):22, 1974.
16. Flagg, G. W., Clemens, T. L., Michael, E. A., Alexander F. and Wark, J. A psychophyisological investigation of hyperthyroidism. *Psychosom. Med.* 27:497–507, 1965.
17. Pelletier, K. R. *Mind as Healer Mind as Slayer: A Holistic Approach to Preventing Stress Disorders.* New York: Dell Publ. Co. Inc., 1977.
18. Antelman, S. M. and Caggiula, A. R. Norepinephrine-dopamine interactions and behavior. *Science* 195:646–653, 1977.
19. Funkenstein, D. H. The physiology of fear and anger. *Sci. Am.* 192(5):74–80, 1955.
20. Miller, N. E. Learning effects on somatic manifestations of stress. Read before the Symposium on Stress and Behavioral Medicine, New York, Dec. 3–4, 1977.
21. Miller, N. E. and Dworkin, B. R. Effects of learning on visceral functions—Biofeedback. *N. Engl. J. Med.* 296:1274–1278, 1977.
22. Lynch, J. J., Paskewitz, D. A., Gimbel, K. S. and Thomas, S. A. Psychological aspects of cardiac arrhythmia. *Am. Heart J.* 93:645–657, 1977.
23. Eliot, R. S. Stress and cardiovascular disease. *Eur. J. Cardiol.* 5(2):97–104, 1977.
24. Brown, B. *Stress and the Art of Biofeedback.* New York: Harper & Row, 1977.
25. Christie, M. J. and Venable, P. H. Change in palmar skin potential level during relaxation after stress. *J. Psychosom. Res.* 18(5):301–306, 1974.
26. Smith, B. M. The polygraph. *Sci. Am.* 216(1):25–31, 1967.
27. Hess, E. H. Attitudes and pupil size. *Sci. Am.* 212(4):46–54, 1965.
28. Beecher, H. K. Relationship of significance of wound to the pain experienced. *J.A.M.A.* 161:1609–1613, 1956.
29. Leff, D. N. Doctors debate brain: Controversy flares over use of endorphins on patients. *Med. World News* 19:86–96, Jan. 9, 1978.
30. Editorial. New findings shed light on acupuncture process. *Dent. Surv.* 53(5):21–24, 1977.
31. Rice, B. The new truth machines. *Psychol. Today.* 12(1):61–78, 1978.
32. Dudley, D. L. and Welke, E. *How to Survive Being Alive.* Garden City: Doubleday & Co., 1977.
33. Glass, D. C. Stress, behavior patterns and coronary disease. *Am. Sci.* 65:177–187, 1977.
34. Rahe, R. H., Ryman, D. H. and Biersner, R. J. Serum uric acid, cholesterol, and psychological moods throughout stressful naval training. *Aviat. Space Environ. Med.* 47:883–888, 1976.
35. Morse, D. R., Martin, J. M., Furst, M. L. and Dubin, L. L. A physiological

and subjective evaluation of meditation, hypnosis, and relaxation. *Psychosom. Med.* 37:304–325, 1977.

36. Morse, D. R., Martin, J. M., Furst, M. L. and Dubin, L. L. A physiological and subjective evaluation of neutral and emotionally-charged words for meditation. *J. Am. Soc. Psychosom. Dent. Med.* 26(1–4): (1979), in press.

37. Schwartz, G. E. The brain as health care system: A psychobiological foundation for stress and behavioral medicine. Read before the Symposium on Stress and Behavioral Medicine, New York, Dec. 3–4, 1977.

38. Benson, H., Dryer, T. and Hartley, L. H. Decreased VO₂ consumption during exercise with elicitation of the relaxation response. *J. Human Stress* 4(2):38–42, 1978.

39. Page, J. D. *Psychopathology: The Science of Understanding Deviance.* Chicago: Aldine-Atherton, 1971.

40. Schlesinger, J., Barzilay, J., Stryjer, D. and Almog, C. H. Life threatening "vagal reaction" to emotional stimuli. *Isr. J. Med. Sci.* 13:59–61, 1977.

41. Radio Shack Catalog No. 289. Pocket lie detector kit. 143, 1978.

42. Oster, P. Technology, Big Brother are invading your privacy. *Philadelphia Eve. Bull.* 1B:10, Jan. 10, 1978.

Part II

The Consequences of Distress

What are the effects of distress? We all know about ulcers and heart attacks. But what about other conditions? And what are the relationships? The answers to these and other related questions are contained in Part II.

Chapter 4 is concerned with the various stress-related symptoms and diseases such as fatigue, weakness, coronaries and ulcers. In Chapter 5, consideration is given to the various stress-related disorders including drug addiction, alcoholism, divorce and suicide. In Chapter 6, the biologic mechanisms of aging are examined along with the effects of distress on aging.

4

Symptoms and Diseases: From Falling Hair to Failing Heart

The reason worry kills more people than work is that more people worry than work.*

CONFESSIONS OF AN AMERICAN YOGURT EATER**

I have some confessions to make. I eat yogurt, and I've suffered from stress-related symptoms and diseases.

It all began when I arrived before the doctor was ready: my mother's "water broke," and I almost drowned. That's how my hydrophobia began. When I was two, I fell out of my crib and my head's never been on straight since. We were a poor family and one of our greatest fears was to have the meterman come to read the gas and electric meters. I remember once we were all huddled on the floor in pitch blackness and utter silence. We weren't allowed to

---

* Robert Frost, *Vogue,* May 15, 1963.
** By Donald R. Morse; not to be confused with DeQuincey's *Confessions of an English Opium Eater.*

talk, breathe or sneeze until the meterman stopped ringing the front bell. I never associated the incident with my asthma attack that evening, but undoubtedly there was a connection (of course, the dust on the floor didn't help either).

While I was growing up, the family suffered several financial setbacks, and I wheezed my way through all of them. I finished college without too much difficulty. By then, I was quite active athletically, doing everything from playing Ping-Pong® to weightlifting. Miraculously, my asthma attacks became a thing of the past.

But then I started dental school. There is a great deal of stress associated with all professional schools, but the stress of dental school is unique.* I responded by working feverishly for A's and was rewarded with facial neuralgia. *That* lasted for the four years of dental school despite lateral skull X-rays and dental, E.N.T., psychological and neurological examinations. As could be expected, upon graduation the neuralgia disappeared.

In the second year of dental school, I got married. It was a happy occasion, and I was really looking forward to the trip to Bermuda for our honeymoon. But beginning at Idlewild Airport (now known as Kennedy), and lasting for the entire trip, I had a pain in the chest (my wife thought I was a pain somewhere else). When we landed in Bermuda, the first stop was the local doctor's office. He assured and reassured me that I had a perfectly healthy heart. The remaining days of the honeymoon were great, and my chest has been fine since.

My career as a dentist began in the U. S. Army. I can't recall any problems during those two years (possibly Uncle Sam suffered the stress for me).

When I opened my first private practice, we already had two young children and a third was on the way. We had a new house with a high mortgage; I wondered whether I would get enough patients to pay for everything. It was fortunate (?) that I didn't start off with a busy practice because I developed a problem with my hands—warts suddenly cropped up on all my fingers. Notwithstanding the many visits to the dermatologist, they kept recurring. But once my practice blossomed, the warts receded (and they've been in hiding for the last 18 years).

---

* If the reader would like more information on dental stress, one good source is *Stress and Relaxation: Application to Dentistry,* by the authors (Charles C. Thomas: Springfield, Ill., 1978).

My last encounter with a stress reaction of note was about six years ago. At that time, there were several simultaneous personal problems related to teaching and practice. This time my lower face and chin got into the act. I started to lose facial hair (alopecia is what the doctor said—you can bet that hearing the diagnosis didn't do much for the condition), and pretty soon I had a face as smooth as a baby's derrière. A multitude of steroid injections helped little, but when my problems were resolved not long afterward, the hair returned (a mixed blessing—shaving is no picnic).

For the past five years I've been an active tennis player and jogger. I've been meditating regularly twice a day and I try to "keep my cool." And I've had no stress-related problems—but it's probably because of the daily yogurt!

INTRODUCTION

In the previous "Confessions," a few stress-induced symptoms and diseases were mentioned (e.g., pain, asthma, alcopecia, warts), but stress is directly or indirectly related to many diseases.*

For each disease there are definitive changes, but there are certain stress manifestations that are common to many diseases. These include chills, weakness, fatigue, pain, high fever, sweating, malaise ("run-down" or queasy feeling), appetite loss, stomach-aches, dizziness and fainting. (Nonspecific management of these manifestations is covered in Chapter 17.)

It is not known why many people may be exposed to the same stress-inducing factors and some escape the development of stress-related diseases. Some people just seem to have better stress tolerance than others. It is also a puzzle why similar stressors result in different diseases for particular individuals. Undoubtedly, all of the factors discussed in Chapters 1 and 2 play a part in the development of stress-related diseases. Some of these factors seem to be

---

* Diseases that are directly related to psychological stressors are called "psychosomatic" illnesses (*psycho* = mind; *somatic* = body—hence, mental disorders causing physical diseases). This term was popularized by the psychiatrist Helen Flanders Dunbar as the result of her examinations of several hundred patients in a New York hospital.[1] But psychosomatic diseases are not the only ones we are concerned with. There are some stress-related diseases in which psychological factors play a small but important part. And there are other stress-related diseases in which physical and social stressors play a prominent role. In our discussion of stress-related diseases we take into consideration all three types; namely, psychological, social and physical stressors.

more important than others. They include: (1) the population and virulence of the microbes or the strength of physical stressors; (2) the frequency of psychological stressors; (3) the occurrence of major life-change events; and (4) the specific makeup of the individual. Let us consider them in a little more detail.

Physical Stressors

The virulence and population of microbes and the potency of other physical stressors—such as air, water and food pollutants— constitute a major determinant in the development of stress-related diseases. For instance, many city dwellers are exposed to low levels of the tubercle bacillus. These organisms may harbor in the lungs for years, and still the individuals do not develop tuberculosis. However, if a group of people came into contact with an overwhelming number of tubercle bacilli, many individuals would come down with tuberculosis. Yet, regardless of the exposure, some individuals would remain free of the clinical disease. Hence, potency of the stressor is only part of the picture.

Psychological Stressors

Another important consideration in certain stress-related diseases is the frequency of psychological stressors. Chronic day-to-day psychological stressors such as worry, anxiety, anger, frustration and guilt seem to be important in the subsequent development of stress-related diseases. However, even with frequent episodes, people who cope well can avoid stress-related diseases (discussed in Part III).

Social Stressors (Life-Change Events)

Although there has been recent criticism about the validity of some of the studies, it does appear that life-change events can predispose individuals to the development of stress-related diseases.[2,3] Holmes and Rahe have been instrumental in the development of life-change rating scales.[4,5] The various life-change events are numerically rated according to their potential for causing disease. For example, death of a spouse equals 100 units, and divorce rates 73 units. These events often antedate physical illnesses such as severe infections, perforating ulcers and heart attacks. The more severe the life-change events and the higher the frequency of such events, the greater the chance for a severe disease to occur.

In addition, the more intense the life-change event, the more likely it is that a serious, rather than a mild, disease will develop. On one of the stress scales, a total of 200 or more units in one year is considered to be predictive of the likelihood of the particular person's getting a serious disease.

One other interesting finding from these life-change stress studies is that a major event may be good as well as bad and still trigger a disease. For example, getting married carries a 50-unit liability. Nevertheless, people vary in their ability to cope with these major stressors, and the most recent evidence indicates that life-change events are just one factor in the tendency toward development of stress-related diseases.[3] The Social Readjustment Rating Scale of Holmes and Rahe is presented in Table 4.1. For later use, the reader should note which of the given events are personally appropriate.

Makeup of the Individual

Of major importance in the susceptibility to stress-related diseases are the following components of the individual's makeup: organ susceptibility; inherited specificity of response patterns; personality; attitudes; age; sex; conditioning; occupation; environment.

H. G. Wolff developed the "weak organ" theory.[6] The theory states that individuals have inherent weaknesses in selected organ systems. Thus, weakness of the gut predisposes one toward ulcers. A weakness of the lungs favors asthma development. And a weak heart does not lead to many love affairs, but inclines one toward getting a heart attack. Somewhat related to this is the tendency for people under conditions of stress to have recurrent episodes of pain in areas of the body that have had previous surgery and have presumably healed. For instance, one of us (DM) had root canal therapy and periapical surgery on the upper left lateral incisor tooth some 25 years ago. The case was considered completely successful, since the bone seems to have healed perfectly. Yet, on occasion, during stressful encounters, a jaw ache occurs at that site.

The investigations of the Laceys have shown that particular people

TABLE 4.1   The Social Readjustment Rating Scale*

RANK	LIFE EVENT	MEAN VALUE
1	Death of spouse	100
2	Divorce	73
3	Marital separation	65
4	Jail term	63
5	Death of close family member	63
6	Personal injury or illness	53
7	Marriage	50
8	Fired at work	47
9	Marital reconciliation	45
10	Retirement	45
11	Change in health of family member	44
12	Pregnancy	40
13	Sex difficulties	39
14	Gain of new family member	39
15	Business adjustment	39
16	Change in financial state	38
17	Death of a close friend	37
18	Change to different line of work	36
19	Change in number of arguments with spouse	35
20	Mortgage over $10,000	31
21	Foreclosure of mortgage or loan	30
22	Change in responsibilities at work	29
23	Son or daughter leaving home	29
24	Trouble with in-laws	29
25	Outstanding personal achievement	28
26	Wife begins or stops work	26
27	Begin or end school	26
28	Change in living conditions	25
29	Revision of personal habits	24
30	Trouble with boss	23
31	Change in work hours or conditions	20
32	Change in residence	20
33	Change in schools	20
34	Change in recreation	19
35	Change in church activities	19
36	Change in social activities	18
37	Mortgage or loan less than $10,000	17
38	Change in sleeping habits	16
39	Change in number of family get-togethers	15
40	Change in eating habits	15
41	Vacation	13
42	Christmas	12
43	Minor violations of the law	11

* Reprinted with permission from *J. Psychosomat. Res.,* 11:213–218, 1967, Holmes, T. H. and Rahe, R. H., The social readjustment scale. Copyright 1967, Pergamon Press, Ltd.

have very stable and consistent autonomic nervous system response patterns.[7] Some people regularly react to stressors with a marked rise in blood pressure; others respond with bronchial constriction; and still others show a dramatic fall in skin resistance level (galvanic skin response). We found similar results in our studies (see Fig. 13.2 in Chapter 13 for an example).

In Chapter 2, sympathetic responders (sympathicotonics) and parasympathetic responders (vagotonics) were mentioned.[8] Sympathicotonics often have high blood pressure and rapid heart rate and are susceptible to cardiovascular diseases. Vagotonics are more prone to parasympathetic-related diseases such as asthma.

Some investigators have considered that for each specific personality type, there is an associated tendency to develop a specific disease.[9] We also touched on this in Chapter 2 when "cancer personality," "ulcer personality," "rheumatoid arthritis personality," "ulcerative colitis personality" and Type A and Type B personalities were mentioned (see Table 2.1). Except for the reportedly high correlation between the competitive achieving nature of the Type A personality and the subsequent development of coronary artery disease, the others are not well documented.

Attitudes and disease were also covered in Chapter 2 (see Table 2.2). These findings are also open to question, but it does seem that people's attitudes (either good or bad) affect the incidence, type and severity of diseases.

Also in Chapter 2, age and stress was discussed. Certain diseases are more frequent during stressful age periods. In old age, immune responses are diminished, and the stress-related diseases such as coronary disease, adult-onset diabetes and cancer become more prevalent.

The connection between the sexes and stress was examined in Chapter 2. One other sex-related stress association is baldness in men. The usual kind of baldness in males is a hereditary condition, but stress can be a factor. The American Heart Association recently revealed that "bald, fat men with hairy chests" had a greater chance of contracting heart disease than men without these attributes.[10] (One tongue-in-cheek remedy for those individuals would be for them to go on a weight-loss diet, and then have hair transplants—with the hairy chest being the donor site.) On the other hand, women rarely become bald, and studies have shown that they have higher blood levels of high-density lipoproteins (HDLs) than men have.[11] HDLs are believed to be protective against coronary heart disease (discussed more fully in Chapters 10 and 11).

Conditioning, occupation and particular environment were also mentioned in Chapter 2. These three factors, which are tied in to individual makeup, are important in the development of stress-related diseases. The level of mental, nutritional and physical conditioning varies with the individual's social status, motivation, financial means and exposure to an education in the sciences.

In a hypothetical example, an average middle-aged American could have a heart attack precipitated by being forced to parachute out of a tumbling plane. A matched individual with respect to age and background who is a well-conditioned, experienced skydiver would probably not even develop a tremor.

Certain occupations—legal and illegal—by their very nature are conducive to stress-related diseases. Consider these: fireman; policeman; air traffic controller; movie stuntman; deep sea diver; soldier; pilot; physician; dentist; musician; accountant; lawyer; criminal; prisoner; stockbroker. People who are always investing in stocks suffer considerable stress. Sewil described a syndrome known as "Wall Street Sickness."[12] The investors develop headaches, stomach troubles and fatigue. They constantly worry and "second guess" themselves. Apparently, as long as they stay in the "market," they continue to suffer from this sickness.

Finally, where one lives can greatly affect the incidence and type of stress-related diseases. Tuberculosis is prevalent in poor, crowded environments. Rickets, which is precipitated by a lack of sunshine, is also frequent in such environments. Stressors of center city living include unsanitary conditions, cramped living quarters and lack of sunshine.

The occurrence of stress-related diseases is linked, in part, to the release of catecholamines and corticosteroids. In some diseases, the catecholamines appear to be more important; e.g., coronary artery diseases. In other diseases, the corticosteroids play a predominant role; e.g., duodenal and gastric ulcers. There are also diseases such as asthma in which acetylcholine release (i.e., a parasympathetic response) is of major importance. A summary of the factors considered to be important in the development of stress-related diseases is given in Table 4.2.

Now that we have examined the stress-related symptoms and the

TABLE 4.2   Factors Important in Development of Stress-Related Diseases

FACTOR OR CONDITION	IMPLICATION
Physical stressors	The greater the potency, the more the disease potentiality.
Psychological stressors	The greater the frequency, the more the disease potentiality.
Social stressors (life-change events)	With greater potency, intensity and frequency, the more and worse are the diseases.
Makeup of individual (Comprises genetic and environmental factors)	
Organ susceptibility	Inherent weakness in different organs for different people.
Inherited specificity of response patterns	E.g., sympathicotonics and vagotonics.
Personality	E.g., "cancer" personality.
Attitudes	Negative attitudes lead to disease.
Age	Increase of disease in old age.
Sex	Bald, fat men tend toward heart disease.
Physical condition	Those in better "shape" tend to get less disease.
Occupation	E.g., fireman and policeman are high stress occupations.
Environment	TB prevalent in crowded spaces.

major factors of importance in the development of stress-related diseases, it is time to explore these diseases.* We begin with a discussion of the cardiovascular diseases.

CARDIOVASCULAR DISEASES

The most important of all the stress-related diseases are those of the cardiovascular system. Cardiovascular diseases include angina pectoris, atherosclerosis (fatty infiltration of the arteries), arteriosclerosis (calcification or hardening of the arteries), cardiac ar-

---

* Obviously, we cannot present here a complete treatise on each disease. Yet, we do feel that given the current consumer approach to health services delivery and the emphasis on home care, the individual should take the opportunity to prevent and to treat (to some extent) stress-related diseases. Hence, it behooves the individual to know something about these diseases. And of all of these diseases, the ones that cause more debilitation and death (by far) are those of the cardiovascular system. Therefore, the most space is allocated to diseases of the heart and circulation.

rhythmias (abnormal heart rhythm), coronary artery disease (coronary thrombosis, myocardial infarction, heart attack), congestive heart failure and cerebral stroke.

Coronary artery disease is the "No. 1" killer in the United States. A recent estimate by the National Heart, Lung and Blood Institute is that in a single year 1.3 million Americans will have coronary artery disease.[13] Of those, about 675,000 will die, with 175,000 of the deaths being premature (i.e., before age 65).

There are many risk factors for coronary heart disease, as may be seen in the following listing: with respect to the sexes, higher incidence in males; age—incidence increased with aging; hypertension (high blood pressure); family history of coronary heart diseases; electrocardiographic (EKG) abnormalities and arrhythmias; smoking (i.e., 20 or more cigarettes daily); high serum lipids (cholesterol, triglycerides, low-density lipoproteins); obesity; diabetes mellitus; gout; high blood uric acid; low vital capacity (decreased ability for lungs to hold oxygen); high salt intake; high sugar intake; excess coffee drinking; alcoholism; lack of exercise; taking of birth control pills by women; Type A personality; psychological and social stressors—the list seems endless.[13-25] A number of these factors are strongly related to stress and are now considered.

The Sexes

In Chapter 2, we mentioned the possible advantage of estrogen in the prevention of heart disease. However, another reason why males have been more prone to heart attacks has to do with the stress associated with being the breadwinner.[26] With more women in the job market, the incidence of job-related stress and heart disease has increased for women.

Race

In Chapter 2, we discussed background and predisposition to certain diseases. Blacks have a higher incidence of coronary artery disease than Caucasians, but it may be primarily related to social and family factors.[9,27]

Age

In Chapter 6, the relationship of stress and aging is considered in detail, but at this point we may note that getting old can be stressful to many people. The stress of aging may help precipitate heart attacks, and with advanced age the incidence of heart attacks increases.

Hypertension

In several animal and human experiments, it has been shown that psychological stressors have caused sustained elevations in blood pressure, or hypertension, which is one of the major risk factors in the development of heart attacks and cerebral strokes. (These studies are discussed shortly when we consider psychological stressors.)

Smoking

Many people smoke as a means of relieving stress. This negative coping method is discussed more fully in Chapter 5. Cigarette smoking has the following effects: (1) increases adrenaline flow; (2) speeds up heart rate; (3)constricts blood vessels; (4) makes blood more likely to clot; (5) increases the blood levels of fatty acids and cholesterol. These effects illuminate the connection between smoking and heart disease.[25,28]

High Serum Lipids

High blood levels of triglycerides and cholesterol (especially low-density lipoproteins) are related in some manner to the incidence of heart attacks and cerebral strokes.[20,29] It is not definite that diet is the key factor. For example, dietary carbohydrates can change within the body to triglycerides, and some people have high serum levels of cholesterol even with a low cholesterol diet.[14,24,25,29]

Nevertheless, studies have shown that stress can raise blood cholesterol levels.[30-32] For example, one study showed that with accountants during tax collection time (i.e., just prior to April 15), blood cholesterol levels rose as much as 100 mg%. The levels tended to remain elevated during the entire period of "time pressure." In another study, medical students had significantly higher blood cholesterol levels at the time of their final anatomy examinations as compared to other nonexam times.

Cholesterol deposits can occur in blood vessels, leading to the condition atherosclerosis. This condition causes a narrowing of the blood vessels, and this narrowing, in turn, increases the resistance to blood flow, which is a factor in inducing high blood pressure. Atherosclerosis of coronary blood vessels can help precipitate coronary thrombosis; and atherosclerosis of cerebral (brain) blood vessels can lead to cerebral stroke.

High Sugar Intake

In some investigations, high sugar intake has been correlated with increased incidence of coronary heart disease.[14,24,29] This effect may be related to the tendency of carbohydrates to form triglycerides (i.e., a form of fat) within the body. The ingestion of sweets is related to stress, since people may eat candies, cookies and rich desserts to relieve stress. High intake of sweets is one of the principal causes of obesity, which can lead to diabetes in a susceptible individual.

Diabetes

The presence of diabetes mellitus increases the risk of a subsequent heart attack. Diabetes is discussed more thoroughly later in this chapter; for now, we can state that although it is primarily a genetic disease, stress does help precipitate diabetic attacks.

Obesity

Obesity is one of the major risk factors in coronary heart disease as well as for diabetes and kidney diseases. (Incidentally, it is also a leading cause of back problems.) Although there are several possible causes, the major reason for overweight is overeating. And one of the main reasons people overeat is to relieve stress.

Lack of Exercise

There are few definitive studies relating lack of exercise to the development of heart disease. Yet, the overall consensus is that lack of exercise does play a role (see Chapter 11). Many obese people have difficulty in touching their toes or even in walking. Unless they become strongly motivated, being heavy (itself a risk factor) inclines them to forego exercise, thereby compounding the risk factors.

High Salt Intake

Animal experiments have provided strong evidence that excess salt intake can lead to coronary heart disease.[20,33] In humans, the evidence is circumstantial, but most investigators believe that salt intake is definitely a factor. Excess sodium (one of the major constituents of sodium chloride, or salt), along with corticosteroids can cause heart muscle damage in animals subjected to physical stressors such as fractures.[28] The fact that high salt intake causes an increase in fluid volume in the body suggests another possible mechanism.[30] The increased fluid can lead to edema, which can cause an overload on the heart muscle.

People often heavily salt their food for taste reasons and from habit. Just as sweets are taken for stress relief, so too are a number of salty products. For instance, munching on potato chips and pretzels is pleasureable and often difficult to stop. (That is, you just can't seem to stop with just one.)

Alcoholism

Studies have shown that in addition to its effects on the liver and brain, alcohol has a toxic effect on the heart that can result in irreversible damage to the heart muscle.*[34] Drinking alcoholic beverages is another negative coping method (covered in the next chapter).

High Coffee Intake

A study reported by Jick and his co-workers showed that coffee drinking increased the risk of heart attacks.[35] Many individuals try to cope by continually drinking coffee (see next chapter).

* Conversely, at a recent symposium, Kenneth Cooper reported that a low level of alcohol intake (one or two drinks daily) increases the blood level of the purportedly coronary-protective high-density lipoproteins (Cooper, K. H. Levels of Physical Fitness and Selected Coronary Risk factors. Presented to the Monmouth-Ocean County Dental Society, Neptune, New Jersey, April 18, 1979). (See also under Lipids in Chapter 10 and Exercise in Chapter 11 for a further discussion of the benefits of high-density lipoproteins.)

Type A Personality

There is a lack of agreement over the strength of the association between Type A personality (discussed in Chapter 2) and incidence of heart diseases. Friedman and Rosenman are the principal proponents of the high risk role of the Type A personality in coronary artery disease.[21,36] Stress and the Type A personality seem to go hand in hand. An individual of this kind is hard-driving and compulsive; he suppresses fatigue and tries to control his environment. The Type A has difficulty in coping with chronic day-to-day stressors (i.e., tends toward anxiety, frustration and worry).

Psychological Stressors

It has been difficult to determine the exact relationship of stress to the incidence of heart attacks because of the many confounding variables. However, stress seems to be a very important factor. In many animal experiments researchers have shown simple physical stressors (e.g., a severe blow to a rat's tail) to be not nearly as effective or consistent in raising blood pressure as psychological stressors.[19,32] The psychological stressors, frustration, and anxiety caused the highest increases in blood pressure, and the elevations were sustained. In human studies, results showed that the previously mentioned tax accountants also suffered sharp increases in blood pressure and faster blood coagulation times during the tax period.[30,32,36] Students' blood pressure levels have been shown to rise before exams, as have soldiers' levels upon entering combat.

Also, as mentioned in Chapter 2, air traffic controllers were found to have developed hypertension four times as frequently as second-class license controllers, and did so seven years sooner in life.[37] High blood pressure occurred earlier in controllers working in busy airports with high-volume control as contrasted to those working in towers with low-volume control.

Psychological stressors have been shown to cause marked rises in blood catecholamine levels (adrenaline, noradrenaline). Studies have shown that catecholamines cause a sustained rise in blood pressure and can also cause unique histopathological changes in heart muscle (ruptured muscle fibers).[19] The latter action can cause sudden death even in an individual with normal coronary blood vessels. In addition, catecholamines tend to cause clumping of blood platelets and accelerate the rate of arterial damage, both of which can lead to coronary thrombosis.[32]

Social Stressors

In Chapters 1 and 2, we discussed life-change events and the subsequent development of serious diseases. In several retrospective and a few prospective studies,* the relationship of recent life changes and heart attacks has been extensively studied.[2-5] Although there is some controversy on this subject, it does appear that severe stress-inducing events such as the death of a loved one or loss of a job can multiply the chances of getting a heart attack or dying suddenly. There is also evidence that many coronary victims have had bouts of anxiety and depression prior to their initial cardiac symptoms.

Summary of Risk Factors

Although the relationship of stress to heart attacks is difficult to express exactly, it can be seen that stress is certainly a factor. And stress is directly or indirectly related to other coronary risk factors such as sex (gender), age, hypertension, smoking, high serum lipids, diabetes, obesity, lack of exercise, Type A personality and the prevalence of psychological stressors. A summary of risk factors for coronary heart disease is given in the self-assessment test of Table 4.3. Standard body weights are given in Table 4.4.

In Table 4.3, the weight given to the various risk factors is an arbitrary one based on the best available information according to our interpretation. Not everyone will agree with us on what constitutes a risk factor or on the emphasis given to the various risk factors. However, this is merely a reasonable attempt at weighing risk factors, and nothing more is intended.

---

* Retrospective studies are those in which subjects are asked to recall events prior to the first manifestations of their diseases. With this method, there is the strong possibility of an individual's not recalling or confusing details as to whether they occurred before or after the onset of the disease. Prospective studies are better in the sense that the population of subjects includes both those who will and those who won't come down with a given disease. Thus the ratios of disease to nondisease can be determined, and the data are collected in the sequence of events in which they occurred—a necessary condition to establish cause and effect. That is, the subjects in a prospective study are interviewed at the beginning of the study and then after a period of time to see what diseases, if any, occur. Unfortunately, this method is both much more time-consuming and expensive.

There are 26 factors and the five-point scales run from values of "0" (the best) to "4" (the worst) for each factor. The reader should take a sheet of paper and number it from 1 through 26. Then he should read the description of each factor in turn and judge where he best fits, being as judicious as possible. The assigned value should be based on the reader's best evaluation of where he belongs on a particular factor. With some factors (e.g., low-density lipoproteins), the reader may not know his values. In those cases, he should select a value of "2." The point score determined from each factor should be placed next to the appropriate factor number (1–26). When all 26 factors are rated, the values are summed, and a total is obtained.

The reader should see where his total score falls according to the following ranges and thus get a rating of his risk for a heart attack:

Very slight risk	Well below average risk	Average risk	Moderate risk	Dangerous risk
1–21	22–42	43–63	64–84	85–104

TABLE 4.3   Risk Factors for Coronary Heart Disease

Group I. Factors *Not* Within Control of Individual

  1. Sex: (Men have greater susceptibility; see Chapter 2)
        _____ (1) Female, before menopause.
        _____ (3) Male; female, after menopause.
  2. Age: (Susceptibility increases with age; see Chapter 2)
        _____ (0) 1–20 years.
        _____ (1) 21–34.
        _____ (2) 34–49.
        _____ (3) 50–64.
        _____ (4) 65 and over.
  3. Race: (Blacks have higher incidence; see Chapter 2)
        _____ (1) Nonblack.
        _____ (3) Black.

Group II. Factors *Partially* Within Control of Individual

  4. Personality Type A or B: (Type A has high risk; see Chapter 2)
        _____ (0) Type B, typical.
        _____ (1) Type B, moderate.
        _____ (2) Between Type A and B.
        _____ (3) Type A, moderate.
        _____ (4) Type A, typical.

5. Heart Disease: (Risk increases if individual or parent[s] had it)
_____ (0) Individual and parents had none.
_____ (1) Individual had none; one parent had it past age 60.
_____ (2) Individual had none; both parents had it past 60 or one before 60.
_____ (3) Individual had none; two parents had it before 60.
_____ (4) Individual had it.

6. Diabetes: (Risk increases if individual or parent[s] had it)
_____ (0) Individual and parents had none.
_____ (1) Individual had none; one parent had it past age 60.
_____ (2) Individual had none; two parents had it past 60 or one before 60.
_____ (3) Individual had none; two parents had it before 60.
_____ (4) Individual has it.

7. Gout: (Risk increases if individual or parent[s] had it)
_____ (0) Individual and parents had none.
_____ (1) Individual had none; one parent had it.
_____ (2) Individual had none; two parents had it.
_____ (3) Individual has it; one parent had it.
_____ (4) Individual has it; both parents had it.

8. Body Weight: (Susceptibility increases with weight; see Table 4.4 for a chart of standard body weights)*
_____ (0) 1–5 lb below standard weight-height-frame values.
_____ (1) ± 5 lb from standard.
_____ (2) 6–15 lb over standard.
_____ (3) 16–29 lb over standard.
_____ (4) 30 lb or more above standard.

9. Blood Pressure: (Risk increases with higher pressure, especially diastolic; i.e., bottom value. If your values fall into two categories, use the diastolic value)
_____ (0) $\frac{100-120}{50-70}$
_____ (1) $\frac{121-130}{71-80}$
_____ (2) $\frac{131-140}{81-90}$
_____ (3) $\frac{141-165}{91-110}$
_____ (4) $\frac{166+}{111+}$

* Kenneth Cooper recently discussed a rapid method to determine an individual's ideal body weight from a coronary risk standpoint. If you are a male, take your height in inches, multiply it by 4.0 and then subtract 128 from the total. If your weight is 9 pounds or more above the ideal weight, you have a significant coronary risk. If you are a female, take your height in inches, multiply it by 3.5 and subtract 108 from the total. If your weight is 7 pounds or more above the ideal weight, you have a significant coronary risk (Cooper, K. H. Levels of Physical Fitness and Selected Coronary Risk Factors. Presented to the Monmouth-Ocean County Dental Society, Neptune, New Jersey, April 18, 1979).

TABLE 4.3 (cont.)

10. Serum Cholesterol: (Risk increases with higher values)
    _____ (0) 120–150 mg%.
    _____ (1) 151–180.
    _____ (2) 181–250.
    _____ (3) 260–350.
    _____ (4) 351+.

11. Serum Triglycerides: (Risk increases with higher values)
    _____ (0) 50–70 mg%.
    _____ (1) 71–100.
    _____ (2) 101–130.
    _____ (3) 131–180.
    _____ (4) 181+.

12. Low-Density Lipoproteins: (Risk increases with higher values)
    _____ (0) 60–100 U/I units.
    _____ (1) 101–141.
    _____ (2) 142–182.
    _____ (3) 183–223.
    _____ (4) 224+.

13. Uric Acid: (Risk increases with higher values)
    _____ (0) 2.7–4.2 mg%.
    _____ (1) 4.3–5.8.
    _____ (2) 5.9–7.4.
    _____ (3) 7.5–9.0.
    _____ (4) 9.1+.

14. Fasting Blood Glucose: (Risk increases with higher values or very low values [i.e., hypoglycemia])
    _____ (0) 70–83 mg%.
    _____ (1) 84–97.
    _____ (2) 98–111.
    _____ (3) 112–125, or 60 or less.
    _____ (4) 126+.

15. Electrocardiographic (EKG) Abnormalities: (Risk increases with arrhythmias and other abnormalities)
    _____ (0) None.
    _____ (1) Very slight and occasional signs.
    _____ (2) Slight but clear abnormalities.
    _____ (3) Normal on resting EKG; abnormal on stress EKG.
    _____ (4) Abnormal on both resting and stress EKG.

16. Heart Rate: (Risk increases with faster rates)
    _____ (0) 50 or less at rest.
    _____ (1) 51–66.
    _____ (2) 70–79.
    _____ (3) 80–94.
    _____ (4) 95+.

TABLE 4.3 (cont.)

17. Life-Change Events: (Risk increases with severe events; see beginning of this chapter)
_____ (0) None within the last year.
_____ (1) One within the last year; "moderate" (e.g., change in residence).
_____ (2) Two "moderate."
_____ (3) One "severe" (e.g., death of a loved one; divorce) or three or more "moderate."
_____ (4) Two or more "severe."

18. Chronic Psychological Stressors: (Increases the risk; see Chapter 1)
_____ (0) None; no frustration, worry, guilt, etc.
_____ (1) Occasional and slight to moderate.
_____ (2) Occasional and severe.
_____ (3) Regular and slight to moderate.
_____ (4) Regular and severe.

Group III. Factors Within Control of Individual

19. Alcohol: (Can damage the heart muscle; see Chapter 5)
_____ (0) None; one glass of wine per day.
_____ (1) One cocktail or two glasses of wine.
_____ (2) Two cocktails or three glasses of wine.
_____ (3) One half-bottle on the average.
_____ (4) Alcoholic.

20. Coffee or Caffeinated Products: (See Chapter 5)
_____ (0) None at all.
_____ (1) Occasional tea or cocoa; decaffeinated products.
_____ (2) 1 or 2 cups of coffee daily; 3-4 cups of tea or cocoa.
_____ (3) 3-4 cups of coffee; 5-6 cups of tea or cocoa.
_____ (4) 5+ cups of coffee; 7+ cups of tea or cocoa.

21. Smoking: (See Chapter 5)
_____ (0) None; no cigarettes, cigars or pipe.
_____ (1) An occasional cigarette.
_____ (2) Less than one pack per day; cigar or pipe regularly; former heavy smoker who quit for at least six months.
_____ (3) One to two packs of cigarettes.
_____ (4) More than two packs per day.

22. Fat Intake: (Animal fats are worse; found in meat, milk and eggs; see Chapter 10)
_____ (0) No animal fats.
_____ (1) 1-10% animal fat of food eaten per day.
_____ (2) 11-25%.
_____ (3) 26-40%.
_____ (4) 41% + .

23. Sugar Intake: (Sugar is worse than starches; see Chapter 10)
_____ (0) None.

TABLE 4.3 (cont.)

_____ (1) Occasionally.

_____ (2) Slight.

_____ (3) Moderate.

_____ (4) High.

24. Salt Intake: (High salt increases susceptibility; see Chapter 10)

_____ (0) None by itself.

_____ (1) An occasional pinch.

_____ (2) Slight.

_____ (3) Moderate.

_____ (4) High.

25. Aerobic Exercise: (Sedentary people are at a greater risk; see Chapter 11)

_____ (0) Daily (e.g., running).

_____ (1) Every other day.

_____ (2) Twice a week.

_____ (3) Once a week or less.

_____ (4) Never.

26. Birth Control Pills: (Women who take them may be at risk)

_____ (0) Never.

_____ (1) Rarely.

_____ (2) Occasionally.

_____ (3) Regularly for one year or less.

_____ (4) Regularly for more than one year.

TABLE 4.4 Standard Weights: WEIGHTS IN POUNDS ACCORD-ING TO FRAME IN INDOOR CLOTHING*

Men of ages 25 and over

HEIGHT (WITH SHOES ON) 1-INCH HEELS FT.	IN.	SMALL FRAME	MEDIUM FRAME	LARGE FRAME
5	2	112–120	118–129	126–141
5	3	115–123	121–133	129–144
5	4	118–126	124–136	132–148
5	5	121–129	127–139	135–152
5	6	124–133	130–143	138–156
5	7	128–137	134–147	142–161
5	8	132–141	138–152	147–166
5	9	136–145	142–156	151–170
5	10	140–150	146–160	155–174
5	11	144–154	150–165	159–179

TABLE 4.4 *(cont.)*

		Men of ages 25 and over		

HEIGHT (WITH SHOES ON) 1-INCH HEELS				
FT.	IN.	SMALL FRAME	MEDIUM FRAME	LARGE FRAME
6	0	148–158	154–170	164–184
6	1	152–162	158–175	168–189
6	2	156–167	162–180	173–194
6	3	160–171	167–185	178–199
6	4	164–175	172–190	182–204

		Women of ages 25 and over		
(WITH SHOES ON) 2-INCH HEELS				
4	10	92–98	96–107	104–119
4	11	94–101	98–110	106–122
5	0	96–104	101–113	109–125
5	1	99–107	104–116	112–128
5	2	102–110	107–119	115–131
5	3	105–113	110–122	118–134
5	4	108–116	113–126	121–138
5	5	111–119	116–130	125–142
5	6	114–123	120–135	129–146
5	7	118–127	124–139	133–150
5	8	122–131	128–143	137–154
5	9	126–135	132–147	141–158
5	10	130–140	136–151	145–163
5	11	134–144	140–155	149–168
6	0	138–148	144–159	153–173

Note: For girls between 18 and 25, subtract 1 pound for each year under 25.

* Copyright 1977, Metropolitan Life Insurance Company.
Courtesy of Metropolitan Life Insurance Company.
From *Metropolitan Life Insurance Statistical Bulletin.* 58:5, October, 1977.

After you have computed your score, if you find yourself a "very slight risk" or "well below average risk," then keep up the good work. If you find yourself to be an "average," "moderate" or "dangerous" risk, you should try to change the factors that are controllable or partially controllable. These are discussed in Chapter 7. One other method that can help in the prevention and treatment of high blood pressure is the use of the relaxation response. This is discussed in Chapters 12–16.

Angina Pectoris

In angina, the coronary arteries are partially occluded. As a result, the heart muscles do not get sufficient oxygen, and severe chest pains can then occur. Angina can be a precursor to a heart attack, or it may follow a heart attack. The angina patient who never develops a full-blown heart attack is believed also to have a Type A personality.[1,9,36] However, he does not seem to have the overwhelming drive of the typical Type A person.

Cardiac Arrhythmias

Patients can have abnormal heart rhythms and not experience a heart attack. However, depending upon the type of arrhythmia, they may suddenly have a heart seizure and die. In reverse, arrhythmias can develop following heart attacks.

Personality traits have also been described for arrhythmia patients.[1,9,38] These people are considered to be fearful, moody and in perpetual mental conflict. They tend to vacillate between feelings of joy and disgust, enjoying friends and mistrusting them, and desiring to win but being afraid to create hostility. Even though distinct personalities have been described for angina and arrhythmia patients, they probably both fit into the Type A personality mold. What has been covered with respect to coronary artery disease generally applies to them as well.

CANCER

The second leading cause of death for all diseases in the United States is cancer, in one form or another. The disease has many possible causes, a large number of which are unknown. Although the relationship of stress to cancer is less well understood than that of stress to heart diseases, the notion of a connection between stress and cancer has been around for a long time.

The second-century physician Galen concluded that women with melancholic dispositions appeared more inclined to develop breast cancer than women of a sanguine temperament;[31] recent evidence indicates that cancer is often preceded by severe life-change events as well as chronic psychological stressors.[39,40] Most of the studies of stress and cancer are based on clinical and personal experiences. The major underlying theme reported is that anxiety, depression, hopelessness and grief are significant precursors of the discovery of the tumors.*

In one long-range prospective study it was found that physicians who developed cancer often were "low-geared," with few outbursts of emotion. Most had feelings that began in childhood of isolation from their parents. (See "cancer personality" in Chapter 2.) Other studies showed that generally there was a major loss of a spouse or a family member just before the appearance of the cancer.[39] Many investigations were undertaken by Lawrence Le Shan in this area.[39] He found that widowed persons had the highest cancer mortality rate, with divorced people being next. In one prospective study, individuals who had significantly higher depression scores in a personality test actually developed a significantly higher incidence of cancer than those people who had a low depression index on the same test.[40]

DEPRESSION

Of all the psychiatric diseases, depression appears to be the one most related to stress. In Chapter 2, the "depression-prone personality" was mentioned. Let us now discuss it further.

Richard Sword, a psychiatrist, has come up with a definition of the "depression-prone personality." He states: "It's a person who works hard, is ambitious, has a high sense of integrity, tells the truth, never gets mad, is very responsible and conscientious, pays bills on time (or at least tries to), is pleasant to everyone, smiles outwardly even when feeling like hell inside, has a strong sense of duty, and sets very high standards of performance for others but even more so for himself."**

---

* Tumors can either be benign (i.e., slow-growing and nonspreading) or malignant (i.e., usually faster-growing, spreading and more apt to kill). Cancer encompasses a group of malignant tumors.

** Sword, R. O., The depression-prone personality: Almost "too good" to be true, *Dental Survey*, 53(3):12, 1977. Copyright© 1977 by Harcourt Brace Jovanovich, Inc.

Has the reader any of these attributes? If so, he should make a note of them for later use in an assessment test.

As mentioned, depression may be of some importance in the development of cancer. It is often a precursor to myofascial pain-dysfunction syndrome (described in the next section), and is a major factor in suicide (discussed in the next chapter).

The connection of stress to schizophrenia and paranoia is not so clear, but stressful incidences may precipitate attacks of these diseases. For example, it is known that breakdown products of adrenaline (produced during stress) can cause hallucinations.[41]

MUSCLE RELATED CONDITIONS

As mentioned in Chapter 3, one of the physiological responses of stress is partial muscle contraction. With chronic psychological stressors such as anxiety, anger, frustration and worry, the involved muscles can form "knots," and pain results.[42] This can occur in the scalp (tension headaches), the oral cavity (clenching, bruxism and myofascial pain-dysfunction syndrome), the neck ("pain in the neck"), the shoulders (shoulder aches) and the back (backaches).

Headaches[6,9,31,40,41]

Tension headaches are the most common of all these muscle-related conditions, often occurring immediately following stressful periods. Migraine headaches occur in individuals who are constantly on the go and then let down completely. (See "migraine personality" discussed in Chapter 2). These headaches tend to occur during the relaxation periods.[43]

The Oral Conditions

Clenching is the act of intense, prolonged contact between teeth in opposing jaws. Bruxing or gritting is similar, but in addition the teeth surfaces grind together. This often occurs at night during fitful periods of sleep. Both of these conditions are believed to be primarily a response to psychological stressors such as anger, and they are correlated with latent aggression. Bruxism is often found in angry, dependent and hostile people.[44] Recent studies have shown that clenching can cause increases in blood pressure for both normal and hypertensive subjects.[45]

Myofascial pain-dysfunction syndrome involves clicking and pain of the temporo-mandibular joint as well as spasms of the masseter muscles of the jaw (see Fig. 4.1). It can follow repeated episodes of clenching and bruxing. Many patients who get myofascial pain-dysfunction syndrome have a history of moderate to severe depression.

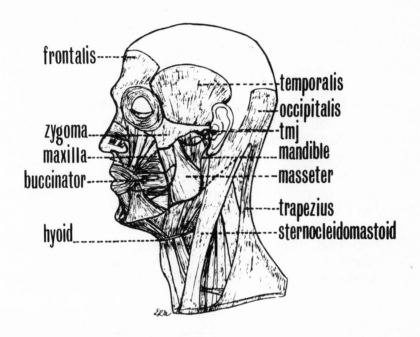

Fig. 4.1 The jaws with associated muscles and joints. The maxilla is the upper jaw, and the mandible the lower jaw. The TMJ (temporo-mandibular joint) is the articulation where the mandible meets the temporal bone. During chewing, only the jaw moves at that joint. The zygoma is the cheek bone, and the hyoid the neck bone. Two important muscles of mastication (chewing) are the masseter and the temporalis. They often become partially contracted in bruxism and myofascial pain-dysfunction syndrome. The frontalis is a muscle in the front of the forehead which often becomes partially contracted during tension headaches. The occipitalis, in the back of the head, also can become partially contracted during tension headaches. The buccinator is a facial muscle that is active during kissing and whistling. The sternocleidomastoid is a neck muscle that can become partially contracted during prolonged tension headaches. The trapezius is a neck and shoulder muscle that also can become partially contracted as a result of psychological stressors.

Shoulder Aches and Neck Pains

Partial muscle contraction as a result of chronic psychological stressors can spread from the jaws to the neck and down to the shoulders, causing intense pain.

Backaches

Backaches, among the most common of all physical complaints, are, in the majority of cases, caused by chronic muscle spasms.[46] Many who develop recurrent backaches tend to be angry, competitive, resentful and apprehensive individuals.[9] They are thought to be constantly on guard but afraid to act.

Bone and Posture Changes

If the muscle contraction is prolonged, there is evidence that it can affect the growth of the bones to which the muscles are attached. A. W. Wilson described a case in which a young man developed an enlarged jaw as the result of stress-induced chronic contraction of the jaw muscles.[47] The overdeveloped jawbone actually prevented him from opening his mouth. Subsequent surgical removal of the excess bone by a dentist allowed the man to regain normal jaw movements.

Graham Fagg presented evidence showing that chronic partial muscle contraction of the neck and shoulder muscles can cause relatively permanent changes in posture and stature.[48] The cringing person (i.e., "fear-hate" posture) tends to lift his drawn-in shoulders and pull his head downward. In contradistinction, the authoritarian person often has a drawn-in chin and a stiffened neck.*

ULCERS

Hans Selye and Neal Miller have shown that rats subjected to physical and psychological stressors develop severe ulcers of the gut.[41,49] As mentioned in Chapter 2, Joseph Brady's studies were with monkeys; the experimental group was designated the "executive" group as distinct from the control group.[50] Both groups of monkeys were

---

* Recently Ken Dychtwald has done extensive investigations on the relationship of personality, attitude and prolonged muscle contraction on postural and other physical bodily changes (Dychtwald, K. *Body-Mind,* Jove Publications, Inc., New York, 1977).

subjected to electric shocks, but only the "executive" monkeys could push a lever that could prevent both animals from getting the shock. As you may recall, it was the decision-making "executive" monkeys who developed the ulcers. This study revealed that decision-making and responsibility can lead to ulcers.

All three studies showed that ulcers occurred more frequently when the stressors were intermittent rather than continuous, and when the occurrence of stress coincided with the natural release of stomach secretions. Moreover, Seligman's work with rats showed that unpredictable shocks were more likely to produce ulcers than were predictable shocks.[51] When the rats were conditioned to a signal that alerted them to a shock that was coming, they had a lower incidence of ulcers.

With humans, studies have shown that gastric and duodenal ulcers often occur in individuals who suffer from such repeated psychological stressors as frustration, guilt, anger and hate.[9,41,52] Duodenal ulcers have been described as following major life-change events (see Chapter 2 for the discussion of the "ulcer personality").[4] Herbert Weiner cites the following personality correlates of the ulcer-type individual: is constantly leaning on others; desires to be fed; seeks close body contact with others; rarely expresses anger; and tends to be prim, tidy, mild, conscientious, inhibited and punctual.[40]

The first definitive evidence that ulcers can be produced in humans by anger came from observations by Stewart Wolf.[52] The esophagus of a man had been so badly burned by scalding hot clam chowder that the surgeon had to make a surgical opening directly into the man's stomach in order to feed him. Thus, it was possible to see the patient getting angry and, at the same time, observe the stomach and acid production, inflammation and finally the formation of a definite ulcer.

During World War II, there was an interesting association reported between stress and ulcers.[6] Veritable epidemics of "air-raid ulcers" occurred in areas of Great Britain under air-raid siege. Immediately following a bombing attack, many people would appear in the neighborhood hospitals with bleeding duodenal or gastric ulcers. Most of them were not physically hurt; apparently they just suffered psychological anguish.

It seems that corticosteroid production is related to the formation of ulcers (as mentioned in Chapter 3). A well-known correlate of this relationship is that latent ulcers can flare up and pre-existent ulcers can become worse when patients are given corticosteroid drugs (e.g., cortisone, prednisone).

DIABETES MELLITUS

Diabetes is one of the top five killers of all diseases in the United States. There are two principal types of diabetes mellitus, juvenile and adult-onset.* The tendency toward getting either is inherited, but the more severe juvenile type is also more related to genetic predisposition.

Adult-onset diabetes can be affected by stress. Remember from Chapter 3 that both corticosteroids and catecholamines cause a rise in blood glucose, which if sustained, could lead to diabetes in susceptible people. The development and exacerbation of adult-onset diabetes has been shown to be preceded in many cases by major life-change events.[4] Juvenile diabetes can be exacerbated by stressful events and psychological stressors. And we already mentioned that diabetes is related to obesity and is one of the risk factors for coronary heart disease.

ASTHMA AND OTHER ALLERGIC DISEASES

Asthma is a serious, occasionally fatal, allergic disease that often is precipitated by stress. With asthma, acetylcholine from the parasympathetic nervous system is a key factor. This disease is opposite to coronary artery disease, in which the release of the sympathetic nervous system catecholamines is instrumental in the disease; asthma is relieved by catecholamines and corticosteroids. With recurrent episodes of asthma, bronchitis and emphysema can develop. Smoking (discussed in the next chapter) can also induce and aggravate these chronic lung conditions.

Other allergic diseases that are stress-related are chronic urticaria (hives), angioneurotic edema (allergic swelling), hay fever and vasomotor rhinitis (allergic cold). In all of these conditions, both chronic psychological stressors and major life-change events have been described as occurring prior to the onset of the diseases.[4] Since

* Another rare type of diabetes is diabetes insipidus. It is caused by a deficiency of a hormone from the posterior pituitary gland known as vasopressin or antidiuretic hormone (ADH).

about 15% of the population have allergies, these stress-related conditions can affect many people.

INFECTIOUS DISEASES

In Chapter 3, we discussed how the body's release of corticosteroids during the stress response causes an interference with the immunological and inflammatory defense systems. This, in turn, allows any microbes or viruses that might be present to disseminate rapidly, gain a foothold and cause the manifestations of the particular disease. In this manner, stress is indirectly related to all infectious diseases.[41] The connection between stress and infection has been shown to be especially true with tuberculosis.

Tuberculosis

The release of corticosteroids paralyzes the phagocytes that keep the tubercle bacilli in check. The microbes are then free to disseminate and cause the overt disease.

When a patient has an infectious disease such as tuberculosis, the disease is exacerbated when the patient is given corticosteroids. In a few studies it has been shown that major life-change events preceded the onset of tuberculosis.[4]

The Common Cold and Influenza

Quite often when a person's resistance is down, he can "catch" a cold or the flu. Stressors often cause a depressed resistance, and when one's resistance is low, the very same or other stressors can cause overt clinical disease. One aspect of this is paraphrased in the common saying, "I opened the window and in-flew-enza (i.e., influenza)."

There is a wonderful song about colds and psychological stressors. It was sung by Miss Adelaide in *Guys and Dolls* and has the appropriate psychosomatic ending:

> In other words, just from waiting around
> For that plain little band of gold
> A person . . . can develop a cold.*

* From "ADELAIDE'S LAMENT" by Frank Loesser
  © 1950 Frank Music Corp., 1350 Avenue of the Americas, New York, NY 10019
  © Renewed 1978 Frank Music Corp., International Copyright Secured, All Rights Reserved, Used by Permission.

HYPERTHYROIDISM

As described in Chapter 3, during the stress response, thyroid hormones (e.g., thyroxine) are released and metabolism increases.[41] Development of hyperthyroidism (one manifestation is exophthalmic goiter—bulging eyes) could be precipitated if the response became chronic. In an animal study, it was shown that a breed of wild rabbits regularly developed hyperthyroidism after being frightened by a barking dog.

In humans, studies have shown that thyroxine levels have markedly increased in: (1) soldiers recalling painful war incidents; (2) hypnotized subjects suggested distressful situations; (3) individuals discussing family problems; and (4) people watching a distressful movie.[53] Furthermore, it has been shown that hyperthyroidism occurs at times following severe psychological or social stressors.[4,41]

RHEUMATOID ARTHRITIS

In Chapter 2, we discussed the "rheumatoid arthritis personality."[31,53,54] Such an individual is purportedly a woman who is unhappy in the traditional female sex role. She is described as being frustrated, self-sacrificing, tidy, orderly, punctual and perfection-minded. Supposedly, such people tend to have inner hostility and feelings of guilt produced by this hostility, and they try to balance the two emotions.

Selye considers rheumatoid arthritis a disease of inadequate adaptive reactions by the body.[41] The reader should recall that the anterior pituitary gland produces both ACTH and STH (growth hormone). If the balance is uneven, this helps in the development of rheumatoid arthritis in susceptible individuals. Rheumatoid arthritis is actually treated with cortisone or ACTH.

ULCERATIVE COLITIS

Ulcerative colitis is an inflammatory disease of the colon (part of the large intestine). The gut bleeds and becomes ulcerated and denuded. The development of this disease might be related to the irritant action on the colon of corticosteroids released continuously during chronic stress.

Ulcerative colitis also has a personality correlate.[31,53,55] Such an individual is described as tidy, prim, mild, well-mannered, conscientious, punctual, inhibited, submissive and overdependent. Supposedly, the ulcerative colitis individual tends to suffer from family and job-related stressors.

Other, less serious afflictions of the colon are constipation and diarrhea. Stress often initiates these attacks.[9] People who suffer repeatedly from constipation have been said to be grim, bored, dejected and depressed. In contrast, individuals with chronic diarrhea are described as being angry and hostile, having guilt feelings and a tendency to panic.

PREMENSTRUAL TENSIONAL SYNDROME

This condition tends to occur in many women just prior to their monthly menstrual periods and for a few days afterward.[41,56] These women have been described as "nervous," depressed, lethargic and irritable. They are also prone to develop migraine headaches, epilepsy, nausea, syncope (fainting), swelling of the face and extremities, backache and joint pains, acne, skin rash, glaucoma, conjunctivitis, styes (i.e., the last three are eye disorders), hypoglycemia, sinusitis, sore throat, mastitis (inflammation of the breast), hemorrhages, and asthma. These clinical manifestations disappear at the onset of the menstrual period (or a few days later), but tend to recur just before the next period. Of course, no one woman has all of these manifestations, and each manifestation varies in intensity.

Selye believes this syndrome may be related to the release of pro-inflammatory hormones during the stress response.[41] As with rheumatoid arthritis, premenstrual tension may result from an inadequate balance of pro- and anti-inflammatory hormones released during stress.

Recent findings have implicated other factors in the etiology of this syndrome. Progesterone (a female hormone) deficiency and a failure in the feedback mechanism between the hypothalamus–anterior pituitary gland and ovaries may be involved (see Fig. 4.2).[56] Not all women develop this syndrome, and there may be psychological components associated with the manifestations. Stress is also a factor in menstrual irregularities such as amenorrhea (lack of menstrual flow).

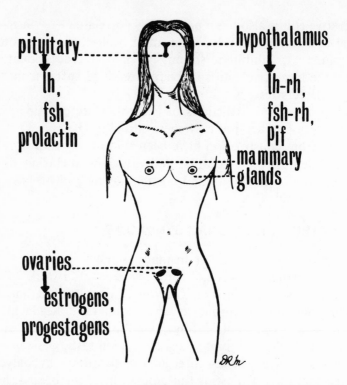

Fig. 4.2 The female hormone system. The female hormone system is geared toward reproduction. Hence, egg release (ovulation), fertilization and impregnation are enhanced by hormonal action. The hypothalamus releases FSH-RH (follicle-stimulating hormone releasing factor), which activates the anterior pituitary gland to release FSH (follicle-stimulating hormone). FSH stimulates growth and development of the ovaries and the ovarian follicles (in which the eggs are found). The hypothalamus also releases LH-RH (luteinizing hormone releasing factor), which activates the anterior pituitary gland to release LH (luteinizing hormone). LH is needed for final development of the mature follicle to cause the release of the egg (ovulation) and to produce the corpus luteum (formed from the follicle after the egg release). Estrogens are formed from the ovarian follicles, and progestagens are formed from the corpus lutea. Estrogens have many functions related to female characteristics and body structure; they are needed for maturation of the follicle, ovaries, corpus luteum, and mammary glands and to maintain pregnancy. Progestagens are essential for the control of reproductive activity, for morphological development of the mammary glands and to maintain pregnancy. During pregnancy other hormones are produced; relaxin from the corpus luteum (prepares tissues for delivery of the fetus) and chorionic gonadotropin (HCG) from the placenta (needed for maintenance of pregnancy). A final hormone released from the hypothalamus is PIF (prolactin inhibitory factor). It turns off the activity of prolactin (PRL, lactotrophic hormone; LTH, luteotrophic hormone). Prolactin is turned on when PIF is not released. This occurs during pregnancy when prolactin is needed for milk formation in the mammary glands. Estrogens and progestagens have feedback activity on the hypothalamus and anterior pituitary to regulate the release of LH and FSH. For example, FSH and LH are turned off by high

THROMBOPHLEBITIS

Thrombophlebitis is an inflammation of the veins that predisposes the veins toward blood clots. The actual development of the clots may be related to the effect of catecholamines (released during stress) on blood platelets, causing them to aggregate.[32] Ex-President Nixon's episodes of thrombophlebitis may have been precipitated by the stressful events that occurred during the Watergate period.

GOUT

Gout is a hereditary disease of uric acid metabolism that can also be precipitated by stress.[41] Uric acid crystals become deposited in and around joints, especially in the joints of the big toe. The disease tends to be exacerbated after stressful encounters. One study showed that uric acid becomes elevated under certain stressful conditions.[57] Gout is also a risk factor for coronary heart disease.[22]

WARTS

Warts are commonly found skin lesions caused by the papova virus, which multiples inside the nucleus of epidermal cells (outer surface of the skin). They frequently crop up after stressful situations. Quite often warts continue to occur despite medical and surgical treatment until the stressful situations are resolved.

MISCELLANEOUS ORAL CONDITIONS

Aside from the previously mentioned oral muscle-related conditions (i.e., clenching, bruxism, myofascial pain-dysfunction syndrome), stress affects the mouth and throat in other ways. Let us consider the resulting afflictions.

---

estrogen and progestin levels produced during pregnancy. (A fertilized egg is present, and no more follicles which have eggs are needed.) This system is active from puberty to menopause. In males, the system is similar except that androgens (e.g., testosterone) are produced by the testes instead of estrogens and progestagens by the ovaries. In addition, sperm are produced instead of eggs.

Dental Caries

One of the physiological effects of the stress response is decreased salivation (xerostomia). Studies have shown that dental decay (caries) increases under conditions of reduced salivation. In research studies, it was shown that animals forced to exercise repeatedly (a physical stressor) had an increased level of caries as compared to immobilized animals.[58]

It has been observed that the period of maximum dental cavities in the average person's life is preadolescence and adolescence.[44] These times are also highly stressful; there is anxiety about family, peer groups, school and "growing up." As the result of cumulative physical and psychological stressors, there are probably diminished salivation (the effect of catecholamines) and impaired immunological responses (the effect of corticosteroids) which can allow the oral microorganisms to multiply and colonize the tooth's surfaces. Of course, if candies and other sweets were eliminated, the bacteria wouldn't stand a chance.

Necrotizing Ulcerative Gingivitis

There are various types of periodontal disease (gum diseases), but the one that may have the closest association with stress is necrotizing ulcerative gingivitis (NUG, Vincent's disease or trench mouth).[44,58] Patients with NUG have been reported to be under severe emotional "strain" just prior to the development of the disease. Students before exams and soldiers during battle have had increased incidence of NUG.

One study showed that patients with NUG had statistically higher sympathetic nervous system activity than unaffected people. They showed higher blood pressure readings, more rapid respiratory rates and greater degrees of pupillary dilation. Other studies have shown patients with NUG to have high scores on anxiety-level tests.[44]

Apthous and Herpetic Lesions

Apthous ulcers are canker sores. These ulcerous lesions can occur anywhere in the mouth, but are often found on the tongue, inside of the cheeks, palate, gums and lips.

Herpetic lesions are cold sores that are caused by a specific virus.

They also can be found anywhere in the mouth, but are more common on the lips. Both canker and cold sores have been shown to crop up immediately after highly emotional periods.[44,58,59] The release of corticosteroids during stress inhibits the body's defense and allows the herpes virus to become activated; then the cold sores appear.

Tics

Ticks are prevalent in dogs and cats—but humans have tics of a somewhat different sort. Human tics are minor muscular twitches that become habitual. The twitches are repetitive and generally purposeless. Tics often begin as voluntary responses to some internal or external stimulus, but in time they become habitual and involuntary.

Tics appear to be anxiety-related and are muscular expressions of psychological conflicts.[44] They are most common in the facial area. Some examples are as follows: twitches of the lips and cheeks; continual throat clearing and spitting out; and uncontrollable coughing, sneezing and hiccupping.

Habits

There are several oral habits that are often induced by psychological stressors such as worry, fear and anxiety. These include thumbsucking, lip-, cheek- and nailbiting and tongue thrusting.

Potpourri

Other oral conditions that are stress-related are metallic taste, glossodynia (burning tongue), gagging, angioneurotic edema (allergic-type swelling), paresthesia (loss of sensation or numb feeling), trismus (difficulty in opening the mouth), atypical facial neuralgia (literally, aching nerves) and cleft palate.[44,59-61] Altered taste sensations can occur in depressed people. Burning tongue has been reported in individuals with emotional conflicts as well as depression. It has been estimated that in over 90% of the cases, gagging is psychological in origin. Many gaggers express fears of suffocation or choking to death.

Psychological stressors have been reported to precipitate

angioneurotic edema, paresthesia and trismus. Atypical facial neuralgia often occurs in depressed postmenopausal females. Although it has not been confirmed for humans, in animal experiments cortisone, ACTH and psychological stressors induced a high incidence of cleft palates.[60]

Summary

The most common of these miscellaneous stress-related oral conditions are dental caries, NUG and canker sores. However, the previously mentioned bruxism and myofascial pain-dysfunction syndrome are also common oral stress-related afflictions.

MISCELLANEOUS DISEASES

There are several other stress-related diseases and conditions including the following: neurodermatitis (a skin rash); Raynaud's disease (a circulatory disturbance of the fingers); wrinkled skin; alopecia areata (loss of hair, baldness); graying of hair; dandruff; arthritis; Cushing's disease (high levels of corticosteroids); liver and kidney diseases (e.g., enuresis, or bedwetting); hypoglycemia (low blood sugar levels); sexual disorders (e.g., impotence, frigidity) and infectious mononucleosis (the "kissing" disease). Although the relationships are not clear, all are apparently precipitated by stressful encounters.[31,41,43,53]

SUMMARY

Of all the stress-related diseases, by far the most important is coronary artery disease. Other prominent stress-related diseases are cancer, depression, muscle-related conditions, ulcers and diabetes. A summary of stress-related diseases and conditions is given in Table 4.5. For later use, the reader should note which of the diseases or conditions he has now or had previously.

It would also be helpful if the reader reviewed Tables 2.1 and 2.2 in Chapter 2, which describe, in part, certain personality correlates and attitudes and their relationship to specific diseases. In the next chapter, we consider the stress-related disorders.

TABLE 4.5   Stress-Related Diseases and Conditions

I. Cardiovascular Diseases
    A. Coronary Artery Disease
    B. Cerebral Stroke
    C. Angina Pectoris
    D. Cardiac Arrhythmias
    E. Hypertension

II. Cancer

III. Depression

IV. Muscle-Related Conditions
    A. Tension Headaches
    B. Oral Conditions
        1. Clenching
        2. Bruxism
        3. Myofascial pain-
           dysfunction syndrome
    C. Shoulder Aches
    D. Backaches
    E. "Pain in the Neck"

V. Ulcers

VI. Diabetes Mellitus

VII. Allergic Diseases
    A. Asthma
    B. Chronic Urticaria (hives)
    C. Angioneurotic Edema
       (allergic swelling)
    D. Hay Fever
    E. Vasomotor Rhinitis
       (allergic cold)

VIII. Infectious Diseases: e.g., tuberculosis and the common cold.

IX. Hyperthyroidism

X. Rheumatoid Arthritis

XI. Ulcerative Colitis

XII. Premenstrual Tensional
    Syndrome

XIII. Thrombophlebitis

XIV. Gout

XV. Warts

TABLE 4.5 *(cont.)*

XVI. Miscellaneous Oral Conditions
   A. Dental Caries (tooth decay)
   B. Necrotizing Ulcerative Gingivitis (NUG; Vincent's Disease; trench mouth)
   C. Apthous and Herpetic Lesions (canker and cold sores)
   D. Tics
   E. Habits (e.g., thumbsucking)
   F. Potpourri (e.g., glossodynia, or burning tongue)

XVII. Miscellaneous Diseases
   A. Neurodermatitis (skin rash)
   B. Alopecia (loss of hair)
   C. Graying of Hair
   D. Dandruff
   E. Arthritis
   F. Cushing's Disease
   G. Hypoglycemia (low sugar)
   H. Infectious Mononucleosis (the "kissing" disease)

REFERENCES

1. Dunbar, F. *Emotions and Bodily Changes.* New York: Columbia University Press, 1954.
2. Rabkin, J. G. and Struening, E. L. Life events, stress and illness. *Science* 194:1013–1020, 1976.
3. Horowitz, M., Schaefer, C., Hiroto, D., Wilner, N. and Levin, B. Life event questionnaires for measuring presumptive stress. *Psychosom. Med.* 39:413–431, 1977.
4. Petrich, J. and Holmes, T. H. Life changes and onset of illness. *Med. Clin. N. Am.* 61:825–838, 1977.
5. Rahe, R. H. and Arthur, R. J. Life changes and illness studies: Past history and future directions. *J. Human Stress* 4(1):3–15, 1978.
6. Wolf, S. and Goodell, H. *Harold G. Wolff's Stress and Disease,* Second Ed. Springfield, Ill.: Charles C. Thomas Publ., 1968.

7. Lacey, J. I. and Lacey, B. C. Verification and extension of the principle of autonomic response stereotype. *Am. J. Psychol.* 71(1):50–73, 1958.

8. Schlesinger, J., Barzilay, T., Stryjer, D. and Almog, C. H. Life threatening "vagal reaction" to emotional stimuli. *Isr. J. Med. Sci.* 13:59–61, 1977.

9. McQuade, W. and Aikman, A. *Stress: What It Is, What It Can Do to Your Health, How to Fight Back.* New York: E. P. Dutton & Co., Inc., 1974.

10. American Heart Association: *Risko: A Way to Alert You to the Risks of Heart Attack.* Columbus, Ohio Affiliate, 1977.

11. Henderson, J. Running commentary. *Runner's World* 13(3):20, 1978.

12. Sewil, C. Those patients with wall street sickness. *Med. Econ.*:102–104, Nov. 10, 1969.

13. Glass, D. C. Stress, behavior patterns, and coronary disease. *Am. Sci.* 65: 177–187, 1977.

14. Morse, D. R. Sucrose: A common enemy. *J. Am. Soc. Prev. Dent.* 2(5):27–28, 1972.

15. Kazan, A. A stressless definition of "stress" and some speculations on its relationship to cardiovascular disease. *Acta Cardiol. T. (Brux.)* 30:331–332, 1975.

16. Jenkins, C. D. Recent evidence supporting psychologic and social risk factors for coronary disease. *N. Engl. J. Med.* 294:987–994, 1976.

17. Hurst, M. W., Jenkins, C. D., and Rose, R. M. The relationship of psychological stress to onset of medical illness. *Ann. Rev. Med.* 27:301–312, 1976.

18. Cassem, N. H. and Hackett, T. P. Psychological aspects of myocardial infarction. *Med. Clin. N. Am.* 61:711–721, 1977.

19. Eliot, R. S. Stress and cardiovascular disease. *Eur. J. Cardiol.* 5(2):97–104, 1977.

20. Mann, G. V. Medical intelligence: Current concepts: Diet-heart: End of an era. *N. Engl. J. Med.* 297:644–650, 1977.

21. Jenkins, C. D., Zyzanski, S. J. and Rosenman, R. H. Coronary-prone behavior: One pattern or several? *Psychosom. Med.* 40:25–43, 1978.

22. Howard, R. B. and Herbold, N. H. *Nutrition in Clinical Care.* New York: McGraw-Hill Book Co., 1978.

23. Rensberger, B. Cigarettes and pill don't mix: The two may spark fatal hemorrhage. *Philadelphia Eve. Bull.*:36, Aug. 23, 1978.

24. McCamy, J. C. and Presley, J. *Human Life Styling: Keeping Whole in the 20th Century.* New York: Harper & Row, 1975.

25. Cooper, K. H. *The Aerobics Way.* New York: M. Evans and Co. Inc., 1977.

26. Colins, A. and Frankenhaeuser, M. Stress responses in male and female engineering students. *J. Human Stress* 4(2):43–48, 1978.

27. Editorial. Hypertension more likely among less educated and blacks. *Med. World News* 19(2):13, Jan. 23, 1978.

28. Editorial: Before they ski stress cardiography *Phys. Sportsmed.* 2(1):22, 1978.

29. Connor, W. E. and Connor, S. L. The key role of nutritional factors in the prevention of coronary heart disease. *Prev. Med.* 1:49–83, 1972.

30. Friedman, M., Rosenman, R. H. and Carrol, V. Changes in the serum cholesterol and blood clotting time in men subjected to cyclic variation of occupational stress. *Circulation* 18:852–861, 1958.

31. Pelletier, K. R. *Mind as Healer Mind as Slayer: A Holistic Approach to Preventing Stress Disorders.* New York: Dell Publ. Co., Inc., 1977.
32. Leff, D. N. Stress-triggered organic disease in this year of economic anxiety. *Med. World News* 16:74–92, 1975.
33. Weinsier, R. L. Overview: Salt and the development of essential hypertension. *Prev. Med.* 5:7–14, 1976.
34. Holt, R. (ed.). *Enlist in the War Against Alcohol.* Nashville: Southern Publ. Assoc., 1974.
35. Jick, H., Miettiner, O. S., Neff, R. K., Shapiro, S., Heinonen, O. P. and Slone, D. Coffee and myocardial infarctions. *N. Engl. J. Med.* 289:63–67, 1973.
36. Friedman, M. and Rosenman, R. H. *Type A Behavior and Your Heart.* New York: Knopf, 1974.
37. Cobb, S. and Rose, R. M. Hypertension, peptic ulcer and diabetes in air traffic controllers. *J.A.M.A.* 224:489–492, 1973.
38. Lynch, J. J., Paskewitz, D. A., Gimbel, K. S. and Thomas, S. A. Psychological aspects of cardiac arrhythmia. *Am. Heart J.* 93:645–657, 1977.
39. Le Shan, L. An emotional life-history pattern associated with neoplastic disease. *Ann. N.Y. Acad. Sci.* 125:780–793, 1966.
40. Arehart-Treichel, J. Can your personality kill you? *New York Magazine* 10:62–67, 1977.
41. Selye, H. *The Stress of Life,* Second ed. New York: McGraw-Hill Book Co., 1976.
42. Brown, B. *Stress and the Art of Biofeedback.* New York: Harper & Row, 1977.
43. Dudley, D. L. and Welke, E. *How to Survive Being Alive.* Garden City: Doubleday & Co. Inc., 1977.
44. Morse, D. R. and Furst, M. L. *Stress and Relaxation: Application to Dentistry.* Springfield, Ill.: Charles C. Thomas Publ., 1978.
45. Burch, J. G. and Abbey, L. M. Preliminary study of changes in blood pressure associated with clenching in normotensive and hypertensive subjects. *J.A.D.A.* 97:54–57, 1978.
46. Norris, C. Is your back biting back? *Dent. Manag.* 17(11):57–60, 1977.
47. Wilson, A. W. Inability to open the mouth: An unusual psychosomatic symptom. *Compr. Psychiat.* 5:271–278, 1964.
48. Fagg, G. The role of habitual movement and posture in psychosomatic disorder. *J. Psychosom. Res.* 9:165–168, 1965.
49. Miller, N. E. and Dworkin, B. R. Effects of learning on visceral functions—Biofeedback. *N. Engl. J. Med.* 276:1274–1278, 1977.
50. Brady, J. V. Ulcers in "executive monkeys." *Sci. Am.* 199(4):95–100, 1958.
51. Seligman, M. Chronic fear produced by unpredictable electric shock. *J. Comp. Physiol. Psychol.* 66:402–411, 1968.
52. Wolf, S. *The Stomach.* New York: Oxford University Press, 1965.
53. Lewis, H. R. and Lewis, M. E. *Psychosomatics: How Your Emotions can Damage Your Health.* New York: Viking Press, 1972.
54. Moos, R. H. and Solomon, R. F. Psychologic comparisons between women with rheumatoid arthritis and their nonarthritic sisters. *Psychosom. Med.* 2:150–164, 1965.

55. Grace, W. J., Wolf, S. and Wolff, H. G. *The Human Colon.* New York: Paul B. Hoeber, 1951.

56. Dalton, K. *The Premenstrual Syndrome and Progesterone Therapy.* Chicago: Year Book Med. Publ. Inc., 1977.

57. Rahe, R. H., Ryman, D. H. and Biersner, R. J. Serum uric acid, cholesterol, and psychological moods throughout stressful naval training. *Aviat. Space Environ. Med.* 47:883–888, 1976.

58. Protell, M. R., Krasner, J. D. and Fabrikant, B. *Psychodynamics in Dental Practice.* Springfield, Ill: Charles C. Thomas Publ. 1975.

59. Ship, I. I. Epidemiological aspects of recurrent apthous ulcerations. *Oral Surg.* 33:400–406, 1972.

60. Rosenzweig, S. Psychological stress in cleft palate etiology. *J. Dent. Res.* (Suppl. 6) 45:1585–1593, 1966.

61. Scialfa, C. T. Electrical stimulation for the treatment of facial paresthesia. *Dent. Surv.* 54(1):42–61, 1978.

5

Stress-Related Disorders: From Alcoholism to Suicide

There is this to be said in favor of drinking, that it takes the drunkard first out of society, then out of the world.*

GOING OUT

"Hi, Jim! Hello, Joan! Come in! Debbie's down in the den." You recognize the sweet pungent odor immediately. No sooner are you seated than you take your first "hit" from the passing "joint." Even though all four of you are respected law-abiding citizens, the legal aspects of marijuana smoking have not deterred you. After a few minutes of pot-induced animated conversation, you decide on a restaurant.

"Hello, Mr. and Mrs. Jones! Welcome, Mr. and Mrs. Brown! We have a fine table by the window for you." After the seating formalities are over, you're greeted with, "Would you like a cocktail for an opener?" Jim and Fred had a rough day at the office; Joan

* Ralph Waldo Emerson, *Journal* (1866).

124

and Debbie had nerve-racking episodes with the kids. The pot was only the prelude—the scotch and martinis put the finishing touches on the daily anxieties.

Being typical middle-class Americans, you enjoy dining out, and you like American food. So it's salad with Russian or French dressing, rolls and butter, a well-garnished steak or lobster, pie-a-la-mode, coffee with cream and, of course, Sweet'n Low® . It soon becomes difficult to stuff anything else down that overused portal. So now you employ the mouth for another stress-relieving function.

Out comes the pack, and the fire-and-smoke ceremony begins. "You know Fred, this time I'm really going to stop—I've already cut back to only a pack a day!" But you continue to puff away, and soon the smoke effectively screens your table from any onlookers. Now that the food has begun to digest, and the lungs have had a tar renewal, only a liquid coating is needed to seal off the inside of the body.

"How about an after-dinner cordial?" the waiter inquires. The hatch opens again, the syrupy liquid glides effortlessly downward, and you all become effectively glued to your seats. But there is still plenty of time, and between the belly and the booze, it's tough to get up. You now have to be stimulated, and caffeine has the last say. Downing the last gulp of coffee, you decide that it's Fred's turn to use the Master Charge—some business *was* discussed, wasn't it!? You drop off the Browns and head for home, a little tired, quite full and a bit woozy. Incredibly, when you get into bed you're wide awake with a million thoughts coursing through your mind. You've got to get up early the next day, and, anyway, one "downer" won't hurt—or will it?

INTRODUCTION

In the previous not-uncommon story, we have portrayed several undesirable methods of coping with stress. If such behaviors became habitual, then the individuals at risk might become alcoholics, overweight, chain smokers, sufferers of caffeinism and drug addicts. In the remainder of this chapter these consequences of maladaptive stress coping behavior are covered, along with accidents, divorce, business breakups and suicide.

ALCOHOLISM

The famous English author G. K. Chesterton (1874–1936) made this statement many years ago: "The dipsomaniac and the abstainer are not only both mistaken, but they both make the same mistake. They both regard wine as a drug and not a drink." Chesterton, himself, was right and wrong at the same time. Regardless of the amount, alcohol *is* a drug. Yet, there is evidence that both the alcoholic and the teetotaler do worse than the person who has one or two glasses of wine daily.

A very interesting prospective study was reported recently by Nedra Belloc.[1] In this study of 7,000 adults, seven personal health-related practices were measured and correlated with mortality rates. We consider this study in more detail later, but for now let us look at practice #6, frequency of drinking alcoholic beverages. Belloc found that alcoholics had a mortality rate two to three times greater than that of abstainers. Abstainers did well, but those who had one or two drinks daily tended to live a little longer—and probably enjoyed life a little more.

Some physicians prescribe a daily glass of wine for its vasodilating action. This drinking practice could conceivably help keep coronary and cerebral blood vessels open. (Question: Would it help prevent heart attacks and strokes?)*

Nevertheless, drinking alcoholic beverages is a poor way of stress management. For the average person has difficulty in managing to drink just *one* glass of wine. And, of course, even one glass of wine can affect some people negatively by giving them a false sense of security. Alcohol interferes with one's ability to handle both physical and psychological stressors. Even in small doses, it destroys brain and liver cells, causes irreversible heart muscle damage and interferes with the body's immune system.[2] Alcohol is a central nervous system depressant, and if it is mixed with other depressant drugs such as barbiturates (or other sleeping pills) and narcotics (e.g., morphine, codeine), the results can be fatal.[3]

It is often reported that someone has died of an apparent heart attack in a restaurant. Recently, it has been found that it isn't the

---

* Although alcohol has a vasodilating action, this action is primarily peripheral (e.g., skin) and may not affect deep blood vessels (such as the coronary arteries). However, as mentioned in the previous chapter, the possible benefit of moderate alcohol consumption could be related to elevation of high-density lipoproteins.

heavy meal that overburdens the heart, but consumption of alcohol is the most likely factor. Alcohol tends to desensitize the mouth and depress the gagging reflex. Thus, someone who has had a couple of predinner cocktails may attempt to swallow a large morsel of food without chewing it first (perhaps a piece of steak or a large shrimp). The chunk of food then becomes lodged in the nasopharynx or trachea (inside of the throat). These attacks have been descriptively named "café coronary" or "backyard barbecue syndrome."[4] To compound the problem, the victim is initially treated as a heart-attack case, and resuscitation procedures may tend to cut off the air supply still further. What is needed at this crucial time is the employment of the Heimlich maneuver to dislodge the obstruction (see Fig. 5.1).

How can one tell whether it is a heart attack or an obstruction? If someone is turning blue (cyanosis) rather than red, then he is directly suffering from an obstruction of his airway. Other signs are choking,

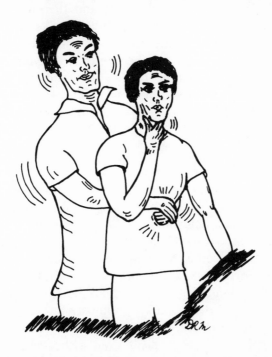

Fig. 5.1 The Heimlich maneuver. As soon as the victim shows signs of choking, the rescuer grabs him from behind. The rescuer's left fist is pressed firmly into the upper abdominal area below the center of the rib cage. This sudden movement should dislodge the obstruction.

grasping of the throat, wheezing, gasping for breath and inability to talk. With a heart attack, one does not usually see cyanosis immediately, and there are other signs such as: (1) the victim can talk and generally complains of severe pain radiating across the chest to the left arm; (2) there is a weak, rapid irregular pulse; (3) the victim's hands are cold and clammy; and (4) there is shortness of breath.[3] In either situation, once emergency treatment has been instituted, a physician should be called.

Alcohol is not even an effective muscle relaxant, according to a recent study.[5] University of Maryland researchers provided 15 students with a predetermined number of alcoholic beverages (gin or whiskey according to their preference). The dose (one to five cocktails) was sufficient to have a discernible effect (as measured by students' reactions as well as Breathalyzer and blood tests). Twelve student controls did not get any drinks. For all of the students, frontalis (forehead) muscle activity was determined by electromyography (EMG) at the start of the experiment and then again 30 minutes later. Although the students who were given drinks reported elevated feelings, there was no discernible change in their muscle activity—nor was there any for the controls. The results of this experiment seem to show that alcohol is not a good muscle relaxant, in contradistinction to the tranquilizer Valium® (to be discussed shortly).

OBESITY

Aside from the satisfaction of nutritional needs and the pleasures derived from it, eating is a means of coping with stressors for many people. However, this is another negative coping method because obesity is the undesirable outcome of compulsive eating. In that aforementioned study by Nedra Belloc, there were three health-related practices concerned with eating: practice #2, eating or missing breakfast; practice #3, snacking or not snacking between meals; and practice #4, maintenance of "normal" body weight.[1] The results showed that those who ate breakfast almost every day tended to live significantly longer than those who consistently missed breakfasts.* Those who snacked between meals lived a shorter time than those

---

* Fifteen years before Belloc's study, the famous American writer John Gunther addressed himself to another possible advantage of eating breakfast. He was quoted in *Newsweek* (April 14, 1958) as saying, "All happiness depends on a leisurely breakfast."

who did not snack. With respect to weight, those whose body weight was within average weight-height adjusted limits had the lowest mortality rates.

As discussed in the previous chapter, six of the risk factors for heart attacks are related to eating. Those factors are: (1) excess fat ingestion; (2) elevated blood cholesterol, triglycerides and low-density lipoproteins; (3) obesity; (4) lack of exercise; (5) high salt intake; and (6) high sugar consumption.

Rather than eating to relieve stress, some people chew gum or tobacco as a stress-relieving mechanism.[6] Even these practices are not without their negative aspects. Chewing sugar-containing gum can lead to dental decay. Sugar-free gum is not 100% safe either. That is, some artificial sweeteners have been implicated as carcinogens (i.e., cancer-inducing agents). Tobacco chewing is not too esthetically pleasing and has associated health-related problems (e.g., mouth cancer). At the other extreme, undereating to the point of starvation may be a response to the stress of growing up. This condition, seen mainly in female teenagers, is known as anorexia nervosa.[7]

SMOKING

People smoke for several reasons. Some smoke because of "peer pressure." It's one of the "in" things for many teen-agers, and rather than not "belonging" many youngsters smoke to comply or to appear grown up. Others simply smoke for the pleasures derived; there is no doubt that many people enjoy the effects of smoking (probably related to the drug nicotine). There are individuals who smoke because of oral gratification; the oral cavity is a primal pleasure zone, and many people love the stimulation produced by smoking. As discussed previously, drinking, eating and chewing are activities that may stimulate the central nervous system. Sucking and biting are other ways of achieving oral gratification. Finally, many people smoke as a means of relieving stress.

Although smoking can serve the purpose of stress relief, there is no doubt that it is detrimental to health. There is now firm evidence of the strong association between smoking and lung cancer. Smoking is implicated in emphysema, and heavy cigarette smoking is one of the important risk factors for coronary artery disease. Additionally, women who smoke and take birth control pills have an increased risk of heart attack and brain hemorrhages.[8] Smoking has also been reported to decrease an individual's ability to cope with stressors. This is related to the finding that smoking reduces the body's stores of vitamin C.[9]

In Nedra Belloc's study, health-related practice #7 was smoking habits.[1] The results showed that smokers had a mortality rate double that of nonsmokers. Heavy smokers who stopped smoking still had a 50% higher mortality rate than nonsmokers.

Marijuana smoking is also associated with "peer pressure," companionship, sheer pleasure and stress release. "Passing the joint," may be today's updated version of "passing the peace pipe." Undoubtedly, there are health-related problems, but the evidence is not as firm as it is for cigarette smoking.

CAFFEINISM

The morning cup of coffee is an American institution. A second institution is the coffee break. In Great Britain, tea is the preferred beverage. Youngsters all over the world imbibe large quantities of cola drinks and eat chocolate bars. And cocoa is a very popular warm beverage. Drinking and eating stimulating beverages and snacks is pleasurable, but they are also ingested for stress-release reasons. The common denominator for all of them is caffeine.

An average cup of coffee contains 100 mg of caffeine; the decaffeinated variety has 3.5 mg; a cup of tea has 50 mg; a cup of cocoa contains less than 50 mg; cola drinks have about 20 mg per glass; and a chocolate bar supplies about 25 mg.[10] Caffeine is the most powerful of a group of stimulating alkaloid drugs known as xanthines. Other xanthines are theophylline (found in tea)* and theobromine (found in cocoa). Taken in moderation (one or two cups daily), caffeinated beverages are effective and pleasurable stimulants. However, for some people even one cup of coffee acts on the kidney as a powerful diuretic (i.e., stimulates urination) and can interfere with sleep.

Coffee drinking has been implicated in several diseases, according

---

* One other product found in tea is tannic acid. Tannic acid has caused tumors in animals and in several countries, tea-drinking populations have had high rates of esophogeal (throat) cancer. One exception is the British, who thanks to the early warnings by the British Medical Association, have added milk to their tea which binds and inactivates the tannic acid (Morton, J. F. Tea with milk. *Science* 204:909, 1979).

to a few recent studies.[10,11] Ralph Paffenberger's group studied 11,000 male college graduates. They found that coffee drinkers had 1.4 times the risk of developing peptic ulcers of abstainers. The common American habit of drinking a cup of coffee and smoking a cigarette increased the risk of subsequently developing ulcers. Philip Cole found that the risk of developing bladder cancer increased with coffee drinking. Jick and his associates, studying over 12,500 patients, found a significant statistical association between coffee drinking and heart attacks. (No such association was found with tea drinking.) However, other studies did not find significant correlations.[11] One disease, though, is directly related to high coffee intake: caffeinism.[10] Symptoms include irritability, headache, nervousness, dizziness and insomnia. Afflicted individuals tend to be extremely anxious and react poorly to stressors.

DRUG ADDICTION

In this "uptight" society of ours, the No. 1 prescription drug is Valium. Valium has proved to be an effective, relatively safe, minor tranquilizer. But as is the case with many drugs, it can be dangerous if its use becomes habitual or if it is mixed with other drugs.[3] Popping pills such as Valium, Librium® , Atarax® , Miltown® and Equanil® is a very common way for Americans to relieve stress. Many a housewife turns to the pillbox when faced with screaming kids; and business executives are well-known users of these anti-anxiety agents. Drugs such as Valium are also excellent muscle relaxants, and they definitely are useful for the release of stress. However, dependency on drugs can be damaging to the mental and physical health of the user.

Barbiturates (known as "downers") are used for sedation and, in higher doses, to induce sleep. Unfortunately, they are habituating and can have serious interactive effects with other drugs (such as alcohol). Taking an overdose of barbiturates is a common method of committing suicide.

When some people are under stress, instead of taking pills to relax themselves, they choose stimulants or "pep" pills (known as "uppers") such as amphetamines, dexedrine, benzedrine and methedrine (known as "speed"). True addiction is unlikely, but psychological dependency (habituation) can occur.

Pain can be extremely stressful, and narcotics often are the only means of controlling it. However, addiction can readily occur, and oftentimes narcotics are then taken even when no pain is present (to avoid the withdrawal discomforts).

Many illegal drugs are taken for pleasure and stress-relief. These include cocaine, lysergic acid (known as LSD) and heroin. They are strongly addictive and often have unpleasant side effects.

Besides the negative effect upon the body's capacity to respond to stressors, people who are dependent upon pills for stress relief tend to develop a false sense of security. However, there is one aspect of taking pills that can be beneficial. Sometimes doctors give their patients pills that contain no known drugs. The pills may be sugar-coated harmless tablets (known as placebos; from "placere"—to please). They are often prescribed when the patient seeks help and automatically expects a prescription. The doctor may not believe that a drug is indicated, but may prescribe the placebo because he is aware that patients often have exaggerated beliefs in the effectiveness of drugs. It has also been shown that when patients believe in their doctors and in the pills they receive, even sugar-coated neutral pills can have physiological effects.

Studies have shown that placebos can decrease stress and pain reactions.[12,13] This effect is probably based on the automatic ability of a person to control his own autonomic nervous system responses. When one believes a pill will work, it may do the job in the sense that the body will respond accordingly. (This concept is covered more fully in Chapter 16, Biofeedback.)

Placebos are also used as controls in experiments of specific drug effectiveness. Sometimes these experiments backfire because the placebos—which trigger responses of the autonomic nervous system—may work almost as well as the established drugs.

ACCIDENTS

There is no question that people who drive while under the influence of alcohol or other drugs tend to cause accidents. In addition, based on the research of Flanders Dunbar (as mentioned in Chapter 2), there appears to be an accident-prone personality.[14] These people are considered to be impulsive doers, those who take on challenges. They tend to be aggressive, angry and hostile.

The accident-prone also may have feelings of guilt and impulses toward self-punishment or even suicide. It has been reported that 20% of all fatal car accidents involve drivers who have had disturbing emotional experiences within the preceding six hours. A second finding indicates that one out of three accident victims is in a state of depression prior to the accident.[15]

DIVORCE AND BUSINESS BREAKUP

Almost one-half of all marriages in the United States either end up in the divorce court or result in separations.[6] There are many reasons for unsuccessful marriages, but inability to manage the stressors of marital life is a key factor. Broken marriages are often related to drinking, smoking and drug problems, obesity in at least one of the partners and inability to manage anxiety, frustration, guilt and depression.

Business associations may break up for similar reasons. Mixing alcohol, drugs and sex at the office can contribute to both marital and business breakups.

SUICIDE

When the stressors of life get to the point where they are perceived to be uncontrollable, then some people decide to give up. Suicide is one of the 10 major causes of death in the United States.[16] Many of the previously mentioned negative coping methods can lead to suicide. Apart from the psychological effects of the chemicals on the mind, the alcoholic, the drug addict, and the grossly overweight may all be tempted to take their own life. Those with a failing marriage or business venture may be similarly inclined. And many accidents may be disguised suicide attempts. A common thread with all these individuals is their mental state; most are in a state of depression. A summary of the stress-related disorders is presented in Table 5.1. The reader should consider the following list of disorders and see which of them are personally appropriate.

In Part III, methods of overcoming these disorders are considered.

SUMMARY

After reading this chapter, the reader might be inclined to repeat the old lament, "Everything I enjoy in life is either illegal, immoral or

TABLE 5.1 Stress-Related Disorders

DISORDER	IMPLICATION
Alcoholism	Brain, liver and kidney damage; high mortality.
Obesity	Risk of heart disease, diabetes and kidney disease.
Anorexia nervosa	Risk of malnutrition.
Smoking	Risk of lung cancer, heart disease and emphysema.
Caffeinism	Extreme agitation; risk of ulcers, bladder cancer and heart disease.
Drug addiction	Risk of overdose and fatal accidents; serious drug interactions; mental breakdown.
Accidents	Driving while intoxicated, "pill popping," can lead to death.
Divorce and business breakup	Related to drinking, smoking, drug addiction, obesity and poor ability to manage stress.
Suicide	Related to depression, alcoholism, drug addiction, obesity and poor ability to manage stress.

fattening," and as Thomas Maugh II (an editor of *Science*) has added, "and hazardous to the heart."[11] However, as is discussed in Part III, there are several positive ways to manage stress and enjoy life. And when these methods are followed, the effects and instances of excessive eating, drinking, drug taking and smoking can be reduced markedly without sacrificing the joys of living. In the next chapter the relationship of stress and aging is covered.

REFERENCES

1. Belloc, N. B. Relationship of health practices and mortality. *Prev. Med.* 2:67–81, 1973.
2. Holt, R. (ed). *Enlist in the War Against Alcohol.* Nashville: Southern Publ. Assoc., 1974.
3. Morse, D. R. *Clinical Endodontology: A Comprehensive Guide to Diagnosis, Treatment and Prevention.* Springfield, Ill.: Charles C. Thomas Publ., 1974.
4. Henderson, J. *Emergency Medical Guide,* Fourth Ed. New York: McGraw-Hill Book Co., 1978, pp. 109–116.
5. Editorial. Relaxation formula: Jogger, si! jigger, no! *Phys. Sportsmed.* 3(10): 16, 1975.
6. Morse, D. R. and Furst, M. L. *Stress and Relaxation: Application to Dentistry.* Springfield, Ill.: Charles C. Thomas Publ., 1978.
7. Offord, D. R. Anorexia nervosa. *Psychosomatics* 8:281–286, 1967.

8. Rensberger, B. Cigarets and pill don't mix: The two may spark fatal hemorrhage. *Philadelphia Eve. Bull.:*36, Aug. 23, 1978.
9. Riccitelli, M. L. Vitamin C: A review and reassessment of pharmacological and therapeutic uses. *Conn. Med.* 39:609–614,1975.
10. Manber, M. The medical effects of coffee. *Med. World News* 17:63–73, Jan. 26, 1976.
11. Maugh, T. H., II. Coffee and heart disease: Is there a link? *Science* 181: 534–535, 1973.
12. Hilgard, E. R. and Hilgard, J. R. *Hypnosis in the Relief of Pain.* Los Altos, Calif.: William Kaufman, 1975.
13. Beck, F. M. Placebos in dentistry: Their profound potential effects. *J.A.D.A.* 95:1122–1126, 1977.
14. Dunbar, F. *Psychosomatic Diagnosis.* New York: Harper, 1943.
15. McQuade, W. and Aikman, A. *Stress: What It Is: What It Can Do to Your Health: How to Fight Back.* New York: E. P. Dutton and Co., Inc., 1974.
16. Resnick, H. L. and Cantor, J. M. Suicide and aging. *J. Am. Geriat. Soc.* 18:152–158, 1970.

6

Premature Aging: The Art of Dying Young

Every man desires to live long; but no man would be old.*

THE ETERNAL QUEST

"I'll take a one-way ticket to The Fountain of Youth." Richard T. Robertson III picks up his ticket from the counter and signals his chauffeur to unload the baggage. An obliging porter tickets the four valises and sends them on their way. Having a half-hour to spare before boarding, Mr. Robertson stops at the VIP lounge. The mellow scotch triggers some memories . . .

The first date, her name was Julie; he had to impress her with his manliness, so it was no sissy filter-tips for him. He smoked a whole pack of a real man's cigarettes—inhaling and all—just like "Bogey." Young Ricky was sick that night, but Julie was impressed, and the habit stayed with him.

* Jonathan Swift, *Thoughts on Various Subjects.*

He recalls the first card game; it was blackjack. That was the evening Richard met his future business partner, Jonathan Slack; he was also introduced to the pleasures of gambling and drinking. "Boy, that first scotch sure tasted bitter," but Richard liked the soothing after-taste and feeling. And the cards fell right, and Jon was a swell guy. That was a long time ago; many scotches have been downed since, and the business venture with Jonathan went up in smoke.

"Passengers are requested to report to Gate 14 for seat assignments for the flight to The Fountain of Youth." The terse announcement interrupts his reveries, and Richard Robertson III has to temporarily forego memory lane for another path.

Business tycoons get nothing but the best, and so Mr. Robertson takes his assigned first-class seat in the forward compartment. The glass of champagne resurrects another incident from the past.

"Finish everything on your plate; think of the poor starving children in China." Richie never could make the connection, but Momma's exhortations did the trick. He learned to love food, any kind of food; taste meant nothing—what he saw, he ate. Poor Richard; he was only being a good boy, but 58 years later he can't climb a flight of stairs, and he hasn't seen his toes in years. The aroma of steak and baked potatoes quickly brings the corpulent Mr. Robertson III back to the present. Of course, he can't refuse second portions and another small glass of champagne.

With a sip still on his lips, Richard reflects again. This time, it's that day in gym, the day of the physical fitness testing. Chubby Richie Robertson was instructed to do push-ups, but he collapsed after barely completing one. Everyone laughed, and as a result Richard shunned physical exercise from that time on. After a while he could afford to be driven anywhere he wanted to go, anyway. Besides, people die from all that exercising and jogging. "Heck, I've even carried a few of my golf- and tennis-playing buddies to the grave!"

However, Richard Robertson III could no longer ignore his present aches and pains. Yet, in retrospect, all those sleepless nights were well worth it. The many quarrels with his "ex," Jane, they didn't matter either; nor did his financial ups and downs. Because, in the end, he had made it—he had reached the top. Mr. Robertson had become Mr. "Big," and money was no object. Now he can well afford this trip. And, he will get "renewed"—he is going to The Fountain of Youth!

The plane begins its decent. The welcoming committee is waiting at the arrival section of the airport at The Fountain of Youth. The passengers get off—but Richard Robertson III has already departed.

INTRODUCTION

It has been said that the best way to live a long life is to choose long-lived parents. Of course, that's an idle thought, but it does point out the importance of genetic factors in determining how long a person may live. Beyond that, there are certain things that people do that tends to shorten their life span. For instance, Richard T. Robertson III was caught up in a significant number of these things. He ate, smoked and drank to excess. Moreover, he didn't exercise, and he had experienced more than his share of personal and business frustrations. In the remainder of this chapter, we examine the effect of these and other factors on the aging process. First, let us consider exactly what is meant by aging.

AGING

Aging can be examined on several levels. There are biological, psychological and sociological aspects to aging. One could also compare chronological age to physiological and psychological ages. Various physiological and psychological changes have been attributed to aging, but recent studies have questioned many of them. Several of the purported aging phenomena may be the result of disease rather than aging per se. But there is no doubt that even without diseases, the human body has a finite existence,* and various tissues do change with time. Let us first examine the biological changes that apparently result from aging.

Biological Aging

Genetic factors are important in aging.[1] Many studies have shown that offspring of long-lived parents tend to live longer than those of

---

* The Bible grants us three score years and ten, while recent research considers the upper limits to be within the range of 110–115 years.[1]

short-lived parents. Although there are some conflicting studies, it appears that the maternal influence is more important. Hence, if an individual's mother lived to be 80 and his father died at 40, the mother's genetic influence would tend to be stronger. As a result, the person might expect to live considerably longer than his father did. One study found that the maternal influence was stronger for sons than for daughters. Another maternally related finding was that offspring of older mothers had a shorter life span than those of younger mothers. The past-40 mother has a high risk for premature births, mongoloid children and those born with other malformations which may result in earlier deaths. Another related finding was that firstborn children tend to live longer. This may be due to the fact that the mother is younger and probably healthier when the first child is delivered and nurtured.

As mentioned in Chapter 2, up to the time of menopause women have a greater resistance than men to infections, cardiovascular diseases and cancer. They also tend to live longer. Females have a lower death rate than males at all ages. There are even more male stillbirths than female. Although the stressors of family, social and business life of the male contribute to his shorter life span, there is no doubt that genetic factors are at work favoring the female. It is generally believed that the female X-chromosomes are not the primary reason for her selected advantage. Rather it may be due to genetically based hormonal differences that cause secondary sex characteristics which result in advantageous behavior, body structure and rate of metabolism.[1]

Although it is not certain that the differences are genetic, actuarial findings have shown that nonwhites tend not to have the longevity of whites. However, the differences are decreasing. For example, in 1900 the life expectancy for nonwhites was 14.6 years less than for whites; in 1963, it was 7.1 years less.[1]

Regardless of how long people live, there are certain biological changes that occur with aging in various tissues and organs.[2-4] These changes are as follows:

1. An increase in collagenous connective tissues that are found in blood vessels, skin, tendons, cartilage, bones and teeth. In addition to increases in amount, cross linkages occur which make the tissues stiffer. Calcium also tends to accumulate within the tissues.

2. A gradual decrease in elastic connective tissues found in blood

vessels and lungs. There is a tendency for hydroxy-apatite crystals (bonelike material) and cholesterol to form on the surface of elastin (an elastic protein) with aging.

3. A decrease in the number of normal functioning cells. As cells die, they often are not replaced. This occurs in connective tissues (fibroblasts), brain tissue (neurones) and various other body tissues. Some of these changes may be due to overwork and abuse.

4. An increase in age pigment (lipofuscin) in the liver, adrenals, heart, the anterior pituitary, and nerve cells in the brain and throughout the body. The significance of this pigment is not really known, although it is believed to be associated with reduced functioning of the involved cells.

5. Other age-associated cellular changes: increases in hydrogen bonds, free radicals, metal ions, aldehydes and peroxides. These changes can result in mutations (mistakes in genetic material) and linkages that affect molecules within cells so that they tend to lose their function and die.

6. An increased amount of fat. This undoubtedly occurs with aging, but it is probably preventable and relates to too high a caloric intake vis-à-vis the amount of exercise done.

7. A decrease in the amount of oxygen taken in by the lungs and used by the tissues. Studies have shown that basic metabolic rate (BMR; oxygen consumed by the body) decreases, as does the amount of oxygen consumed by the brain. Nutrients tend to be delivered more slowly to tissues, and waste removal from tissues becomes impaired. Older people tend to become fatigued more readily. Undeniably some of these changes are part of the aging process, but apparently some are caused by the lack of exercise and poor nutrition of the aged.

8. A reduction in muscular strength. Skeletal muscle tissues are greatly reduced in mass in aged individuals. There is probably loss in muscle fibers as well as decrease in actual size (muscle atrophy). Again, a good part of these changes could be due to the inactivity of aged people.

9. Decreased functioning of endocrine glands (those that produce hormones). With old age, partial involution of the thyroid gland has been found. Some of its clinical consequences in the aged are: dry skin and scalp; loss of hair; increased susceptibility to infections; muscle weakness; reduced speed of mental performance; slower

reaction time. One study showed a decrease in ACTH production by the anterior pituitary gland with aging; this could result in less efficient stress responses. The pancreas appears to be less effective in the production of insulin with aging; this may be one reason for the higher incidence of diabetes in the aged. Recent findings show that one reason for the decreased efficiency of hormones is that, with aging, there is a decrease in the number of hormone receptors on various cells.[5] Part of these changes may be related to lack of exercise and mental withdrawal that occurs in many of the aged.

10. With aging, there is decreased functioning of the immune system (spleen, thymus, lymphocytes, plasma cells). The result is diminished resistance to infection, poorer repair potential and increased susceptibility to cancer. It also appears that there are more mistakes made by the body's immune system with aging, so that the individual's immune cells (lymphocytes, plasma cells) may perceive the body's own cells as foreign, and rejection reactions occur (known as auto-immune responses). In aging, there is a great increase in auto-immune diseases. If an individual lives long enough, there is no doubt that the immune system will show signs of decline, but many physically and mentally active octogenarians show little evidence of immunological deficiency.

11. An increase in amyloid formation with aging.[6] Amyloid is a protein found in aged tissues. Its significance is unknown, but some scientists believe amyloid results from the body's rejection of its own cells (auto-immunity).

In addition to these general changes, three important organs and systems show age-related changes. These are the heart and circulatory system, the brain and nervous system and the kidneys and genital-urinary system. With aging, there is a reported decrease in the amount of blood pumped by the heart at rest. The heart muscles' contractions are prolonged, and the heart tends to hypertrophy with age. Human hearts become thicker with age according to a recent report.[7]

There are also circulatory disturbances that may be related to the decreased elasticity of the arterial walls and increased cholesterol and calcific deposits within blood vessels. There is a slowing down of the blood circulation which apparently results from a reduction in cardiac (heart) output.

The diminished circulation leads to a reported lowering of skin temperature of the elderly as compared to young subjects. Poor circulation and hormonal changes can lead to reduction in number of skin capillaries, dry and rough skin and a lessened ability to dissipate excess heat.

Pulse rate has been reported to increase less rapidly after exercise in the aged as contrasted to younger people. However, exercise causes greater increase in blood pressure for the aged as compared to the young. Some of these reported changes may be the result of atherosclerotic heart disease and lack of exercise, and therefore would not be true age changes. But the heart and circulatory system does become less efficient with age.

With respect to the brain and nervous system, reported aging changes are decreases in size and loss in number of neurons (nerve cells). The nerve cells also accumulate calcium, which inhibits their function. Other types of cells (glia) proliferate, and the nervous connections (synapses) decrease. Large vacuoles, age pigment and amyloid also appear in the aging brain. The brain appears to shrink as its metabolism decreases in old age. There is a gradual increase of water as the neurons decrease and change. One finding shows a decrease in fats, protein and oxygen consumption in the brain of the aged. Some investigators believe that these morphologic changes in the brain and central nervous system result in some of the supposed impaired mental functioning of the aged; that is, loss of recent memory, slow learning, rigidity of knowledge, inflexibility, decreased perception and slower mechanical responses.[2]

Yet, many people have active minds well into their nineties. Undoubtedly, aging affects the brain and central nervous system, but some of the deleterious effects are caused by atherosclerosis, alcoholism, lack of exercise and decreased use of mental faculties. The kidneys lose functioning cells and units with aging. There are also circulatory changes which tend to interfere with function. The circulatory changes may result partially from the sedentary life of the elderly. The sexual organs also decrease in function with aging, but this change does not have to interfere with sexual enjoyment.

There are other organs and structures affected by aging. Vision, hearing, taste, smell, touch and speech, other sensations and perceptions (i.e., integration of the senses) decline with age. Recent findings show that as the result of structural eye changes, the colors blue, green and violet are more difficult for older individuals to distinguish. Hearing loss with age is primarily in the upper frequencies. Taste buds in the mouth decline with age, especially after age 70. The teeth become less sensitive as the result of calcification of the pulp ("nerve") canals.[8] The sense of smell diminishes markedly with age. Touch, pressure and pain show age-related decreases. In terms of perception, the elderly require more time to receive and interpret complex figures. The way people feel when they age is the subject of the next section.

Psychological Aging

Certain behavioral patterns and attitudes apparently accompany aging.[2,3,9,10] They include the following:

1. A memory loss for recent events, but an accentuated recall of past events. Although previous studies indicated that intelligence decreases with aging, recent studies in which adequate time is given for responses have revealed that older people are not less intelligent than younger individuals.

2. A self-assertive attitude. This may be related to fears of being considered wrong. The elderly also don't care so much about possible consequences. They've lived long, and the attitude might well be, "What more could happen anyway except death?"

3. Anxiety about death, diseases, bodily changes, economic security, lack of friends and indifference of family.

4. A turning inward which can border on paranoia.

5. Feelings of loneliness and isolation which can lead to depression.

6. More conservative attitudes about people and events (i.e., being opinionated).

7. A lack of energy. This is probably more the result of poor conditioning than a biologic phenomenon.

8. Feelings of a loss of attractiveness (related to hair loss, graying, wrinkles, elongation of ears and nose, flabby muscles and stooping).

9. Some older women trying to act "young again" as a reaction to aging and the loss of responsibility for the family; some older men letting their hair grow longer and trying to act as if they are part of the "in" crowd.

10. On the other hand, the possibility that decreased sexual capacity will lead to severe anxieties and depression.

11. The tendency to act emotionally unstable. The elderly may laugh or cry at the slightest provocation.

12. Carelessness in appearance, lack of sanitary considerations and poor manners, all of which can occur as a result of lack of interest in life. Many of these altered appearances and attitudes are the result of diseases, poor nutrition, lack of mental stimulation and a sedentary life style. Foremost among the diseases are: atherosclerosis, hypertension, coronary artery disease, arthritis, osteoporosis (brittle bones), glaucoma, cancer and mental diseases (e.g., paranoia, schizophrenia, manic-depression). Recent findings by the National Institute of Mental Health (NIMH) have revealed that many of the psychological aging phenomena could be prevented with proper medical and sociological support.

Let us now consider the sociological aspects of aging.

Sociological Aging

Just as there are genetic factors that predispose individuals toward longevity, there are environmental factors that do the same thing.[1,2,10-12] They are as follows:

1. Married people tend to live longer than single people.* This may be related to better nutrition, emotional support and superior medical care.

2. Overeating and unbalanced diets are life-shortening. Ethnically related food preferences could negatively influence life span (e.g., consider the mountains of Italian pasta and Jewish potato pancakes one eats at a sitting).

3. People who work in higher-status occupations tend to live longer than those employed in lower-status positions.[1] The higher-status positions are usually less hazardous to health, the health benefits are generally superior, and the individuals are often better educated and more concerned with health. Higher income also helps in the procurement of better food, clothing, shelter and medical care.

4. Educated people tend to live longer. A Metropolitan Life Insurance study showed that college graduates from eight eastern col-

---

* With respect to married men and living longer, one wag has suggested: "It is not that they live longer; it just seems longer."

leges had a better life expectancy than the general white male popula-tion.[1] The honor students had the longest life expectancy. A recent *Who's Who In America* (a listing that is considered to be of intellec-tually superior people) showed that for ages 45-64, the mortality of the *Who's Who* group was less than half that of the general popula-tion. Within the *Who's Who* listings, the longest life expectancy was for scientists, and the shortest for journalists. Scientists are presumably knowledgable about medical advances, a fact that is probably reflected in their greater longevity. It also may be that their occupations are among the least hazardous.

5. Where people work and live influences their longevity. In the United States, people living in the agricultural states of the Midwest where the population density is the lowest lived the longest in the study cited. White farmers had the lowest mortality rates of all the occupations.[1]

Apart from these factors, there are certain sociological changes which usually occur in older age that can cause negative responses. These changes are related to forced retirement, the lack of respect for the aged in the Western world and the economic insecurity and loss of power and status that occur with diminished income and loss of an income-generating position.

If people do not develop hobbies and interests, retirement can be frustrating. People used to routine work may find the relaxation and recreation available during retirement to be unbearable. They also may become unhappy because their direction or counsel is no longer heeded; their friends are retiring, leaving or dying; their family ties are loosening; and they are feeling the infirmities of old age.

There is a great interplay among the biological, psychological and sociological aspects of aging. For instance, forced retirement can lead to social isolation that generates depression, which, in turn, causes the person to eat poorly, not exercise and disuse his mental faculties. The last three factors can intensify cardiovascular changes, which then can lead to either senility, a stroke or a heart attack. But much of this is preventable. Don't forget the old maxim, "You are only as old as you feel"—and, we would add, "and act." A sum-mary of aging phenomena is given in Table 6.1. In Chapter 17, methods of reducing and reversing these phenomena are considered.

Let us now consider more specifically how stress can affect the ag-ing process.

TABLE 6.1 Aging Phenomena

BIOLOGICAL

A. Increase in collagen, calcium and cross-linkages in tissues.
B. Decreased elasticity of blood vessles and lungs.
C. Decrease in cells, especially neural (brain) cells.
D. Increase in fat deposits.
E. Increase in age pigment (lipofuscin).
F. Increase in peroxides, free radicals, etc.
G. Decrease in metabolism.
H. Decreased waste removal.
I. Decreased oxygen intake.
J. Decreased muscular strength.

K. Decreased activity of hormones.
L. Decreased function of immune system.
M. Increased amyloid.
N. Thicker and less efficient heart, slower pulse rate, higher blood pressure.
O. Poorer circulation.
P. Decreased function of brain and nervous system.
Q. Decreased function of kidneys and genital organs.
R. Decline in vision, hearing, taste, smell, touch, pressure, pain and speech.

PSYCHOLOGICAL

A. Memory loss for recent events; better recall for past events.
B. A self-assertive attitude.
C. Anxiety about death, disease, body changes, security, etc.
D. A turning inward.
E. Loneliness and isolation.
F. Conservatism.

G. Lack of energy.
H. Feeling of loss of attractiveness.
I. Trying to revert to younger behavior.
J. Depression.
K. Emotional instability.
L. Carelessness in appearance.

SOCIOLOGICAL

A. Loss of job.
B. Loss of family ties.
C. Loss of friends.

D. Economic insecurity.
E. Loss of power and status.
F. Lack of respect by others.

STRESS AND AGING

All of the negative coping responses described in the previous chapter (e.g., drinking to excess, overeating) lead not only to diseases and disorders but to premature aging and death.

For example, Nedra Belloc's study on health-related practices and mortality rates was reviewed above.[13] The results of the seven practices may be summarized as follows:

1. People who slept eight hours per night had a 50% lower mortality rate than those who slept six hours nightly. The eight-hour sleepers also tended to live longer than the nine-hour or more sleepers (the latter may have tended to sleep longer because of illness).

2. People who ate breakfast regularly had a lower mortality rate than those who routinely skipped breakfast.

3. Those who snacked between meals died sooner than those who did not snack. (Snack foods are often junk food, which is considered to be unhealthy.)

4. Obese people had a higher mortality rate than those considered to be normal in weight.

5. Those who exercised regularly lived longer than those who rarely exercised.

6. Chronic alcoholics died earlier than abstainers or "one-drink-a-day-ers."

7. Smokers had a mortality rate double that of nonsmokers.

Such stress-related diseases as hypertension, coronary heart disease, atherosclerosis, diabetes and asthma can result in altered body tissues, changes that in effect result in premature aging and early mortality.

As people age, they are faced with many physical, social and psychological stressors. These stressors have been discussed previously, but to reinforce the concept, let us reconsider the major stressors of aging.

Physical stressors for the elderly are similar to those of younger people, but responses are slower or less effective. The aged are usually not as strong; they can't lift as much; their hearts don't pump as efficiently; they don't tolerate heat, cold or radiation as well; they become fatigued more readily; and their reaction time is slower. Social stressors are as follows: forced retirement from work; loss of family, friends, business associates; change in residence (e.g., to a nursing home or to a room in one of their children's homes); coming down with a major disease (e.g., heart attack, stroke, cancer); death of a loved one; and, with illness or retirement, sudden change in income.

Psychological stressors include: anxiety about death, sickness, finances, loneliness and loss of family ties; feelings of inferiority related to decreased sexual prowess, memory loss and loss of physical attractiveness; grief as a result of the death of a loved one; guilt as a result of review of past mistakes and regrets; and anger at society for forced retirement, family for neglect, and God or nature for diseases and the inevitability of death.

Hans Selye considers that after years of repeated exposure to stressors, the aging individual's resistance breaks down (see Chapter 3, General Adaptation Syndrome).[14] Something is used up, which Selye calls adaptation energy.*

This adaptation energy is, in large part, genetically determined. Selye says that once the energy is lost, it can't be replaced. To quote:

"Life is essentially a process which gradually spends the given amount of adaptation energy which we inherited from our parents. Vitality is like a special kind of bank account which you can use up by withdrawals but cannot increase by deposits—each exposure leaves an indelible scar in that it uses up reserves of adaptibility which cannot be replaced—since we constantly go through periods of stress and rest during life, just a little deficit of adaptation energy every day adds up—it adds up to what we call 'aging'."**

There is, of course, no Fountain of Youth and we cannot regain "adaptation energy," but we can slow down its loss so that aging can be a very gradual, pleasant and rewarding process of life—we can age gracefully. In Chapter 17, we discuss coping strategies for the aged.

SUMMARY

In these last three chapters, Part II, we examined how stress can negatively affect our health, our relationships with others and the aging process. In Part III, the management of stress is covered.

REFERENCES

1. Bell, B. and Rose, C. L. The interdisciplinary study of life span. *In* Spencer, M. G. and Dorr, C. J. (eds.), *Understanding Aging: A Multidisciplinary Approach.* New York: Appleton-Century-Crofts, 1975, pp. 40–66.
2. Wolff, K. *The Biological, Sociological, and Psychological Aspects of Aging.* Springfield, Ill.: Charles C. Thomas Publ., 1959.

* When a person is frightened, a popular response which he may give attests to a loss of something that results in premature aging. The response is: "You just took 10 years off my life."
** From *The Stress of Life* by Hans Selye. Copyright © 1956, McGraw-Hill, New York, p. 274. Used with permission of McGraw-Hill Book Company.

3. Kasterbaum, R. (ed). *Contributions to the Psychobiology of Aging.* New York: Springer Publ. Co. Inc., 1965.
4. Sinex, F. M. The biochemistry of aging. *In* Spencer, M. G. and Dorr, C. J. (eds.), *Understanding Aging: A Multidisciplinary Approach.* New York: Appleton-Century-Crofts, 1975, pp. 21–39.
5. Greenberg, L. H. and Weiss, B. B-Adrenergic receptors in aged rat brain: Reduced number and capacity of pineal gland to develop supersensitivity. *Science* 201:61–63, 1978.
6. Hendin, D. Protein fibrinoid in pregnancy may shed new light on amyloid function in aging. *Biomed. News*:6, Nov., 1971.
7. Kolata, G. B. The aging heart: Changes in function and response to drugs. *Science* 195:166–167, 1977.
8. Morse, D. R. *Clinical Endodontology: A Comprehensive Guide to Diagnosis, Treatment and Prevention.* Springfield, Ill.: Charles C. Thomas Publ., 1974.
9. Dibner, A. S. The psychology of normal aging. *In* Spencer, M. G. and Dorr, C. J. (eds.), *Understanding Aging: A Multidisciplinary Approach.* New York: Appleton-Century-Crofts, 1975, pp. 67–90.
10. Butler, R. N. and Lewis, M. I. *Aging and Mental Health,* Second Ed. St. Louis: C. V. Mosby Co., 1977.
11. Sweetser, D. A. Sociological perspectives on aging. *In* Spencer, M. G. and Dorr, C. J. (eds.); *Understanding Aging: A Multidisciplinary Approach.* New York: Appleton-Century-Crofts, 1975, pp. 91–104.
12. Marble, B. B. and Patterson, M. I., Nutrition and Aging. *In* Spencer, M. G. and Dorr, C. J. (eds.), *Understanding Aging: A Multidisciplinary Approach.* New York: Appleton-Century-Crofts, 1975, pp. 195–208.
13. Belloc, N.B. Relationship of health practices and mortality. *Prev. Med.* 2:67–81, 1973.
14. Selye, H. *The Stress of Life,* Second Ed. New York: McGraw-Hill Book Co., 1976.

Part III
Coping with Distress and Promoting Eustress

Now that we know all about stress, how do we cope with it? We have heard about meditation and hypnosis. But what of other methods—and how are they related to stress? The answers to these and similar questions are contained in Part III.

In Chapter 7, an overview is presented. Chapter 8 deals with the mental methods of avoidance, evasion, goal selection, solo coping and consultation. Chapter 9 reviews the diversion methods of handling stress.

The subject of nutrition and stress management is examined in Chapter 10. Exercise and other physical methods of massage, heat and cold are considered in Chapter 11. The effects of sleeping, napping and relaxing constitute the subject matter of Chapter 12. The relaxation response is introduced in Chapter 13.

Specific examples are then examined in the next three chapters. Chapter 14 deals with self-hypnosis; in Chapter 15, the topic is meditation; and biofeedback is evaluated in Chapter 16. In Chapter 17, the focus is on the use of various management methods for the aged and people with specific diseases. Finally, in Chapter 18, the topic is coping strategies to be employed with doctors and hospitals.

7

An Overview of Stress Management

As a cure for worrying, work is better than whiskey.*

Work, for Thomas Edison, may have been a method to overcome distress and promote eustress. Edison was a great inventor, and his work was so varied that it was almost as if he had a series of hobbies. For many people, however, work is tedious and boring; thus they turn to whiskey to relieve the stress. Unfortunately, as we've said, alcohol gives a false sense of security and power, and its long-term effects are harmful to health and life.

There are many other ways to deal with stress. Just as personality differences determine how stressors affect various people, so do personality differences determine how different people manage stress. For example, as discussed in Chapter 15, meditation is not effective for everyone.

Stress management can be divided into two phases; the first is cop-

* Thomas A. Edison, Interview on Prohibition, from the *Home Book of Humorous Quotations,* A. K. Adams (ed.), New York: Dodd Mead and Co, 1969.

ing with stress and the second is counteracting the stress response. There are five major methods of coping with stress.

AVOIDANCE

The first way to cope with stress is *not* to cope with stress. In other words, the best way to manage stressors is to avoid or prevent stress.

Consider this. One of us (DM) used to live in Smithtown, Long Island. He drove to New York several times a week via the Long Island Expressway. The expressway, which has been described as the world's longest parking lot, was a great generator of stress because of the traffic. So DM decided to do the logical thing—he would avoid this stress by no longer driving; he would go to New York by the Long Island Railroad. The idea was a good one, but unfortunately there were often delays and a variety of other problems with the railroad. Thus, instead of being a means to avoid stressors, this was a trade of one set of stressors for another. But though the railroad trip was stressful at times, it was less stressful than driving. The train ride provided an opportunity for reading, writing or sleeping, all of which are stress-reducing methods. (Avoidance is considered further in Chapter 8.)

EVASION

Rather than simply avoiding potential stressors, one may sidestep or evade them.[1] For instance, one could abstain when asked to vote on a controversial issue. However, as discussed further in Chapter 8, evasion may only postpone the stressful decision.

DIVERSION

The third major way to manage stress is to distract one's mind. In other words, diversion is a means of sidetracking stress. This method is somewhat similar to avoidance; but with avoidance the particular stressors are never met, while with diversion, one knows the stressors must be met eventually, but perhaps at a later time when one is rested or fortified.

Diversions can take many forms; e.g., regularly going to shows, movies, restaurants or sporting events and having rewarding hobbies such as photography, painting, needlepoint, writing and reading.

Diversions also include going on trips and vacations. Sometimes they do not serve the intended purpose, particularly if they are combined with business. Conversely, some avocations may interfere with true vocations. (This is the subject matter for Chapter 9.)

PREPARATION

A fourth major way to manage stress is to be prepared for it. There are three basic means of preparing oneself: the mental, the nutritional, and the physical.

Mental Preparation

It is surprising how easy many exams become when you study for them. Although Americans have a fetish for ad-libbing comics, many of the "spontaneous" gag-lines have been well rehearsed. When you mentally consider the various possibilities of a potentially stressful situation, this helps to reduce the stress. (Mental preparation is elaborated on in Chapter 8.)

Nutritional Preparation

The old adage "You are what you eat" makes good sense. Vitamins, minerals, proteins, carbohydrates, fats and fiber all play a role in stress management. (Nutritional preparation is discussed further in Chapter 10.)

Physical Preparation

In order to manage physical encounters well, it is necessary to be "in shape." And even though there are jogging and tennis fads in evidence now, being in shape is more than just dabbling in these two activities. (Exercise in its many forms is presented in Chapter 11.)

EUSTRESS RESPONSES

The fifth and last major way to manage stress is to change the stress response from distress to eustress.[2] There are two main ways to do this: the mental and the physical.

Mental Attitude

How do you address the stressful situation, and how do you react to it? Consider the following hypothetical example. Your husband had a rough day at the office, and you have had a trying day at home with the kids. Apparently, he lost two accounts, his stenographer quit, and his boss "blasted" him. He comes home late, snarls at the kids, impugns your cooking abilities, and flings his coat on the floor after kicking the dog. Should you respond with a verbal barrage, or should you smile, give him a kiss and just let it all "boil over"?

Maybe the former alternative is initially easier and more direct, but it can only give you distress as a reward. The "smile" response, on the other hand, could conceivably change potential distress to eustress. However, this might only work for some women. If it were contrived, one might smile outwardly but churn inwardly, a situation that would be even more distressful.

A possible compromise would be polite evasion. For example: "I'm really sorry you had such a difficult day—I did too—but I am not to blame. I'm going out now; if you want something else to eat, there's food in the refrigerator. I'll be back in a half hour, and we can talk it over." (Further discussion of eustress mental responses is found in Chapter 8.)

Physical Response

The second main way to change distress to eustress is physical, for as was discussed in Chapter 3, there are physiological as well as psychological components to the stress response. Although exercise tends to cause a stress response, with a proper mental set the results can be extremely beneficial. Remember, forced exercise is no more than a physical stressor and as such tends to be distressful. Just as "Beauty is in the eyes of the beholder," so is the nature of the stress response in the attitude of the exerciser. (The role of exercise is amplified in Chapter 11.)

COUNTERACTING THE STRESS RESPONSE

The second major division in stress management is counteracting the stress response. During the stress response, the adrenal cortex is activated with the production of corticosteroids.[3] Also activated is the sympathetic division of the autonomic nervous system with the release of catecholamines (adrenaline, noradrenaline).[4] In addition, the opposite autonomic nervous system division, the parasympathetic branch, may be deactivated. Thus, to counteract the stress response one tries to select means of damping down the activities of the adrenal cortex and the sympathetic branch and increasing the parasympathetic activity.

These objectives are achieved in part when we relax, take a nap or have a restful sleep (discussed in Chapter 12). A better and more predictable method is by initiating the relaxation response. There are various techniques that may be employed to elicit the relaxation response, including self-hypnosis, meditation and biofeedback. These subjects are covered in Chapters 13–16.

Table 7.1, gives a summary of the various stress management methods just described. The relationship of stress management to the stress and relaxation responses is shown in Fig. 7.1.

People who suffer from chronic diseases and the elderly have special problems when it comes to coping with stressors; stress

TABLE 7.1   Stress Management: Coping with Stress and Counteracting the Stress Response

COPING WITH STRESS

1. Avoidance

2. Evasion

3. Diversion
   a. Going out to shows, movies, etc.
   b. Having hobbies such as photography, etc.
   c. Taking vacations

4. Preparation
   a. Mental
   b. Nutritional
   c. Physical

5. Change Response from Distress to Eustress
   a. Mental attitude
   b. Physical (exercise)

COUNTERACTING THE STRESS RESPONSE

1. Sleeping, Napping, Relaxing

2. The Relaxation Response
   a. Self-hypnosis
   b. Meditation
   c. Biofeedback
   d. Others: e.g., Yoga; Zen

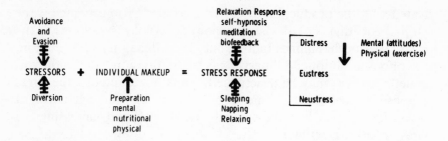

Fig. 7.1 Stress management in relationship to the stress and relaxation responses. ↑ and ↓ (lined) = overcomes by prevention or counteraction; ↑ and ↓ = reinforces by strengthening or changing.

management for these individuals is discussed in Chapter 17. Many people are ill at ease when they go to a physician, dentist or hospital; the way to cope in these stressful situations is the subject matter of Chapter 18.

REFERENCES

1. Mischel, W. *Introduction to Personality,* Second Ed. New York: Holt, Reinhart and Winston, 1976.
2. Selye, H. *Stress Without Distress.* Philadelphia: J. B. Lippincott Co., 1974.
3. Selye, H. *The Stress of Life,* Second Ed. New York: McGraw-Hill Book Co., 1976.
4. Kopin, I. J. Catecholamines, adrenal hormones and stress. *Hosp. Pract.* 11:49–55, 1976.

8

Mental Methods: The Plus And The Minus

Delay is the best remedy for anger.*

WITHIN THE WALLS

The man opens his eyes and finds that he is sitting in an empty, dark room. All is quiet. He sees that the walls are closing in and that there is no exit through a door or a window.

How did he get there? What did he do to be in such a predicament? He has no idea. But he *is* there and the walls are advancing toward him at a slow, steady, unrelenting pace. At that rate he figures that he has about 30 minutes to live unless he can find a way out. What can he do? What *does* he do?

His first mental response is *denial*. He closes his eyes again and says to himself, "It's only a bad dream." But when he reopens them, the walls are still in motion. As he pinches himself to make

* Seneca The Younger (4 B.C.–A.D. 65), *De Ira.*

sure he's awake, another thought comes to mind—it's not a dream, it's a hallucination! But he can't recall ever experiencing anything like this before, and he doesn't remember having drunk or eaten anything recently. And he *knows* he wasn't hypnotized.

The man becomes terrified. Often, people *regress* when they panic. So this man behaves like a child and starts to cry. In the long past, his mother would have soothed his fears and wiped his tears, but now she's not around—and the walls won't stop their inexorable advance.

This man is physically strong, so he resorts to brute force. But the pounding and pushing only serve to weaken him while the walls march on. And it's *really* happening; this is no mental aberration.

The man now reviews his life and begins to *rationalize*. "Oh God, why is this happening to me?" He reflects on his many past misdeeds and decides that he is being punished. But he'll repent, and God will forgive him; prayer is the answer. So he prays . . . and neither God nor the walls seem to be paying any attention whatsoever.

At this point, realizing that death is not far away, he carefully considers a *plan of action*. After a few minutes, he's ready. Slowly and methodically he covers every inch of the room—he looks, he feels, he listens.

"Ha!" One spot sounds hollow. Using his pocket knife, he is able to force open a section of one wall. "Quick, quick, the other walls are now perilously close." Spotting a new electric wire, he proceeds to cut it—there's a flash and . . .

The man opens his eyes and finds he is sitting on a fleecy, white cloud. All is deathly quiet.

INTRODUCTION

The previous story has a moral to it: Sometimes even with the best planning and preparation, death is still in the offing. The story also serves to introduce a few of the various ways to cope mentally with stressful situations. Denial, regression and rationalization are just a few of the defense mechanisms that may help temporarily but often in the long run are self-defeating. Preparation and then effective action is the best course to take, even if in the end it sometimes fails.[1,2]

In the remainder of this chapter, we cover the above methods along with avoidance, evasion, goal selection, other solo coping methods and consultations. Perhaps the reader may regard as obvious the suggested alternative behaviors, but oftentimes it is the very simple things that escape us.

AVOIDANCE AND EVASION

In Chapter 7, we introduced avoidance and evasion as ways of preventing stress reactions. However, most stressors usually have to be confronted sooner or later. With respect to avoidance, the reader should analyze his work situation and home life in trying to figure out how he might avoid potentially stressful situations. Let us pose some hypothetical examples.

If Chinese pepper steak always gives you a stomach ache, why relieve the acid indigestion with patented pills? You might consider eating a pizza instead—making sure you don't burn your palate. Does listening to the evening news depress you? This may be a time when ignorance pays—change to a music station, or try some light reading.

The method of evasion is like a balancing act—it may take some fancy footwork. Sometimes it is better to face the stressors immediately; at other times, evasion permits preparation. Two examples follow.

You have to make a decision about buying a car. You want economy, style, power and longevity. You've looked at 10 cars so far, and each has its advantages and disadvantages. You would like to wait another month to see the new issue of *Motor Trend Magazine*. But your present car is a gas-guzzling, oil-burning catastrophe—and the waiting and looking are not helping your blood pressure. Hence, make the decision now, and avoid the stress of indecision.

Consider another case: You just got a "hot" tip about a stock. It's selling at $10 a share, and "they" expect it to zoom rapidly. Gambling in all its forms is one of the most stressful avocations, and the stock market is no expection. You are a novice when it comes to stocks. Should you wait and investigate the company, or should you take the plunge? You decide not to buy, and it later develops that, in this particular situation, investigation would have reinforced your decision, since the stock price fell. The chances are that had you acted out of ignorance, it would have cost you money. Not purchasing that particular stock at that time saved you both money and a few points on your blood pressure. The decision in this case was to postpone or evade the situation that called for a decision in the face of uncertainty. It is worthwhile to remember that no matter which way you decide, it is difficult to avoid or evade stress where gambling is concerned.

GOAL SELECTION

Each of us is unique. There has never been anything like us on the face of the earth before, and there never will be again. Every individual is far more complicated than the most sophisticated computer, and each should be proud of his own uniqueness. Everyone should look within himself and recognize that his likes, dislikes and wants are his alone. Awakened to this realization, one should be careful and selective about goals and regard each one in its proper perspective.

A tennis pro is usually not a trained scientist; and a good scientist usually would not have the time to become a tennis pro even if he had the capacity. This may appear obvious, but with the many current sports crazes, people who will never "make it" are setting unrealistic goals for themselves in competitive sports such as tennis and running.

When one has attainable goals, frustrations are greatly diminished. In Chapter 1, under the discussion of frustration, it was seen that each choice was beset with possible frustration. With respect to the choice between personal goals and interpersonal relationships, the best way to manage is by being selective. In the case where a specific goal is of paramount importance—e.g., a matter of life or death as in a combat situation—then it might take precedence over interpersonal relationships. For instance, it is foolhardy to observe democratic voting procedures when the enemy is just over the horizon. On the other hand, if the goal is not primary or "pressing," it is only human to consider other people first. One must "Look out for Number One," but should not have to step on others along the way. (See "Eustress Mental Responses" in the next section.)

There is something else to keep in mind with respect to goals. Even within your own field of expertise, it takes time to attain objectives.

Impatience only engenders stress. Conversely, procrastination also induces stress. Thus, if a long-range goal is not reasonably attainable, then one should consider abandoning it. Many people who are presently successful changed goals and careers when they found that their original aspirations had lost their appeal or were not within reach. For instance, Casey Stengel started as a dentist and wound up as the legendary manager of the New York Yankees. One could point to numerous other examples.

There is one other consideration with respect to changing goals: Monotony is stressful. This is one of the problems of specialization. Specialists learn more and more about less and less; and while this process may be the hallmark of efficiency, it tends to produce boredom.

One study of 23 occupations disclosed that assembly-line workers had the highest degrees of irritation, physical illness and depression.[3]

Hence, if your particular field of endeavor is tedious, try adding variety. Perhaps you should consider changing fields or your career if your best efforts would be to no avail. However, frequent career changes are, in themselves, stressful (e.g., the stressors of moving and facing unknown situations).

A final thought. Life is a series of compromises. To keep stress within bounds, one should not expect everything to go his way. Even if you were always satisfied or content, that too would be stressful. Or as George Bernard Shaw said, "But a lifetime of happiness! No man alive could bear it: It would be hell on earth."*

SOLO COPING

Once a person is face to face with a stressful situation that he cannot avoid or evade, he is forced to cope. There are certain stressors that are unavoidable and cannot be evaded, including: aging and death (inevitable), taxes (must be paid sooner or later) and the weather ("Everybody talks about it, but nothing can really be done about it").

There are a variety of coping behaviors, ranging from defense mechanisms to effective action. Of course, the preferred behavior is effective action.

* George Bernard Shaw, *Man and Superman,* Act 1.

Effective Action

Familiarity breeds contempt—so the saying goes—but in another sense, familiarity greatly diminishes stress. One of the most entrenched fears is fear of the unknown (as illustrated in the introductory story).

When a person is forced to deal with a situation that he has never met before, he has no experience to fall back on, and he is more likely to become severely stressed. That is why, if it is at all possible, when faced with a new situation a person should plan and rehearse his actions before he acts. Vigilance is the key. All of the senses should be employed to the maximum.

It is surprising how often people miss things that are "right in front of their noses." This happens oftentimes because they are not used to looking at a particular place or because they assume something is not there when it is not in its usual spot. (This phenomenon is known as negative hallucination; see Chapter 14, Hypnosis.)

People often don't hear because they are preoccupied. It is amazing how much more one hears when he looks at the person who is speaking. The sense of smell accommodates rapidly so that if one doesn't concentrate on an odor, it will quickly disappear. Touch is another important sense modality that can give many clues and is often overlooked.

One other important aspect of mental preparation is to be unbiased in weighing the available information. A person should be "calm, cool and collected" in his observations. Unfortunately, prejudice too often affects one's judgment. For instance, many individuals are convinced that if something is published, it must be the truth. Even in highly respected journals, erroneous information has been printed. And, of course, advertisements are based on selective presentation of the facts, which allows contrary information to be purposefully neglected. Everything cannot be thoroughly investigated, but at least an attempt should be made to glean the facts. When a person is prepared in this way, the stress is lessened, and the situation may become bearable.

Insulation

Sometimes the best response is to do nothing. If one knows from previous experience that a particular situation will be stressful, then the best response may be no response. For example, every time you talk with a friend about politics, you have a violent disagreement. Although you feel that you are in the right, and you get the better of the arguments, you really lose because you have "upped" your stress levels (e.g., raised your blood pressure, triggered another ulcer). So the next time that your friend starts a political battle, just don't offer any comments, or you might politely change the subject.

Eustress Mental Responses

In Chapter 7, the concept of eustress mental responses was introduced. As Selye has shown, the same stressors yield opposite responses in different individuals.[4] The difference lies in whether the stressor is perceived as being positive or negative and how the individual reacts.

For instance, in an American household it is considered to be good manners to finish everything that is put on one's plate. An American housewife might become upset if her guest left a portion of his dinner uneaten. Recently, a friend of ours married a young woman from Thailand. She was invited to her fiance's house for dinner and according to Thai customs left a portion of the food on her plate to show that she was satisfied. In Thailand, this is a sign of good manners; in the United States, it usually is not. Perception is different in the two cultures, and distress would have been avoided had the Americans known about the Thai custom.

Interestingly, when our same friend went to Thailand to visit his wife's home, he ate everything on his plate. The Thai hostess, thinking that he was not satisfied, refilled his plate three times. Finally, after the third refill he gave up in despair and said that he was full and the food was excellent. In the discussion that ensued, the two possible interpretations of good manners emerged, and the situation was resolved.

In a similar vein, a postmeal belch might embarrass the guest and distress an American hostess, but this is a sign of contentment in China; the Chinese hostess would experience eustress when her guest belched.

In terms of facing stressors, people often react poorly, since they tend to magnify a stressful situation way out of proportion. For instance, winning a tennis match becomes a life-and-death struggle, and arriving late at the theater or a restaurant is a catastrophe.

Part of the eustress mental response is not to "make mountains out of molehills." Yes, it's nice to win and preferable to see a performance from the start—but it's not worth an ulcer or a migraine.

There are many serious life-change events that are unavoidable and quite stressful. These we have to face with *all* our coping abilities, but the minor things should be left as minor. One should just try to smile and learn to forget. As Shakespeare said, we should smile at grief.*

Many of us set standards for ourselves and others that are much too high. We expect perfection in an imperfect world. Going into a situation *not* expecting the best is another good way to decrease the chances of frustration, anxiety and other causes of distress.

Selye says that we should act with "altruistic egoism" to "earn our neighbors' love."[5] In order to do this we have to change our values. Success and self-satisfaction are important but not at any cost. "It's nice to be important, but it's more important to be nice." If we achieve our goals by stepping on others and raising our own stress levels in the process, we have achieved distress—not eustress. On the other hand, if we respond to criticism positively rather than emotionally, and if we replace anger with joy, it is possible to have a beneficial eustress response rather than a pathogenic distress response. (See Chapter 17 for a discussion of how positive attitudes may help in the cure of serious diseases such as cancer.)

Mental Repetition and Rehearsal

When considering how to act, it is important to look at past actions if reviewing them helps in the current situation. However, it is damaging to dwell on previous inappropriate behavior. Rehashing the past or "crying over spilled milk" only increases psychological stressors such as anxiety, frustration, guilt and anger. Worrying about what will happen in the future is just as bad. Going over and over the same things prevents effective action in the present.

An illuminating example is found in the game of tennis. Timothy Gallwey stressed the perils of dwelling in the past and worrying about the future.[6] He found that fewer errors are made when one concentrates on breathing or on seeing the ball rather than when one

* "Smiling at Grief," William Shakespeare, *Twelfth Night,* II, IV, 112.

makes a mental replay of the previous point or worries about what will happen if the present point is lost.

A somewhat similar situation occurs when a person has "pressing" problems on his mind and can't concentrate on the present situation. It is important to put those distressing thoughts out of one's mind for the present. Later, when the individual feels up to it, the problems can be tackled again, possibly with new insight gained during the delay.

One way to relieve disturbing thoughts temporarily is to find a quiet room and meditate or practice self-hypnosis (see Chapters 14 and 15). Another way is to try to concentrate on opposite thoughts. For instance, if your head is filled with images of "pink elephants," then concentrate on thoughts about "blue elephants." The basic principle invoked is that one cannot think of two opposing things at the same time. As is discussed later, if a person is relaxed (e.g., after a meditation session), that individual cannot simultaneously be anxious.

Defense Mechanisms[1,2]

The coping mechanisms of avoidance, evasion, effective action, insulation and eustress mental responses involve flexibility and choice, while, in contrast, defense mechanisms involve behavior that is rigid and automatized and are, by and large, neurotic ways of handling frustration and conflict. The unconscious utilization of defense mechanisms is a common reaction to stress that is shared by normal and disturbed persons. These defenses are useful in preserving self-esteem, averting personality disorganization or restoring some sort of equilibrium.

Generally, the more intense the stressors are, the greater the use of defense mechanisms is. In time, these mechanisms become more persistent, less appropriate in relation to the person's recent experiences, less controlled and more severe, incapacitating and disturbing to the individual. Let us now consider some of the more common and important defense mechanisms.

Denial. Denial is a perceptual blindness that temporarily protects the individual from the necessity of facing intolerable stressors. For instance, the shock of a personal loss is an occurrence in which denial as a defense is frequently employed. Typically, physicians who smoke or drink heavily tend to deny their excesses—the "it can't happen to me" syndrome. Obviously, this kind of denial is dangerous and can lead to serious diseases and early death.

Projection. Another common defense that protects a person against anxiety-producing impulses is projection, which disguises the source of conflict by ascribing one's own motives to someone else. For example, if a student has a strong desire to cheat on an examination but is unwilling to admit it to himself because of his moral code, he may become unduly suspicious of others and accuse them of cheating when in fact they are innocent. In the extreme form, triggered by strong stressors, such projection is the mark of the behavior disorder called paranoia.

Regression. Regression is a retreat to an earlier or primitive form of adaptation (e.g., the man who resorted to crying in the introductory tale). It takes the form of a childish, rather than an adult, reaction to frustration. The stressors of extreme frustration can be expected to produce regression in otherwise normal people.

Rationalization. Another defense against the anxiety aroused by conflict is known as rationalization. There is an invention of "good" reasons to discount failures or to engage in experiences that might otherwise be perceived as damaging. Thus, disappointments may be softened by "sour grape" rationalization; and personal defects and misfortunes may be converted into blessings in disguise ("sweet lemon" rationalization). For instance, you may have encountered the individual who boasts of his fabulous income and of all the wonderful places he has visited. Oftentimes, the boasting is only a rationalization for his boring business, which he detests. Sooner or later, he'll have to face the business stressors directly or else suffer the consequences of distress.

Displacement. Displacement is another kind of defense against anxiety-provoking situations. In displacement, the real source of anxiety is disguised by placing it on some object or circumstance. For instance, the man who gets angry at his boss but is afraid to tell him off may bawl out his wife or kick the family dog.

Reaction Formation.   A person may disguise his conflict by believing that his motive is exactly the opposite of his real motive. The defense mechanism of reaction formation may be seen in the case of the daughter who unconsciously hates her mother but appears to be oversolicitous of her mother's health and comfort. The common quotation from Shakespeare "The lady doth protest too much, methinks," refers to this disguise.

CONSULTATION

There are times when people find that they cannot face a situation alone; they need support or help. Many people are unwilling to admit they are "sick" or are so proud that they don't want to seek aid. This is part of the American ethic of strength and "being a man," but it is a distorted view.

Most people who find themselves in difficult situations need others for moral support at least. When people are angry, sad or upset, they need someone to listen with empathy. Even happiness should be shared. This old maxim is certainly appropriate today: "A shared grief lessens, a shared joy increases."

The mere act of talking with someone is cathartic and therapeutic. Shouting at others to vent anger may be preferable to bottling up the feelings, but it makes for increased hostility.[7] A far better method is to replace "anger with joy" as was discussed under "Eustress Mental Responses." Talking to one's self, whistling or singing in time of trouble can be helpful, but talking to others is usually more beneficial. In group sessions, chanting and screaming (e.g., Primal Scream Therapy) can be a beneficial means of stress release. Laughing and crying are responses to stressors, which can be of benefit when one is alone, but may be even more effective when someone else is around to give empathetic support. It is better not to inhibit the laughing or crying responses; otherwise there may be a build-up of psychological stressors which may cause distress.

Another strange but interesting way to release stress is by sneezing. One case was reported in which the person did not talk, shout or scream when faced with situations that caused resentment—he sneezed instead.[8]

Once a person decides he needs help, he should begin with his family and friends. If they are not helpful, then he should try his clergyman (if he has one) or perhaps the family physician or dentist. Should none of these avenues prove beneficial, then he should consider seeking professional assistance. Admitting to one's self that help is needed is not a sign of weakness, any more than seeking dental care to relieve a toothache is an admission of "weak" teeth.

Psychologists and psychiatrists are trained to deal with stress; hence, their professional expertise should be sought.* Some psychotherapeutic methods that have been employed to cope with anxiety and depression include psychoanalysis, client-centered psychotherapy and behavior therapies such as assertiveness training and behavioral modification.

For some people, group therapy is a more effective way of dealing with stress. Some individuals are more comfortable in sharing their problems with others who have similar problems. There are many approaches, ranging from group psychotherapy to eclectic encounter groups. The various groups and courses combine in some manner such techniques as relaxation, exercise, sensory deprivation, assertiveness training, transactional analysis, "brainwashing" and "touching and feeling."

Some of the popular offerings are: Gestalt; Esalen; Reality; est (Erhard Seminar Training); Psychocybernetics; Rational-Emotive; Psychodrama; Silva Mind Control; Bioenergetics; and Primal Scream Therapy. Another approach, helpful to some, is family therapy, in which the individual shares his concerns in sessions with his family members and the therapist.

Several of these approaches, methods and procedures may be scientifically questionable, besides being unusually demanding.**

FACING SOCIAL STRESSORS

When a person becomes aware of a stressor, he may choose to avoid it, evade it or confront it. If he chooses to meet it directly, he can either confront it appropriately, or he can take some halfway measure. At the very least, he is now aware and can plan a strategy based on available evidence.

* Confidential referrals may be made by the family physician, dentist or local professional societies and schools.

** Before becoming involved, it is advisable for an individual to seek guidance from an appropriate professional society.

When a severe social stressor strikes someone unawares, it can often leave that person in a state of shock. One of the most severe life-change events occurs when a loved one is killed in an accident. There is really no time for preparation; hence, one must fall back on the resources previously built up. No one can really tell a person how to react when tragedy strikes. All that can be said is that it is normal to grieve—up to a point.

Without meaning to sound unfeeling, after an appropriate interval, life must go on much as before if a double tragedy is to be avoided. Some people can cope well during these trying times. Perhaps the deeply religious and the fatalists are best equipped. In the final analysis, each of us must rely on our own resources. Expressing emotions through crying and embracing, seeking the company and support of others, as well as professional assistance, are appropriate behaviors during the period of mourning.

As far as less severe social stressors go—such as loss of a job and change of residence—effective action and rethinking of goals are important. Feeling sorry for oneself may feel "sweet," but it solves nothing. Keep in mind that there are many niches "out there." Although it may take time and effort to find an appropriate one, a person must keep on trying if he is to survive with dignity in this demanding world.

A summary of the various mental methods is presented in Table 8.1. The reader should identify the ones he generally employs to cope

TABLE 8.1   Mental Methods of Stress Management

I. Avoidance	To prevent stress reactions.
II. Evasion	To postpone stress reactions.
III. Goal Selection	Must be individually tailored.
IV. Solo-Coping	The first line of defense is to help oneself.
A. Effective action	Entails mental preparation.
B. Insulation	A "no" response to prevent distress.
C. Eustress mental responses	Change distress to eustress.
D. Mental repetition	Self-defeating.
E. Defense mechanisms	Rigid and automatized.
1. Denial	Telling oneself that it is not happening.
2. Rationalization	Telling oneself that it is all for the best.
3. Regression	Reverting to childlike behavior.
4. Projection	Blaming it all on others.

5. Displacement	Turning toward an alternate target.
6. Reaction forma- tion	Reaction in the opposite direction.
V. Consultation	If self-help fails, seek others.

A. Methods
1. Talking, shouting, whistling and singing (solo as well as consultation).
2. Chanting (solo as well as consultation).
3. Screaming (Primal Scream Therapy).
4. Laughing (solo as well as consultation).
5. Crying.

B. Groups (small and large)

1. Family.	5. Psychologists.
2. Friends.	6. Psychiatrists.
3. Clergymen.	7. Encounters (e.g., Gestalt; Esalen; Reality; est;
4. Family physician or dentist.	Psychocybernetics; Rational-Emotive; Psycho- drama; Silva Mind Control).

with stressors. If he discovers that he tends to use mental repetition and rehearsal and relies on defense mechanisms, then he should actively try to use the other more positive approaches. Change comes slowly, so one should not expect to be able to cope well immediately and under all circumstances.

SUMMARY

There is no one made-to-order method to manage stress mentally. If one knows that a situation will be stressful, it would be best to avoid or evade it if at all possible. If the stressors must be faced eventually, then the best way to cope is to be prepared mentally and then to take effective action.

Whenever possible, one should try to see the bright side of things, to convert anger to joy and to choose praise over criticism. Finally, if a person finds that he cannot handle it alone, then he should seek personal or professional help, perhaps as part of a group.

In Chapter 9, we turn to another way to relieve stress, diversion.

REFERENCES

1. Krech, D., Crutchfield, R. S., Livson, N. and Krech, H. *Psychology: A Basic Course.* New York: Knopf, 1976.

2. Mischel, W. *Introduction to Personality,* Second Ed. New York: Holt, Rinehart and Wilson, Inc., 1976.

3. Pelletier, K. R. *Mind as Healer Mind as Slayer: A Holistic Approach to Preventing Stress Disorders.* New York: Dell Publ. Co., Inc. 1977.

4. Selye, H. *The Stress of Life,* Second Ed. New York: McGraw-Hill Book Co., 1976.

5. Selye, H. *Stress Without Distress.* Philadelphia: J. B. Lippincott, 1974.

6. Gallwey, T. *The Inner Game of Tennis.* New York: Random House, 1974.

7. Varro, B. What's this? Don't vent our anger? *Philadelphia Eve. Bull.* A:17, Aug. 8, 1978.

8. Lewis, H. R. and Lewis, M. E. *Psychosomatics: How Your Emotions Can Damage Your Health.* New York: The Viking Press, 1972.

9

Diversions: Getting Away From it All

A man travels the world over in search of what he needs and returns home to find it.*

ESCAPE

DR. GRIMES: (Only 26 days, 5 hours and 22 minutes to go. Oh the bell! It's the Anderson brat. He's not going to get me today. This time I'm protected. Heck, I've got on gloves, safety glasses, a mask and ear plugs.) "Hi, Jimmy! Come right in! How's my favorite patient?" (Martinique, I need you *now*.)

NANCY: (That darn phone never stops ringing.) "Hello, Mrs. Carmen. Yes, your appointment is for 10:30. We'll see you then. Bye!" (Let's see, what was I doing? Oh yeah! The check book, paying the Deal account. He should have hired a bookkeeper. Gee, I'm supposed to do everything—make appointments, order

* George Moore, *The Brook Kerith*.

supplies, greet patients, type letters, balance the books, and of course, always smile, smile, smile. Oh, the bell! Here comes Mrs. Anderson with her "charming" child.) "Hello, Mrs. Anderson! Hi, Jimmy! We'll be right with you. How was your summer vacation?" (It's going to be one of those days—but wait, tonight's the music fair. Oh great, I almost forgot, and my favorite rock group will be there!)

MRS. CARMEN: "Jimmy, hurry up or we'll be late for our appointment with Dr. Grimes." (Oh, that brat is going to give me an ulcer, he's so slow and lazy. Let's see, after this appointment I've got to go food shopping and then to the bank. And let me see, Kathy wanted to play tennis. If it wasn't for the tennis I think I'd go crazy.) "James, let's go *now*!"

Three different people are involved with Jimmy and his appointment. All three are faced with cumulative stress, and each has a particular escape mechanism. Dr. Grimes is anxiously looking forward to a vacation on the island of Martinique. His receptionist, Nancy, is anticipating that evening's musical extravaganza. Mrs. Carmen uses tennis as a means of daily escape.

These are just three ways of breaking away from the routine. In the next section we consider these and other methods of diversion.

METHODS OF DIVERSION

Whether one is a housewife or a business executive, many chronic stressors must be dealt with each day. Even if an individual uses mental coping methods successfully, the constant coping may produce mental fatigue and sluggishness. "All work and no play makes Jack a dull boy." An old cliché—but how true!

Hans Selye has formulated a stress quotient that permits an individual to determine when a diversion or complete rest is indicated.[1] Selye's stress quotient is as follows:

$$\frac{\text{Local Stress In Any One Part}}{\text{Total Stress In The Body}}$$

If it is found that a person has too much stress in any one part of the body, then diversion should be sought. For instance, if one has spent hours scrutinizing detailed material, then a different activity should follow (e.g., taking a swim). On the other hand, if the person is physically or mentally exhausted (i.e., total stress in the body), then rest and relaxation are called for (discussed in Chapters 12-16).

There are many methods of diversion, and each individual should do what suits him best. How can one tell? One good way to "know thyself" is to try a variety of things. For instance, people whose daily work is largely sedentary and unexciting may elect activities such as water skiing, scuba diving, mountain climbing, sky diving, hang gliding or riding on rollercoasters. Others, who have active and exciting jobs, might choose to relax with a book. Some people like the classics; others escape into science fiction; still others prefer detective stories or romantic novels; and some are inclined toward self-help books.

If you like Mah Jong, bridge or poker, then play them, but don't force yourself just because the other guys are doing it. You might prefer solitaire.

Various sports and athletics are fine for diversion, but if you'd rather watch than play, then do just that. (The beneficial aspects of exercise and athletics are covered in Chapter 11.) "Eating out" is a wonderful diversion, especially for the harried housewife, but don't eat yourself into a heart attack. And don't go to restaurants every day because then that too becomes routine.

To many people, diversion means being entertained. It may be that for such people it is the opposite of work; for when they work, they work hard. Diversion, then, may mean they want to do "nothing" or as little as possible. Perhaps the best thing for them is to play the role of the spectator or simply to lie on the beach.

Movies, shows, theater, opera, sporting events and television are great forms of entertainment. But even these can become addictive and less than beneficial. Continually viewing shocking and frightening programs and movies can raise a person's stress level.

Watching the "tube" is probably the most common daily diversion in the United States. There are many fine programs on television, but there are also violence, sex and inanity. Too much TV watching can cause eyestrain and hearing loss (more likely from constantly listening to loud music such as rock-and-roll), and there are radiation effects from sitting too close to a color set. Among other unhealthy effects of constantly being "glued" to the TV, people tend to snack a lot, talk too little and get no exercise.

An article in the *Detroit Free Press* showed that TV watching can also be quite addictive.[2] Newspaper representatives approached 120 families in the Detroit area and offered to pay them $500 per family if they would agree to have no television for one month. Of the families approached, 93 refused the offer. Twenty-seven families accepted, including five that had their sets temporarily disconnected. Some of the results were as follows: One man spent almost every day reading newspapers; two individuals became chain smokers; several children became very cranky and repeatedly begged to have the sets turned back on. And, conversely, some families became more tightly knit, there was a renewal in reading, visits with other families increased, and some took more vacations.

The sex act may be considered an effective diversion. However, it can either be boring (i.e., doing the same thing with the same partner for many years) or exciting (e.g., employing varied techniques). Masturbation is another sex outlet. While it still may be thought of as evil and a damaging practice, some experts believe that it is an appropriate form of stress release.[3]

An affair may also be considered a diversion. According to Morton Hunt in his book *The Affair,* some people can manage an affair in a way that it can even be helpful to their marriage.[4] However, engaging in an affair is like handling a double-edged sword. On the one edge, it may be a way to relieve the day-to-day boredom of home and business life. Meeting someone in clandestine places can be exciting and stimulating. A noted philosopher once said: "Sex without guilt is a bore." But the other edge of the sword may be more damaging: Often there is guilt about the secret relationship; anguish about finding the time; anxiety about the possibility of disease (syphilis, gonorrhea) and bringing it home; fear of being caught; worry that one's marriage is in jeopardy with repercussions affecting the children; doubt about one's ability to measure up sexually; embarrassment about one's physical appearance which the years have not helped; torment about what excuse to use for being absent; concern about being financially able to afford the relationship; and, for the religious, fear about drawing the wrath of God ("Thou shalt not commit adultery"). Hence, before engaging in this form of diversion, a person should think twice and perhaps a third time. Group sex may also be considered as a diversion, but it is even more fraught with potential distress.

It is important to have daily diversions as well as take regular vacations. But when that trip is taken or that oil painting is created, it is essential that one's daily business is not taken along for the ride. Some people tend to work hard and to play hard, but this typical behavior should be left behind. For instance, if there are problems at home or work, mulling them over while on vacation is self-defeating. The idea is to remove oneself from the troubling environment so as to take advantage of peace and quiet. Interestingly, when one gets back, things don't appear quite as black or hopeless. It may be that a new perspective was all that was needed.

Another important aspect of getting away is that you should have faith that the home or business won't fall apart in your absence. Perhaps we need to feel indispensable, but on balance it is to our advantage to let someone else carry the burden for awhile. It is far better to have someone else do the work even if it is not up to your standard. You don't want to be the most efficient employee or businessman in the grave. Does it really matter that you have the cleanest household in the neighborhood if you are not around to enjoy it? Take a trip and enjoy.

During vacations it is important to have rest as well as activity. A person should not program his vacation in the way that he plans his business or home life. The vacation should be free-floating, and should be a combination of pure relaxation along with invigorating exercise. And there shouldn't be any "time pressures" about when to do what.

Yet, vacations may be detrimental for some people. An active individual may find relaxation is not tolerable. He finds it necessary to be engaged in something, whether it be fishing, hunting or skiing. For people who suffer migraine headaches, relaxation may precipitate an attack, and cerebral strokes have occurred during periods of relaxation rather than during active periods.[5]

In the introductory story, the diversions were presented as a way to escape from the stressors of daily life. However, if one is really to manage life well, there should be only a few daily stressors. Thus, if work or home life produces repeated anxieties and frustrations, if it is dull and boring with few challenges, then it is time to change the daily routine.

For instance, one could go back to school, take new courses, read the literature in one's chosen field and try to incorporate some of the latest advances. If it is reasonably possible, one could consider different hours, another position or even a new career. Nowadays it is accepted that a housewife might think of herself for a change and perhaps look into business opportunities.

Remember that vacations and hobbies are great, but if the working hours are not sufficiently rewarding, then one spends much of his day in thinking about escaping. And then if the escape doesn't live up to expectations, the frustrations may be compounded.

A summary list of methods of diversion is given in Table 9.1. The reader should identify his preferred methods and add any that might have been missed. Given this base, he should expand both his daily and longer periods of diversion as required.

TABLE 9.1   Methods of Diversion in Stress Management

I. Solo-Active

  A. Reading.
  B. Writing.
  C. Photography.
  D. Art (e.g., painting, drawing, sculpting).
  E. Playing a musical instrument.
  F. Solitaire.
  G. Collecting (e.g., stamps, coins, antiques, etc.)
  H. Running.
  I. Hobbies (e.g., knitting, wood-carving, etc.)
  J. Sex (e.g., masturbation).
  K. Vacations.

II. Group-Active

  A. Sports (e.g., tennis, bowling, golf, etc.)
  B. Games (e.g., Mah Jong, bridge, poker, etc.)
  C. "Eating out."
  D. Sex (i.e., with one's own partner).
  E. Affairs (Note: can do more harm than good).
  F. Sex orgies (Note: not to be recommended).
  G. Vacations.

III. Solo-Passive and IV. Group-Passive

  A. Television.
  B. Movies.
  C. Shows and Theater.
  D. Listening to music (e.g., radio, records, tapes, etc.)
  E. Concerts, opera.
  F. Sporting events (e.g., baseball, football, basketball, hockey, etc.)
  G. Vacations.

In addition to mental coping with stress and escaping from stress, there are two other major ways of help in managing stress: one is nurturing the body; the other is physically preparing the body. The nurturing aspect (nutrition and stress) is covered in the next chapter. This is followed by the physical methods (including exercise) covered in Chapter 11.

REFERENCES

1. Seyle, H. *The Stress of Life,* Second Ed. New York: McGraw-Hill Book Co., 1976.
2. Bricklin, M. This year make time for fun. *Prevention* 30(1):32–42, 1977.
3. Sharpe, R. and Lewis, D. *Thrive on Stress: How to Make it Work to your Advantage.* New York: Warner Books Inc., 1977.
4. Hunt, M. *The Affair.* New York: New American Library, 1973.
5. Dudley, D. L. and Welke, E. *How to Survive Being Alive.* Garden City: Doubleday & Co., 1977.

10

Nutrition: From Chicken Soup to Vitamin C

We never repent of having eaten too little.*

THE ANTISTRESS COCKTAIL

"Let's see. One teaspoon of brewer's yeast, a tablespoon of wheat germ, two bone meal tablets, one half cup of rose hips powder, a teaspoon of soy lecithin and two tablespoons of carob powder. Great! It's all in there now. What's next? Oh, yeah! A glass of skim milk and three tablespoons of natural malt. Okay, in it goes. Now blender, do your thing."

"Wow! That sure doesn't taste like tomato juice. I can feel it in my toes already. Boy, I'm not gonna be uptight tonight. I'm rarin' to go."

INTRODUCTION

Wouldn't it be great if all we had to do was drink a nutritional blend as just described and then be able to face any stressors without dis-

* Thomas Jefferson (1743–1826), *Writings.*

tress! Unfortunately, that is not reality, and even health food advocates will admit that probably there is no mixture that will make one impervious to the damaging effects of stress. Yet, nutrition can be a factor in stress management. It does appear that optimum levels of vitamins, minerals, carbohydrates, lipids, proteins and fiber are necessary in order to cope adequately with stressors.*

Controversy exists over what constitutes an optimum level and under what conditions. There is also controversy over the effects of large doses of nutrients on stress and diseases. There are three basic reasons for these controversies: One is that results of animal experiments are not readily transferable to humans. The second is that there is great biochemical variability among people, which is related to each individual's specific makeup. That is why average daily requirements of vitamins and minerals may be well below—or well above—the amount needed by a particular individual. The third reason for controversy is that many of the studies claiming beneficial results either have been poorly controlled or are based on uncontrolled clinical observations and testimonials. With these limitations in mind, let us begin the discussion with the vitamins, starting with vitamin C.

VITAMIN C

An absolute deficiency of vitamin C (ascorbic acid) leads to scurvy, a disease in which hemorrhages occur in the skin, mouth, muscles and joints. Other effects are anemia, debility and increased susceptibility to infection.[1-3] In the normal individual the highest levels of vitamin C are found in the adrenal glands, the liver and the white blood cells.[4] Under stressful conditions, there is an excessive outpouring of vitamin C from the adrenals into the urine. Some investigators believe that vitamin C acts as a coenzyme (i.e., helps speed up the reaction) for the manufacture of cortisone. Hence, more vitamin C would be needed in times of stress.

Detoxification of foreign substances in the liver has been proposed

---

* Although there is currently no specific nutritional blend that can "turn off" stress, recent findings have revealed that there may be natural substances produced by the brain that can act as tranquilizers. These substances, known as purines, may bind at specific anti-anxiety sites in the brain to induce tranquility. Anti-anxiety drugs such as Valium also appear to act at these sites (Schmeck, H. M., Jr. Researchers tracking brain's own tranquilizers. New York Times. C1, 4, April 13, 1979).

as another role for vitamin C. Certain white blood cells (polymor-phonuclear leukocytes and the larger macrophages) destroy bacteria and viruses, in part, by phagocytizing (engulfing) them. Vitamin C appears to help in activating white blood cells so that their phago-cytizing ability is enhanced.

Linus Pauling, the famed Nobel Laureate, is the principal advo-cate of the use of megadoses of vitamin C to prevent colds and other viral infections.[5] The most recent findings on the effects of mega-doses of vitamin C are of interest.

One Canadian study showed that the vitamin C–supplemented group experienced slightly fewer colds and fewer days of cold symp-toms than did a placebo-control group.[6] Aside from this cold-related finding, the results showed that the vitamin C–supplemented group had significantly fewer days of any illness and significantly fewer doctors' visits than the placebo group. This prompted the in-vestigators to ask the question: "Did the large intake of ascorbic acid exert a specific anti-viral (or anti-bacterial) effect or was the mechanism involved a non-specific one responding to any type of acute illness, or indeed to any acute stress?" The answer given was: "Our data cannot provide a clear answer to this question, but the fact that general rather than local symptoms were the most strongly influenced, and that different types of illness appeared to be equally affected, would seem to favor a relatively non-specific mechanism. The high concentration of ascorbic acid (and its depletion at times of stress) may be relevant to this question."*

Another interesting study with respect to the role of vitamin C in stress was reported by Robert Hodges and his co-workers.[7] In this experiment, six prisoners were deprived of vitamin C and were then given varying doses of the vitamin, including a small amount that was radioactively tagged (so that it could be identified later). Then, from the amount of radioactivity present in the urine, it was deter-mined that each prisoner used approximately 3% of the existing body pool of vitamin C, irrespective of the dose given.

Two of the six prisoners escaped on the fifty-fourth day of the study. The cell-mate of the escaped pair was continually interrogated until he "cracked," and it is reported that he "admitted full knowledge of the escape and he 'told all' to the authorities." As a

---

* Anderson, T. W. et al. Vitamin C and the common cold: A double blind trial. Originally published in *CMA Journal* 107:503–508, 1972.

result, the three remaining prisoners threatened to kill the "squealer," who for the next two weeks suffered considerable distress. He was apprehensive and tremulous—and not without cause; he looked pale and could barely sleep. After another two weeks, the warden informed the agitated and distraught prisoner that as a reward for his cooperation, he would be pardoned immediately at the conclusion of the experiment. Within minutes, the prisoner quieted down and became relaxed and calm.

During this entire time, the testing involved in the experiment had continued. The interesting results showed that for the two-week stress period, the harried prisoner's utilization of vitamin C increased almost threefold. After the warden's intervention, it returned to the normal baseline.

H. Howland, a Swiss researcher, gave 13 athletes—who exercised on a bicycle ergometer—1,000 mg (1 gram) of vitamin C per day. It was found that the athletes had an increased work capacity in comparison with the work capacity they had when they did not take the vitamin C supplementation.[8] In another Canadian study on incidence of colds, it was found that those in the vitamin C group as compared with those in the control group showed fewer and less severe stress-related symptoms such as headache, fatigue, nausea and fever.[9] Measurements made on soldiers under battlefield combat stress conditions showed that they had drastically reduced vitamin C levels in their blood.[9]

Based on the results of these studies, it would appear that vitamin C is needed in higher doses during stressful periods.

Vitamin C has also been used to overcome the results of a physical stressor—the toxic pollutant lead. In a recent clinical study, 22 workers in a battery plant where there were high levels of lead in the air, were given 2,000 mg (2 grams) of vitamin C and 60 mg of zinc daily.[10] The workers' blood lead levels were measured before and during the study. After 24 weeks, the average blood lead levels had dropped 26%.

The possible role of vitamin C in protecting against heart attacks is discussed later is this chapter under the heading lipids (fats).

An average dose of 500 mg vitamin C daily for the day before and a few days afterward has been used successfully by the author (DM) for dental surgical procedures on his patients. A similar dose is suggested for potentially stressful situations. The preferred form is a time-release capsule, which would tend to prevent one possible complication of high vitamin C intake, crystalluria (kidney stones).*

Very high doses of vitamin C (2 grams or more daily) have been recommended by some authorities.[5] Aside from the possiblity of kidney stones, there is some evidence that excess vitamin C could cause destruction of vitamin B_{12}.[11] The B_{12} deficiency might lead to anemia (insufficient oxygen-carrying capacity of the blood). However, most investigations have shown that excess vitamin C is eliminated by the kidneys, and no permanent damage occurs.[1-4]

Let us now look at the vitamin B complex.

VITAMIN B COMPLEX

There are 10 important members of the vitamin B complex: B_1(thiamine), B_2 (riboflavin), B_3 (niacin), B_6 (pyridoxine), B_{12} (cobalamine), pantothenic acid (pantothenate), folic acid (folacin), choline, biotin and inositol.

Vitamin B_1

Vitamin B_1 is the best-known B vitamin. An absolute deficiency leads to the disease beriberi with manifestations of weakness, lack of energy, fatigue, irritability, paralysis, constipation, headaches, chest pains and heart failure.[1-3] There is some questionable evidence that extra amounts of vitamin B_1 can improve the functioning of the central nervous system. Experiments have shown learning and intelligence to be increased under a vitamin B_1 regimen.[9]

Vitamin B_2

A vitamin B_2 deficiency leads to ariboflavinosis with such manifestations as cracking of the lips at the corners (cheilosis), inflammation of the tongue (glossitis) and vascularization of the cornea ("bloodshot" eyes).[1-3] As is the case with vitamin C, vitamin B_2 is needed in higher doses during the stressors of surgery and injury.

Vitamin B_3

An extreme deficiency of vitamin B_3 results in pellagra, which has the following signs and symptoms: fatigue, headache, backache,

---

* A typical preparation is Cevi-Bid® (Geriatric Pharmaceutical Corp).

sore mouth, diarrhea, dermatitis (skin rash), dementia (severe mental disease) and, finally, death.[1-3] High doses of vitamin B_3 have been used to treat mental stress-related diseases such as schizophrenia.[12]

Vitamin B_6 *

Pyridoxine deficiency causes nerve and muscle pains, tics, tremors, twitches, vomiting, weakness, dermatitis, cheilosis and sluggish antibody production.[1-3,9] Vitamin B_6 has been used to overcome women's depression associated with the taking of birth control pills.[13]

Vitamin B_{12}

Deficiency of vitamin B_{12} leads to pernicious anemia with such manifestations as pallor, inflamed tongue, unsteady walk, mental depression and paralysis.[1-3,9] Vitamin B_{12} has been used for the treatment of simple fatigue (a stress-related symptom) in patients not having pernicious anemia or any other diagnosed disease. A British study showed that there was a statistically significant improvement in mood and feeling in the patients given B_{12} in comparison with those patients receiving a placebo.[14]

Pantothenic Acid

Pantothenate deficiency results in such signs and symptoms as headache, nausea, vomiting, malaise, cramps, stomach-aches and sluggish antibody production.[1-3,9] Pantothenate is converted in the body to coenzyme A (CoA); and one of the functions of CoA is to activate the adrenal corticosteroids.[15] (Chapter 3 covered the role of the corticosteroids in the stress response.)

There have been a few animal studies affirming the role of pantothenic acid in stress.[15,16] In one study, a group of rats were prefed with pantothenate, while a comparison group did not get the vitamin supplementation.[15] The pantothenate-supplemented rats swam an average of 62 minutes in cold water, while the nonsupplemented rats only averaged 16 minutes.

In a second study, Group A mice received a pantothenic acid supplement, and Group B mice did not get the supplement. Otherwise,

* Researchers determined that B_4 and B_5 are not true vitamins; hence, they are no longer listed.

both groups had identical diets. It was found that the Group A mice had an average life span of 653 days, while the Group B mice averaged 550 days.[17]

In a third study, two groups of 50 mice each were exposed to total body X-irradiation. Group A mice were pretreated for one week with pantothenate, while the Group B mice had no pretreatment. The results showed that Group A mice had a 200% longer survival time than group B mice.[18]

There do not seem to be any definitive relationships between stress and the other B vitamins. Let us now consider vitamin E.

VITAMIN E

It is difficult to produce vitamin E (mixed tocopherols) deficiency in humans, but long-term deficiencies can lead to anemia.[1-3] There have been many exaggerated claims describing the use of megadoses of vitamin E. It has been prescribed for heart disease, acne, ulcers, muscular dystrophy, sexual impotence, habitual abortions and menopausal disorders. Vitamin E has also been used to improve muscle functioning and delay aging.[9] Chemically, this vitamin acts as an antioxidant. Lipid peroxides accumulate in aging cells (see Chapter 6), and vitamin E may play a role in the removal of these peroxides.[19]* The Shute brothers—heart specialists—have claimed good results for vitamin E in treating and preventing heart disease,[20] but others dispute their findings.[1-3] For instance, one study showed that high doses of vitamin E could produce coagulopathy (disturbances in blood clotting) in humans.[21]

As far as stress is concerned, there have been a few animal studies involving vitamin E and various stressors. In one study, three groups of rats were fed varying amounts of vitamin E over a period of eight weeks.[15] The rats were then exposed to high concentrations of the atmospheric pollutant ozone. Significantly less lung damage was found in the high vitamin E–supplemented rats as compared to the low vitamin E–supplemented rats. Another similar study showed that vitamin E–supplemented animals lived 50% longer than an E-deficient group.[22]

In a third study, another environmental pollutant, lead, was fed to

* Recent findings have shown that high intake of unsaturated fats (discussed later) can form lipid peroxides which are also implicated as cancer-producing agents and can lead to gallstone formation. Vitamin E may also help in this aspect (Broad, W. J. NIH deals gingerly with diet-disease link. *Science* 204:1175–1178, 1979).

laboratory animals.[22] These subjects were fed large amounts of lead and varying doses of vitamin E. The results showed that those animals given the lowest doses of vitamin E had the highest levels of lead in their tissues. This seemed to show that vitamin E can prevent lead absorption and, therefore, decrease its toxic effects.

In a final study reported, two groups of rats were placed in a maze that contained food in one corner.[22] Group A rats were supplemented with vitamin E (100 mg per day), whereas Group B rats did not receive the supplementation. Both groups of rats were continually blocked in their attempts to get at the food. After eight days of frustration, the rats were sacrificed and examined. It was found that the vitamin E–supplemented rats had significantly fewer gastric ulcers than the nonsupplemented group. This study seems to show that vitamin E has the capability of protecting against a psychological stressor (e.g., frustration) and its deleterious results (e.g., ulcers).

There is experimental evidence supporting the use of wheat germ oil in coping with physical stressors. Wheat germ oil contains high amounts of vitamin E as well as the vitamin B complex. A clinical study by Thomas Cureton, Jr.—a renowned physical educator— showed that athletes who took wheat germ oil supplementation prior to their exercises did significantly better and evidenced less fatigue than a control group who did the same exercises without the supplements.[23]

Let us now look into vitamin A and its role in stress.

VITAMIN A

Vitamin A (retinol) deficiency leads to night blindness. Other signs and symptoms of deficiency in vitamin A intake are rashes, dry skin, corneal ulcers, loss of appetite and dry and brittle hair and nails.[1-3,9] Vitamin A is required for soft tissue repair (epithelialization) and plays a role in stress.[24] In one recent study, it was shown that when mice were given a sarcoma virus along with other physical stressors, they had a greater number of, and more severe tumors than when they were only given the virus.[25] However, when other similar mice were pretreated with vitamin A and then given the combined sarcoma virus and physical stressors, they had a significantly lower incidence and severity of tumors. Hence, at least with mice, vitamin A can be protective against physical stressors, including viruses.

In a clinical study, it was reported that twice-daily administration of vitamin A (50,000–100,000 IU) given to burn patients reduced the incidence of intestinal ulcers. The vitamin A–supplemented patients had less than one-third the ulcer incidence as compared to a similar group of burn patients who were not given vitamin A supplements.[26]

It has also been stated that vitamin A may play an important role in detoxification of toxic substances (i.e., physical stressors) such as pesticides and carbon tetrachloride. However, there are no controlled studies to back up this claim.

The last vitamin to be considered as an antistress vitamin is vitamin D.

VITAMIN D

A deficiency of vitamin D (calciferol) leads to the bone disease rickets (and, in adults, osteomalacia). Vitamin D is needed for bone metabolism, and supplementation might be necessary following surgery in which bone healing is required.[24] For instance, in periodontal and periapical disease, bone has been lost beneath the gingiva and alveolar mucosa (i.e., under the gum tissue and beneath the end of the root). Vitamin D works along with parathyroid hormone and other metabolites to help restore the bone following periodontal and endodontic (root canal) surgery. Although there are no controlled studies to support this, it seems reasonable that vitamin D supplementation just before and for a few days following surgery would be helpful; the recommended dose is about 1,200 IU per day.

Let us now consider the role of minerals in stress.

MINERALS AND STRESS

There are many minerals required by the body, including sodium, chloride, potassium, calcium, phosphorus, magnesium, iron, copper, iodine, selenium, chromium, cobalt, manganese and fluoride.[1-3,9,24] Deficiencies of some of these minerals can affect the stress response.

Sodium and Chloride

Sodium and chloride are needed for water metabolism and to help control homeostasis (i.e., the balance of the internal environment of the body). Too much salt (sodium chloride) is a risk factor for coronary heart disease. Sodium is also needed for nerve transmission.

Potassium

Potassium is required for nerve transmission, and deficiencies can lead to hypoglycemia (low blood sugar), muscular weakness, paralysis and degenerative effects on the heart.

Calcium

Calcium is essential for nerve conduction, muscle contraction, bone and teeth formation and blood clotting; and it is claimed that calcium can act as a tranquilizer. It has been used as a sedative and hypnotic (sleep-inducing) agent. The relaxing effect of a warm glass of milk, which seems to promote sleep, has been attributed to its calcium content.[9] However, milk also contains tryptophan, one of the essential amino acids. Tryptophan is linked to the internal release of serotonin, which appears to have a sleep-inducing effect on the brain.[27]

Phosphorus and Magnesium

Phosphorus is also necessary for nerve conduction, bone and teeth formation and energy reactions. Magnesium is required for nerve conduction, muscle contractions and bone and teeth formation. Magnesium deficiency has been associated with such reactions as "nervousness" and irritability.[28]*

Other Minerals

Zinc is required for the repair of wounds. There is also some evidence that zinc can play a role as a scavenger of lead (antipollutant effect), and act as a protective agent against esophageal (throat) cancer.[29]

---

* Kenneth Cooper recently reported on a newly discovered function of magnesium. That is, the control of heart muscle irritability. Abnormal heart rhythms (arrhythmias) which can lead to fatal heart attacks may be related to low serum magnesium levels. Cooper stated that many Americans have a magnesium deficiency. He recommends a daily dietary intake of 350 mg. Good sources of magnesium are found in seeds and nuts (Cooper, K. H. Levels of Physical Fitness and Selected Coronary Risk Factors. Presented to the Monmouth-Ocean County Dental Society, Neptune, New Jersey, April 18, 1979).

Iron is needed for oxygen transport and muscle functioning (lack causes iron deficiency anemia). Copper lack also leads to anemia.

Iodine is necessary for the formation of the thyroid hormones (e.g., thyroxine), which are important in the stress response (see Chapter 3 for the role of thyroxine in metabolism).

Selenium works along with vitamin E for antioxidation; and manganese is required for normal bone formation, as is fluoride. Fluoride also makes teeth more resistant to decay.

As is the case with vitamin C, during periods of anticipated stress such as surgery, there should be higher doses of the mineral, zinc, the vitamin B complex and vitamins A, D and E.*

Aside from the vitamins and minerals, effective stress management requires an adequate intake of proteins, carbohydrates and lipids (fats), together with water.

PROTEINS, CARBOHYDRATES, LIPIDS AND WATER

Proteins

Proteins are essential for growth and repair of injuries and wounds and replacement of cells.[1-3,9,24] Hence, an adequate intake of proteins is necessary, especially following the stressors of trauma and surgery. Proteins consist of twenty amino acids, including eight that are essential: threonine, leucine, isoleucine, valine, lysine, methionine, phenylalanine and tryptophan. Complete proteins are needed for repair, and include all eight essential amino acids. These are found in meat, milk and milk products, and eggs.

In general, vegetables do not contain all eight amino acids. That is why vegetarians may suffer from malnutrition. Proteins may also be used for energy, once carbohydrates and fats have been depleted. One gram of protein yields four calories of energy. The average American ingests about 85 grams of protein daily.[30]

Carbohydrates

Carbohydrates, which are the main source of energy, comprise about 50% of the average American's caloric intake.[1-3,9,30] The typical American ingests about 280 grams of carbohydrates daily. As is true

---

* Typical preparations are: Albee® with C and Z-Bec® (A. H. Robins); Stresstabs® 600 (Lederle); B-C-Bid (Geriatric Pharmaceutical Corp.); and Alpha-E® (Barth Vitamin Corp.). Vitamins A and D are found in supplemented cod-liver oil and milk.

for protein, one gram of carbohydrate yields four calories of energy. Carbohydrate in the form of glucose (a simple sugar; monosaccharide) is used by the body for energy, and is the only form of energy usable by the brain, nerves and lung tissues.

Refined sugar (sucrose) is a double sugar (disaccharide), which is converted in the body to glucose. However, sucrose is very damaging to teeth. Also, excess sugar has been considered to be a risk factor for coronary heart disease as well as a predisposing factor for diabetes.[31,32] High sugar intake is also thought to cause irritability and distorted thinking. It can lead to hypoglycemia, which causes fatigue, irritability and depression.[9,32,33]

Cheraskin and his associates investigated the social habits (i.e., tobacco, alcohol, coffee/tea consumption, exercise) and the dietary intake (i.e., fats, sugar, protein, vitamins, minerals) of 579 subjects and correlated these factors with the subjects' incidence of sickness and diseases.[34] The factor that had the highest correlation with sickness and disease was high intake of refined carbohydrates (dietary sugar). In another study, these investigators found that the ability of white blood cells to phagocytize (ingest) bacteria is diminished in subjects with high blood sugar levels.[35]

When simple carbohydrates (saccharides) are complexed, they form starches (polysaccharides). Examples of foods rich in polysaccharides are bread, spaghetti and potatoes. Excess carbohydrates (of all types) can be converted within the body to triglycerides (a form of fat), which are implicated in coronary heart disease. Generally, an active person burns carbohydrates readily; hence, this conversion is less likely. There is also some evidence that even when there is an increased triglyceride level from carbohydrate ingestion, it is only temporary and levels off in a couple of weeks.

Under ordinary conditions, it might be advisable to increase the daily intake of carbohydrates (starches rather than sugar) at the expense of fats. Some authorities suggest that carbohydrates should be increased from about 280 grams to approximately 390 grams per day, or from about 50% to about 75% of the total caloric intake.[30] The average American takes in about 2,400 calories per day.*

* A lot of publicity has recently been given to a dramatic new high-carbohydrate, low-sugar, low-fat, low-protein diet. It was developed by Nathan Pritikin, director of the Longevity Research Institute in Santa Barbara, California. Its use purportedly greatly diminishes the occurrence of heart attacks (Pritikin, N. and McGrady, P. M., Jr. *The Pritikin Program for Diet and Exercise.* New York: Grosset & Dunlap, 1979).

There is no doubt that we would all be a lot better off with a lot less sugar. On the other hand, it is advisable to supplement proteins and carbohydrates following stressful procedures such as surgery.*

Lipids

Lipids (fats) are required in the body to absorb and transport the fat-soluble vitamins (A, D, E and K**).[1-3,9] Moreover, fat is needed to form a layer of tissue to cushion and protect the internal organs.[36] Fats are also the most concentrated form of energy; but although one gram of fat yields nine calories of energy, carbohydrates are a more efficient energy source and are used first by the body.

Excess fat is stored in the body and is detrimental to health. The average American takes in about 105 grams of fat daily, most of which is animal fat. Usual fat intake is about 40% of the total calories. Animal fats are saturated (e.g., cholesterol) and have been implicated as one of the risk factors in coronary heart disease. The average American ingests about 800 mg of cholesterol per day. One egg yolk alone contains around 240 mg. Saturated fats come primarily from beef, pork, lamb, bacon, ham, milk and milk products and eggs. Lean meats, veal, turkey, chicken and white (meat) fish contain less saturated fat. Vegetables usually do not contain saturated fats. Notable exceptions are coconut oil, palm oil and cocoa butter.

Unsaturated fats are found in vegetables, nuts and grains. Linoleic acid, which is unsaturated, is now considered to be the only essential fatty acid. It tends to lower serum cholesterol, but evidence for this use in preventing heart attacks is inconclusive. Although fats are needed, we should all cut down on their consumption and try to limit the amount of fat, especially of the high-cholesterol type. Some experts estimate that the maximum total daily intake of fat should be about 55 grams or about 20% of the daily calories.[30] This should be primarily of the unsaturated vegetable type. The maximum suggested daily intake of cholesterol is 100 mg (keeping in mind that one egg yolk contains about 240 mg).

However, it should be recognized that dietary cholesterol is not the only source of high blood cholesterol—it can be formed in the body without an outside source. Recent findings have shown that the

* Typical vitamin-mineral food supplements are: Nutrament®, Instant Nutrament®, Meritene® and Carnation Instant Breakfast®.
** Vitamin K is important in blood coagulation.

type of cholesterol may be significant. Cholesterol found in the blood as low-density (beta) lipoproteins is believed to be more damaging than cholesterol found as high-density (alpha) lipoproteins.[36,37] The type of cholesterol found in the blood is related to genetics, diet and amount of exercise. Most low-density lipoproteins are believed to be diet-derived. (The role of exercise and types of lipoproteins are discussed in the next chapter.)

There is some evidence that lecithin can decrease the blood levels of low-density lipoproteins and raise the blood levels of high-density lipoproteins, and thus possibly have a protective effect against coronary heart disease.[38] Lecithin, a phospholipid, contains choline and inositol (considered to be B vitamins), phosphorus and unsaturated fats (primarily linoleic acid). A good source is soybeans. It has also been reported that vitamin C can raise the blood levels of the protective high-density lipoproteins.[39]

Water

Another essential of stress management is water. All cells and tissues require it for metabolism, and extra salt and water are needed when one is faced with the stressors of high heat and humidity. With respect to water, warm noncaffeinated beverages such as Postum® (made from cereal grains), herbal teas and soup (e.g., Heinz®, Campbell's® or Momma's chicken) are soothing and relaxing for many people.[40] Some prefer decaffeinated coffee (e.g. Sanka®).

Apart from satisfying its nutritional needs with vitamins, minerals, proteins, carbohydrates, lipids and water, the body requires nonnutritional roughage (i.e., fiber), which also has a role to play in stress management.*

FIBER AND STRESS

Indigestible carbohydrate is called roughage or fiber. It adds bulk to the diet and helps in moving food along the intestinal tract.[1-3] Foods rich in roughage include bran, leafy vegetables, rice and fruits.

---

* Recently, a new term has been coined that encompasses much of what we have discussed regarding nutrients and stress management. The term *orthomolecular medicine*, was created by Linus Pauling. It is defined as the maintenance of good health and treatment of disease by providing the body with optimum levels of vitamins, minerals, trace elements, amino acids, hormones and other nutrients (Williams, R. J. and Kalita, D. K. *A Physician's Handbook on Orthomolecular Medicine*. Defiance, Ohio: Huxley Institute for Biomedical Research, 1979).

Fiber appears to play a role as a protective agent against intestinal disease such as appendicitis, diverticulitis (an inflammatory disease of the large intestine), gastrointestinal tract cancer and peptic ulcer. As we previously pointed out, stress and peptic ulcers are strongly related.

There is an interesting story with respect to fiber and ulcers. During World War II, American prisoners of war in Japanese prison camps were given a large supplement of rice polishings, which had a high fiber content (derived from the rice kernel).[41] In three prison camps, containing 13,000 prisoners, only one case of ulcers was reported in the year investigated. After that year, the prisoners were moved out of Japan, and the rice-polishings supplement was discontinued. As a result, ulcers became rampant. Conversely, American prisoners who were kept in Hong Kong did not receive rice polishings, and they had a high incidence of ulcers. When those prisoners were subsequently transferred to Japan, they were given unmilled grains and bran supplements. The rate of new ulcers then rapidly decreased.

A summary of possible relationships of nutrients and stress is given in Table 10.1.

TABLE 10.1   Nutrients and Stress

NUTRIENTS	POSSIBLE STRESS-RELATED ROLE
Vitamins	
C (ascorbic acid)	To prevent and treat colds; lead detoxification; increased work capacity; reduces stress symptoms; post-surgical repair; increases high-density lipoproteins.
B₁ (thiamine)	Improved functioning of central nervous system.
B₂ (riboflavin)	Postsurgical repair.
B₃ (niacin)	To treat schizophrenia.
B₆ (pyridoxine)	To treat depression of women taking birth control pills.
B₁₂ (cobalamine)	To treat fatigue.
Pantothenic acid (pantothenate)	Activates corticosteroids.
E (mixed tocopherols)	Acts as an antioxidant.
A (retinol)	Soft tissue repair.
D (calciferol)	Bone repair.
Minerals	

Sodium	Nerve transmission; water metabolism; homeostasis.
Chloride	Water metabolism; homeostasis.
Potassium	Nerve transmission.
Calcium	Nerve conduction; muscle contraction; blood clotting; bone formation; use as a sedative.
Phosphorus	Nerve conduction; bone formation; energy reactions.
Magnesium	Nerve conduction; bone formation; muscle contraction; heart rhythm.
Zinc	Repair of wounds; lead detoxification; possibly prevents throat cancer.
Iron	Oxygen transport; muscle functioning.
Copper	Oxygen transport.
Iodine	Thyroxine formation.
Manganese	Bone formation.
Fluoride	Bone formation.
Selenium	Antioxidation, along with vitamin E.
Foods	
Proteins	Repair of injuries and wounds.
Carbohydrates	Energy.
Fats (lipids)	Energy; absorb and transport fat-soluble vitamins; cushion internal organs.
Lecithin	Decreases low-density lipoproteins; increases high-density lipoproteins.
Water	Supports metabolism of all tissues.
Roughage	
Fiber (not a nutrient)	Aids in moving food along in the intestines; prevents ulcers and possibly cancer.

SUMMARY

Thomas Jefferson was correct—our big problem is not eating too little, but rather eating too much and not wisely. There are real dangers associated with obesity, but one can also undereat and eat incorrectly. It is considered important for stress and health management to have a balanced diet, including adequate protein (on the average about 85 grams a day), carbohydrate (between 300 and 400 grams a day, depending upon how active a person is), fat (55 grams a day or less), fiber (about 5 grams daily) and vitamin and mineral supplements during periods of anticipated stress—which may be every day for most Americans.

The best sources of protein are poultry and fish. Fruits, vegetables, flour and cereal products are the preferred sources for carbohydrates. Fats should be reduced in the diet as much as possible, and fish and vegetable sources are preferred (e.g., the white fishes such as white fish and flounder, and cottonseed, soy and sunflower oils).*

An excellent way to burn off excess carbohydrates and fats is by exercising, which is also an effective means of coping with stress. The subject of exercise is considered in the next chapter.

REFERENCES

1. Mitchell, H. S., Rynbergen, H. J., Anderson L. and Dibble, M. V. *Nutrition in Health and Disease,* Sixteenth Ed., Philadelphia: J. B. Lippincott, 1976.
2. Robinson, C. H. and Lawler, M. R. *Normal and Therapeutic Nutrition,* Fifteenth Ed. New York: Macmillan, 1977.
3. Williams, S. R. *Nutrition and Diet Therapy,* Third Ed. St. Louis: C. V. Mosby Co., 1977.
4. Riccitelli, M. L. Vitamin C: A review and reassessment of pharmacological and therapeutic uses. *Conn. Med.* 39:609–614, 1975.
5. Pauling, L. *Vitamin C, The Common Cold and the Flu.* San Francisco: W. H. Freeman and Co., 1976.
6. Anderson, T. W., Reid, D. B. and Beaton, G. H.: Vitamin C and the common cold: A double blind trial. *Can. Med. Assoc. J.* 107:503–508, 1972.
7. Hodges, R. E. The effect of stress on ascorbic acid metabolism in man. *Nutr. Today* 5(1):11–12, 1970.
8. Sheehan, G. Medical advice: Update on vitamin C. *Runner's World* 10(5):38, 1975.
9. Rosenberg, H. and Feldzamen, A. N. *The Doctor's Book of Vitamin Therapy: Megavitamins for Health.* New York: G. P. Putnam's Sons, 1974.
10. Editorial. Nutrients that team up against pollution. *Prevention* 30(8):123–131, 1978.
11. Herbert, V. and Jacob, E. Destruction of vitamin B_{12} by ascorbic acid. *J.A.M.A.* 230:241–242, 1974.
12. Ross, H. M. Vitamin pills for schizophrenics. *Psychol. Today* 7(4):83–88, 1974.
13. Feltman, J. The B vitamin that's something special. *Prevention* 30(8):74–79, 1978.
14. Elis, F. R. and Nasser, S. A pilot study of vitamin B_{12} in the treatment of tiredness. *Brit. J. Nutr.* 30:277–283, 1973.

* The authors are not nutritionists; these recommendations are based on personal experiences, discussions with nutritionists and physicians and review of the literature. It is important that anyone with a particular medical problem see his physician before contemplating any change in his diet. Also, people on special diets or who are engaged in strenuous occupations may have radically different nutritional requirements.

15. Feltman, J. A nutritional shield against the arrows of stress. *Prevention* 28(9):88–93, 1976.
16. Editorial. Pantothenate—The "anti-stress" vitamin. *Prevention* 29(11):127–132, 1977.
17. Williams, R. *Nutrition Against Disease: Environmental Prevention.* New York: Pitman, 1971.
18. Szorady, I. Pantothenic Acid: Experimental results and clinical observations. *Acta Paediatr. Acad. Sci. Hung.* 4:73–85, 1963.
19. Marx, J. L. Aging research (I): Cellular theories of senescence. *Science* 186:1105–1107, 1974.
20. Shute, W. E. and Taub, H. J. *Vitamin E for Ailing and Healthy Hearts.* New York: Pyramid House, 1970.
21. Corrizi, J. J., Jr. and Marcus, F. I. Coagulopathy associated with vitamin E ingestion. *J.A.M.A.* 230:1300–1301, 1974.
22. Editorial. Nutrients that team up against pollution. *Prevention* 30(8):123–131, 1978.
23. Cureton, T. K., Jr. *Physical Fitness and Dynamic Health,* Second Ed. New York: Dial Press, 1973.
24. Morse, D. R. *Clinical Endodontology: A Comprehensive Guide to Diagnosis, Treatment and Prevention.* Springfield, Ill.: Charles C. Thomas Publ., 1974.
25. Seifter, E. Of stress, vitamin A, and tumors. *Science* 193:74–75, 1976.
26. Chernov, M. S., Hale, H. W., Jr. and Wood, M. Prevention of stress ulcers. *Am. J. Surg.* 122:674–677, 1971.
27. Wiley, D. B. Sleep: Too much or too little, it's a problem. *Philadelphia Eve. Bull.* A:37, 42, Aug. 17, 1978.
28. Kinderlehrer, J. Improve your moods with better diet. *Prevention* 25(2):79–87, 1973.
29. Rodale, R. The healthful touch of zinc. *Prevention* 30(6):25–30, 1978.
30. Connor, W. E. and Connor, S. L. The key role of nutritional factors in the prevention of coronary heart disease. *Prev. Med.* 1:49–83, 1972.
31. Morse, D. R. Sucrose: A common enemy. *J. Am. Soc. Prev. Dent.* 2(5):27–28, 1972.
32. Cheraskin, E., Ringsdorf, W. M. and Clark, J. W. *Diet and Disease.* Emmaus, Pa.: Rodale books, 1968.
33. McCamy, J. C. and Presley, J. *Human Life Styling: Keeping Whole in the 20th Century.* New York: Harper & Row, 1975.
34. Cheraskin, E., Ringsdorf, W. M., Michael, D. W., Hicks, B. S. and Wright, W., Jr. The pluses and minuses of the syndrome of sickness. *J. Am. Soc. Prev. Dent.* 1(12):26–48, 1971.
35. Ringsdorf, W. M., Jr., Cheraskin, E. and Ramsay, R. R., Jr. Sucrose, neutrophilic phagocytosis and resistance to disease. *Dent. Surv.* 52(12):46–48, 1976.
36. Howard, R. B. and Herbold, N. H., *Nutrition in Clinical Care.* New York: McGraw-Hill Book Co., 1978.
37. Schaeffer, E. J., Anderson, D. W., Brewer, H. B.,Jr., Levy, R. I., Danner, R. M. and Blackwelder, W. C. Plasma-triglycerides in regulation of H.D.L.-cholesterol levels. *Lancet* 2:391–393, 1978.

38. Feltman, J. Lecithin cleans up cholesterol's dirty work. *Prevention* 30(6):52–57, 1978.
39. Editorial. Vitamin C, HDL and a healthier heart. *Prevention* 30(2):86–90, 1978.
40. Wheeler, A. C. Try a tisane for tranquility. *Prevention* 24(6):142–146, 1972.
41. Siegel, S. *Dr. Siegel's Natural Fiber Permanent Weight-Loss Diet.* New York: Dial Press, 1975.

11

Physical Methods: Exercise, Massage, Heat and Cold

It is better to wear out than to rust out.*

INTERVIEWS

Q. Why do you work out? A. To get big muscles.
Q. And what good are big muscles? A. It impresses the girls.
Q. Is that all? A. I like to look at myself in the mirror.
Q. And what else? A. I'm not afraid of anybody. I'm strong you know!
INTERVIEWER: Thank you.

Q. Why do you work out? A. I feel so good afterward.
Q. Any other reasons? A. I love the feel of my tensed muscles. And I impress people with my strength.
Q. Anything else? A. I'm proud of my body and lots of my friends are jealous of how I look and what I can do.

* Richard Cumberland in Boswell's *Tour to the Hebrides*.

INTERVIEWER: Thank you.

Q. Why do you work out? A. Because it's healthy. I can also eat what I want to without getting fat.

Q. What makes exercise healthy? A. I don't get headaches, I rest and sleep well, and things don't "bug" me.

INTERVIEWER: Thank you.

Q. Why do you run? A. I run for my life.

Q. What do you mean? A. Running opens up my blood vessels so that I won't get a heart attack.

Q. Are you sure? A. I read it in a magazine.

INTERVIEWER: Thank you.

Q. Why are you jogging? A. It gets rid of my stress.

Q. Always? A. Almost always. Whenever I feel down in the dumps, I feel good after a run. And it's better than screaming at the wife.

INTERVIEWER: Thank you.

Q. Why do you run? A. I run because it puts me on another plane, my head gets lost in the clouds, and my worries melt away.

Q. Do you enjoy running. A. Not always, but it feels great afterwards.

INTERVIEWER: Thank you.

These interviews are fictitious, but they incorporate statements frequently made by people who exercise regularly. Exercise as a means of stress release was a common theme in all the discussions. Many people believe that exercise improves their chances of avoiding a heart attack and also makes them better able to face the rigors of life.

In the remainder of this chapter we consider the roles of exercise in great detail, along with the other physical methods of massage, heat and cold.

EXERCISE

Major Benefits

Exercise has a dual role in stress. It is, in itself, a physical stressor; and by the proper use of exercise one is able to cope with physical stressors. Exercise is the contemporary transformation of the beneficial fight-or-flight response. Not only is there advantageous release as a result of the muscular work in exercise, but strengthening of the body's muscles, tendons and bones results in an increased capacity to deal with stressors.

The evidence is growing that regular, strenuous exercise is of major importance in decreasing the incidence of stress-related diseases and in prolonging life. However, for the person who is out of shape, sudden, severe exertion can result in a life-threatening stress response.

Longevity. In Nedra Belloc's study that was considered in Chapters 5 and 6, it was shown that exercise is one of the most important factors in longevity.[1] Belloc found that men who participated regularly in active sports such as swimming and jogging had the lowest mortality of all the subjects. The rate was even lower than that of individuals who never smoked but did not exercise. It was found that people who rarely exercised had twice the mortality rate of the active exercisers, regardless of age. Women who exercised regularly also had a much lower mortality rate than those who never exercised.

Heart Attacks. Ralph Paffenberger reported on an important study at the annual meeting of the American Heart Association (1977).[2-4] In the early 1960s, Paffenberger sent a questionnaire to approximately 36,000 Harvard alumni. It included questions about types of sports and exercises engaged in, frequency of participation and incidence of other severe activities (e.g., climbing stairs). About half of those surveyed responded. In 1972, the respondents or their survivors were sent a second questionnaire. Results showed that 572 alumni had had heart attacks, including 257 fatal attacks. Concerning exercise, it was found that those who exercised casually (i.e., burning less than 2,000 calories per week) had a 64% greater risk of coronary artery disease than those who exercised regularly and vigorously.*

Paffenberger found that the strenuousness of the exercise was a much more important factor than other risk factors such as obesity,

---

* Some examples of caloric expenditure are as follows: A 154-lb man walking on a level road at 2.5 mph burns about 144 calories per hour;[5] a man over 200 lb in weight burns about 150-160 calories per mile; and while an average man burns about 100 calories per mile, an average woman consumes about 80-90 calories per mile.[6]

hypertension, smoking or family history of heart disease. Exercises that he found to be especially effective were running, swimming, handball, squash and basketball—if played for an hour or more each day. Tennis was found to be effective if the individuals played a good, stiff, competitive game of singles. (Both the authors play primarily baseline rallying types of tennis, which are beneficial in terms of cardiovascular fitness but can be awfully boring for spectators to watch.)

At the heart association meeting, Paffenberger also reported on another study: a 22-year analysis of longshoremen.[2] Results showed that longshoremen who engaged in heavy strenuous work had only half the number of fatal heart attacks that longshoremen who engaged only in light activities suffered.

The best documented study on risk factors in heart disease was the one conducted in Framingham, Massachusetts.[7] As part of this study, it was found that sedentary people had over twice as high a death rate from heart attacks as active individuals had.

In a study in Great Britain, physicians examined the diet, exercise patterns and heart disease rate of 337 working men who had jobs such as bank clerk and bus driver.[3] They found that those who consumed the greatest number of calories and exercised the most were least likely to suffer heart attacks. Another study showed that London bus drivers (i.e., who were relatively inactive) had twice as many heart attacks and much higher blood-lipid levels as compared to bus conductors who regularly moved around in the (double-decker) buses.[8]

Other study results are: (1) Sedentary Kibbutz workers in Israel had 2 to 4½ times the number of fatal heart attacks suffered by active workers; (2) sedentary office railroad workers (i.e., clerks) in the United States had a heart attack rate almost twice that of men working the yards; (3) postal clerks had a heart attack risk 1.4 to 1.9 times that of letter carriers; (4) North Dakota farmers who were vigorously active for one hour or more each day had a coronary heart disease incidence less than one-fifth that of those who were active for less than one hour each day; (5) postmortem examinations in Great Britain of 3,800 apparently noncoronary deaths showed that those who had active lifetime occupations had fewer coronary occlusions than were found in the hearts of the sedentary workers;[5] (6) Masai warriors exercise regularly and are considered to be free of coronary artery disease, but it was found that even in cases where atherosclerosis was present, exercise apparently produced an enlargement of the coronary arteries so that nutrient and gaseous exchange increased;[9] and (7) in seven different countries, individuals who engaged in occupations that required strenuous physical work had the lowest incidence of coronary heart disease among all the occupations studied.[9]

In all of these studies, there may have been other factors besides exercise—e.g., diet, occupation—that could have influenced the results. Nevertheless, the evidence is fairly strong that exercise may help prevent cardiovascular disease. On the other hand, there is flimsy evidence for the prevention of other diseases through exercise.

Cancer.   Two recent animal studies show that exercise may help in the prevention of cancer.[10] In the first study, there were three groups of mice that were prone to develop liver cancer. Mice in Group A had free access to an exercise wheel in each cage. Group B mice had no access to an exercise wheel. Members of Group C had access to an exercise wheel, but the mice were kept in colonies of five so that each of the mice had to take turns. After sacrifice, it was found that the mice of Group B—no use of exercise wheel—had a 60% incidence of cancerous livers. The mice in Group C—moderate exercise—had a 35% incidence of cancerous livers. Finally, the mice in Group A—high exercise—had the lowest incidence of cancerous livers (23.5%).

In a second study by the same investigators, the cancer-inducing chemical, benzidine, was given to two groups of mice. The mice in Group A were active exercisers, while those in Group B were low exercisers. The mice of Group A had a 63% incidence of cancer, while those in Group B had a 93% cancer incidence.

Advantages of Exercise.   Exercise enables a person to cope with stress and prevent stress-related diseases.[4-6,10-12] A listing of the physiological and subjective benefits of exercise includes the following:

1. Decreased heart (pulse) rate with vigorous exercise done over a period of several months or more.

2. Reduced blood pressure with prolonged and vigorous exercise.

3. Increased cardiac stroke volume (blood output per heartbeat).

4. Increased oxygen intake and improved breathing efficiency.

5. Decreased serum cholesterol (primarily the low-density lipoproteins) and triglycerides.[5] One study at Kent State University showed that there was a 25% reduction in blood cholesterol levels over a period of months from following a regular exercise program.

6. Increased high-density lipoproteins (HDLs)—believed to be protective against coronary artery disease. Peter Wood and his co-workers at Stanford University compared middle-aged male runners with their nonrunning peers.[4] They found that the runners had a 50% higher level of HDLs than their more sedentary contemporaries had. Two hundred twenty Norwegian male skiers had their HDLs measured against a comparable group of nonskiers. The skiers' HDL levels were significantly higher.[13]

7. More effective utilization of carbohydrates.

8. Less adrenaline and noradrenaline released by the body in response to psychological stressors (as compared to someone who is not physically fit).

9. Lowered likelihood of clot formation inside blood vessels.

10. Possibly increased formation of collateral blood vessels in the heart (emergency short circuits in case of blockage of main coronary arteries).[5,12]

11. Increased flexibility of blood vessels so that they have a decreased tendency to get atherosclerotic patches.[12]

12. Possibly increased diameter of existing coronary arteries.[5,12]

13. Improved muscular strength: skeletal; smooth (internal); and cardiac (heart) muscles. Animal experiments have shown that when excess sodium and corticosteroids are given prior to physical stressors, such as fractures, the result is cardiac muscle necrosis. However, when regular exercise precedes the stress situation, there is a tendency to protect the heart against muscle death and damage.[14]

14. Increased muscle flexibility and tone.

15. Improved physical endurance (stamina).

16. Increased gaseous and nutrient exchange at the tissue level.[15,16]

17. Improved digestion.

18. Better overall physical appearance as a result of either weight loss or gain.

19. Decreased appetite, which helps in loss of excess weight.

20. Improved complexion, probably as a result of better circulation.

21. Better posture.

22. A better attitude and frame of mind.
23. Feelings of euphoria, tranquility and relaxation.
24. Subsequent muscle relaxation.[17]

Cardiovascular Fitness Programs

Exercises geared to prevent heart disease tend to promote cardiovascular fitness. Two well-known programs that follow this principle are: (1) Kenneth Cooper's program, *Aerobics*[12] (also followed by the Royal Canadian Air Force program); and (2) the West Point fitness conditioning program.[18] The premise behind these programs is that the heart and lungs must be effectively stimulated.

According to Cooper, the exercise should be of sufficient intensity to raise the heart rate to an average minimum of 150 beats per minute. This value varies with age, sex and condition. The beneficial results generally begin within five minutes of the start of the exercise. Cooper states that a sufficient aerobic training effect will occur if the individual attains an average heart rate of 150 beats per minute, maintains it for ten minutes and does this four times per week (e.g., by stationary bike riding).

If the heart rate doesn't go up to the average minimum, but is still demanding of oxygen, the exercise should be continued for considerably longer periods. The actual time depends upon the amount of oxygen used. As this cannot be determined without elaborate testing, most physical educators use the pulse rate as an indication of the severity of the exercises. Again, Cooper states that with a maximum heart rate of 130 beats per minute, the exercise should be continued for 30 minutes, and done four times weekly (e.g., stationary bike riding).

Some running experts consider that the minimal time that Cooper advocates for strenuous exercise is too little to get maximum cardiovascular benefits from exercise.[19] However, Cooper has done extensive investigations and so far has not found any difference in heart attack risk if the minimum 30 points is followed per week (discussed shortly) or if it is increased to 50, 75, 100 or more points (as could be obtained from slow, long distance running). Running experts also contend that the mental effects (e.g., feelings of euphoria and dissipation of depression) do not occur unless one runs for at least 30 minutes and often not unless one runs at least an hour.[19-23] Since mental benefits cannot be substantiated as readily as physiological benefits, this controversy cannot be easily resolved.

Still, attesting to the mental role of running, several psychologists and psychiatrists are now using running as a form of psychotherapy, and they report encouraging results in the treatment of anxiety and depression.[23] Basing the results partly on the low heart attack rate of marathoners, the American Medical Joggers Association (members are physicians who also run) and other running experts state that running six miles a day four times weekly is protective against getting a heart attack.[19-22]

According to the West Point Program, the exercise should raise the heart rate to approximately 70% of the maximum rate for the particular age.[18] For example, 134-142 for ages 18-29, and 99-105 for ages 70-79. The individual's condition determines the length of the exercise period. If the heart rate is kept between 60 and 70% of maximum for the age group, then the exercise can be continued at that pace until the person feels winded (generally between five and twelve minutes).

Regardless of the length of the exercise period, it is essential that a gradual warm-up period of calisthenics precede any vigorous exercise. There should also be a gradual tapering off period. Good strenuous exercises are: running, jogging,* swimming, rowing, cross country skiing, stationary bike riding, and rope jumping. Participant activities and sports that include sustained periods of strenuous exercise are: basketball, volleyball, handball, squash, racquetball, soccer, hockey, lacrosse, vigorous singles tennis, and dancing.

Cooper has assigned aerobic ratings to various activities. For men, he suggests working up to a minimum of 30 points per week with his system. For women, the value is 25 points per week. For a 45-year-old man, some examples of activities that yield approximately 30 points are: (1) swimming 800 yards within 16½ minutes, four times weekly; (2) running two miles within 21 minutes, four times weekly; (3) running in place for 15 minutes at 80-90 steps per minute, four times weekly; (4) cycling six miles within 23½ minutes, five times weekly; (5) walking three miles within 43 minutes and 15 seconds,

---

* There is continual controversy over the difference between running and jogging. Some say that if you do a mile in less than eight minutes, then it is running; if more, then it's jogging. Others say that a runner keeps track of time while a jogger doesn't give a darn. It appears to be simply a question of semantics; both are variations on the same theme.

four times weekly; and (6) playing handball, racquetball, squash, soccer, hockey or lacrosse for 45 consecutive minutes, four times weekly.

It is important that all adults over age 35 have a thorough medical examination before beginning any vigorous exercise program. Most physicians suggest that this examination include a cardiovascular stress test.

The Stress Test

The condition of the heart, blood vessels and the respiratory system can be evaluated by the use of the cardiovascular stress test. People generally first see their family physician or internist who gives them a preliminary medical examination (usually including blood tests, blood pressure and chest X-ray). They are then referred to a testing center where a cardiologist re-examines them before beginning the stress test.* The tests used include a resting electrocardiogram (EKG), heart rate and blood pressure.

People who take the stress test generally fall into the following categories: (1) patients suspected of having heart disease; (2) people over 35 years of age who want a determination of their cardiovascular condition before undertaking a vigorous exercise program; and (3) individuals who are just interested in having their physical fitness tested.

In the more elaborate setups, four measures of fitness are taken: (1) EKG; (2) heart rate; (3) blood pressure; and (4) energy expenditure—oxygen (O_2) consumption and carbon dioxide (CO_2) elimination (only the more sophisticated setups make this determination).

The patient is "hooked up" and he walks on a treadmill (which usually runs between 2 and 3.3 miles per hour) or pedals a stationary exercise bicycle (bicycle ergometer). The treadmill is generally considered to be superior to the ergometer for these reasons: (1) people may not be able to pedal to full capacity; (2) many people are not used to riding a bike and their legs may give in before they attain sufficient aerobic stimulation; (3) the treadmill is not difficult to walk on; and (4) the resistance on the treadmill is easily and gradually increased by raising the incline.

* A list of Stress Testing Centers is given in Jan./Feb. 1978 issue of *Jogger* and is reprinted in, *The Aerobics Way* by K. H. Cooper (New York: M. Evans and Co., 1978).

While the individual is exercising, his responses are fed into recording and viewing devices. (See Fig. 11.1 for an illustration of a

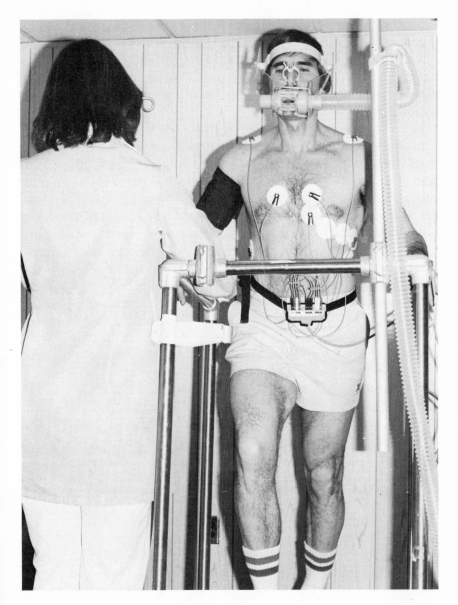

Fig. 11.1 The treadmill stress test. The author (DM) is seen undergoing a stress test, which includes measurements of blood pressure, EKG, heart rate and energy expenditure. (From Morse, D. R. and Furst, M. L., *Stress and Relaxation: Application to Dentistry,* 1978. Courtesy of Charles C Thomas, Publisher, Springfield, Illinois.)

subject undertaking the stress test.) The cardiologist pays attention to both the patient and the instruments. As the test continues, the treadmill is gradually inclined to increase the resistance and challenge the individual. With the bicycle, the resistance is increased so that the pedaling becomes more strenuous.

The stress test is continued until the individual achieves a target heart rate of 75-90% of his predicted maximum. (In some testing centers the target rate is considered to be 70-85%.) Cooper's results indicate that some abnormalities will be missed if one doesn't get close to the maximum heart rate.[12] The predicted maximum is based on values found on a chart keyed to age and sex. An easy way to determine your predicted maximum heart rate is to take 220 and subtract your age (in years). For example, the predicted maximum heart rate at age 45 for males is 175. However, this is only an average value, since it is possible, for instance, for a 50-year-old male to have a maxiumum heart rate of 195. Conversely, a 30-year-old male could have a maximum of only 168. The average maximum attainable heart rates and target zones for various individuals based on the 75-90% range are shown in Fig. 11.2.

Depending on the individual's condition and an evaluation by the

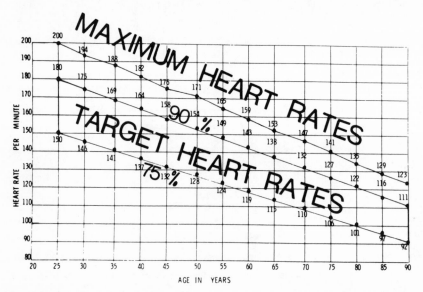

Fig. 11.2 Maximum heart rates and target heart rates. This figure shows that with increasing age, the highest heart rate attainable during all-out effort falls. See text for further discussion. (Adapted from Zohman, L. R.: Beyond diet . . . exercise your way to fitness and heart health. *CPC International, Inc.,* 1974.)

cardiologist, the test is either continued or terminated. Some circumstances that may signal the cardiologist to end the test are: (1) the heart rate exceeds 90% of maximum; (2) the O_2 retention of the lungs falls to 3% or less (about 5% is considered normal); (3) the individual shows signs of cyanosis (extreme pallor), which is associated with falling O_2 levels; (4) the blood pressure increases too much (a gradual increase is considered normal); (5) EKG abnormalities are detected (some apparent abnormalities occur in well-conditioned runners, but cardiologists are generally aware of this);[24-26] (6) the individual's legs become fatigued (e.g., he may begin to stagger); and (7) the individual gives up (usually the result of shortness of breath, dizziness, chest pain or fear of getting a heart attack).

The monitoring is continued as the test is gradually ended; and it is expected that the blood pressure and pulse rate should return nearly to normal within five minutes. The stress test results are used to determine the possible presence of heart disease, and the test is generally a good diagnostic tool for this purpose, although some diseased individuals may "pass" the test, and some healthy people occasionally may show abnormalities. The test results are also used to show the level of cardiovascular fitness, which can then be the basis of tailoring a specific exercise training program.

For best results, the test should be given in two sessions. At the first session, the individual fills out forms, answers diagnostic questions and gets acquainted with the sophisticated equipment. The combination of the treadmill (or bicycle ergometer), the blood pressure cuff, the EKG wire leads and the respiratory mask can induce anxiety and raise resting values; the preliminary visit helps overcome apprehension and helps control for psychological artifacts. Including the two visits, the complete testing usually takes about two hours. The cost varies; in the Greater Philadelphia area, it is approximately $200. Comprehensive medical plans often cover much of the fee.*

Other Benefits

In addition to the cardiovascular value of strenuous exercise, moderate activity offers other benefits, such as the following:

* Some of this information was supplied by: Ted Quedenfeld, Administrative Director of Sports Medicine Center, Temple University Hospital; Albert Paolone, Director Adult Fitness Program, Temple University; and Joan Carter and the staff of the Anthropometrics Heart Clinic, 56 Haddon Avenue, Haddonfield, New Jersey.

1. Prevention and treatment of minor back, shoulder and neck problems.[15,27-29] Exercise can relieve the partial contraction and muscle "knots" that develop from chronic psychological stressors (e.g., anxiety, anger, frustration). People in occupations in which they bend too much should do exercises to maintain good posture and counteract the tendency to bend.

2. Providing opportunities for good companionship. For instance, some sports—golf, bowling, doubles tennis and fishing—are not particularly effective for cardiovascular fitness, but permit the players to interact in pleasant and relaxing ways. On the other hand, there may be some factors that offset the benefits; e.g., waiting for hours to tee off at municipal golf courses and the libations at the "nineteenth hole."

3. Prevention of cramps, pooling of blood and varicosities that may result from sitting or standing for long periods of time.

4. Increased strength of muscles, tendons and bone that comes from doing strength-building exercises such as weightlifting. Thus, greater ability to cope with physical stressors is possible, which helps in the "fight" phase of the stress response.

5. Increased strength of muscles, tendons and bone that decreases the body's vulnerability to injury.

6. Improved fast reflex activities that comes from becoming adept at sports such as Ping Pong® , judo and karate. Thus, one can escape physical stressors, a help in the "flight" phase of the stress response.

7. Better support for internal organs which comes from strengthening abdominal muscles. Weak abdominal muscles are also a cause of back problems.

8. Increased energy and reduced fatigue. This permits an individual to accomplish his daily mental and physical work and still feel refreshed at the day's end.

9. Helping people get to sleep and sleep better. In the morning, simple stretching helps in the awakening process.

10. Improved thinking, since there is increased cerebral (brain) circulation as a result of exercise. The increased circulation to all parts of the body permits generally improved functioning. (The relatively new running psychotherapy has already been mentioned.)

11. Provision of a basis for acquiring a skill in a particular activity or sport. Besides ego-enhancing benefits, the person may become part of the circle of people who identify with a given activity.

TABLE 11.1   The Benefits of Exercise

1. Provides stress relief.
2. Helps prevent coronary artery disease and possibly other diseases.
3. Delays the aging process.
4. Improves breathing efficiency.
5. Stengthens muscles, tendons, and bones (i.e., preparation for the "fight" stress response).
6. Increases muscle flexibility, tone and reflexes (i.e., preparation for the "flight" stress response).
7. Increases stamina.
8. Improves digestion.
9. Increases energy and reduces fatigue.
10. Enhances physical appearance including complexion and posture.
11. Decreases appetite.
12. Results in better mental attitudes and frame of mind.
13. Results in improved thinking.
14. Promotes feelings of euphoria, tranquility and relaxation.
15. Promotes muscular relaxation.
16. Provides a method to prevent and treat minor back problems.
17. Allows for good companionship.
18. Prevents varicosities.
19. Results in better support for internal organs.
20. Allows for easier and better sleeping.
21. Provides a self-enhancing skill in a particular activity or sport.
22. Builds self-esteem and reinforces self-image.

12. Building of self-esteem and reinforcement of self-image that may be a beneficial consequence of body-building exercises (e.g., weightlifting, isometrics).

A summary of the benefits of exercise is given in Table 11.1.

Summary

It almost seems as if exercise is "good for everything that ails you." But this is really not the case. As we have been emphasizing throughout this book, people vary, and "one man's food is another man's poison." Although the statistics with respect to exercise seem to show that heart disease and possibly other diseases may be prevented, and aging may be delayed, there are numerous examples of people who rarely exercised and still lived a long, healthy life. Undoubtedly, heredity was the major factor for them.

It is also true that some people detest certain exercises and activities such as calisthenics, weight training and running. At this time it is not clearly known what it would take to get people to engage in the various exercises and activities. Some suggestions to motivate them are:

1. Avoid the unpalatable exercises and substitute others of a comparable nature that are found to be pleasurable.
2. Try to exercise or run in the company of others.
3. Participate in group exercise classes.
4. Experiment with different times of day and various locations (especially true for running).
5. Refer oneself to a trained counselor.
6. If nothing seems to do it, give up and take your chances.

Then, if you do suffer a heart attack—and survive—you might become motivated enough to engage in an exercise program.

Finally, each sport and activity has potential physical problems. For instance, runners can get bad feet, shin splints and joint problems, and tennis players can develop "tennis elbow" and "tennis toe." On balance, exercise is clearly favored. Most people find that exercise makes them feel and look good, and it brings them a little closer to that ideal known as health.

In Chapter 15, we consider another role of exercise, its combination with meditation. In the next section, the physical method of massage is briefly considered.

MASSAGE

Massage is a physical method in which the muscles, tendons, joints, skin and fat tissues are manipulated. Its main purpose is to relieve partial muscle contractions and thereby induce muscle relaxation.[30] The various methods of massage include the following: Swedish massage; use of hand-held vibrators; facial massage; scalp massage; hydromassage (water under pressure); shower massage (e.g., The Shower Massage by Water Pic®); massage built into reclining chairs (e.g., Contour® by Contour Chair Lounge, Inc.); concentrated foot massage (reflexology); and rolfing (a dramatic form of deep massage developed by Ida Rolf).

Some believe that foot manipulation, because of the relationship of feet nerves and blood vessels to other parts of the body, can relieve aches and pains in various sections of the body;[31] this approach, however, is not supported by the general medical community. Many physicians believe that chiropractic is nothing more than a form of massage. An unbiased review of the literature seems to show that chiropractic can help in relieving pain and discomfort related to abnormalities of alignment and muscle functioning. (As far as other purported claims, they are left for the experts to substantiate.)

In general, most people find massage to be relaxing, and it often helps in inducing sleep. However, there are many kinds of massage, and some forms of deep massage can be painful. Not everyone is willing to suffer the "treatment" in order to be helped. One kind of massage may, in fact, turn out be more stimulating than relaxing: massage by a member of the opposite sex (e.g., that given at a "massage parlor").

Let us now turn to heat.

HEAT

High heat is a severe physical stressor, but moderate heat for short periods of time can act to relax an individual. The most popular means of employing heat are a warm bath, a "bubble" bath (together with a good book and background music), a steam bath and a sauna bath, and the "new", old Roman-style hot water tub.

It is believed that use of the steam and sauna baths has some health value. For instance, their use can help ease the pain of stiff and sore muscles. A sauna is a well-known remedy for a hangover, and its use often generates feelings of well-being. It is also felt that the heat from a steam or sauna bath causes loss of excess salts, toxins and metabolic products.[32] However, there can definitely be dangers from the high temperatures involved.

Prolonged exposure to heat can result in dizziness, ringing in the ears and fainting. It is also dangerous for people with heart and respiratory conditions. A recent study showed that the high heat in saunas may possibly cause newborn infant nervous system malformations.[33] (Hence, the investigator advises pregnant women either to avoid steam and sauna baths or to stay in a sauna no longer than five to seven minutes.) An excellent combination of moderate heat and gentle massage is found in the Jacuzzi® whirlpool bath.

COLD

Strange as it may seem, cold can also relax an individual. Cold probably shocks the system, thus permitting subsequent relaxation. For instance, the cold shower is popular after a workout. The Finns are famous for their romp in the snow following a sauna.

Going from hot to cold or vice versa is a stimulating and relaxing experience for many people. However, this procedure may be dangerous for the cardiac or potential cardiac patient.

SUMMARY

Of the physical methods, exercise is of far greater importance than massage, heat and cold. Exercise prepares one to cope with stressors, is an excellent means of stress coping in itself and permits subsequent mental and physical relaxation. The proper uses of massage, heat and cold are refreshing and relaxing.

Sleeping, napping and relaxing are considered in the next chapter.

REFERENCES

1. Belloc, N. B. Relationship of health practices and mortality. *Prev. Med.* 2:67–81, 1973.
2. Editorial. Medicine: Coronary curb: Bully for the strenuous life. *Time* 110(24):80, Dec. 12, 1977.
3. Editorial. New Rx for a healthier heart: 2,000 calories of sweat a week. *Exec. Fitness Newsletter,* Sample Issue 1–2, 1978.
4. Henderson, J. Running commentary. *Runner's World* 13(3):20, 1978.
5. Fox, S. M., III and Naughton, J. P. Physical activity and the prevention of coronary heart disease. *Prev. Med.* 1:92–120, 1972.
6. Bricklin, M. What readers want to know about fitness, figure and physique. *Prevention* 30(6):32–40, 1978.
7. Kannel, W. B., Gordon, T., Sorlie, P. and McNamara, P. M. Physical activity and coronary vulnerability: The Framingham study. *Cardiol. Dig.* 6:28–40, June, 1971.
8. Morris, J. N., Kagan, A., and Pattison, D. C. Incidence and prediction of ischemic heart disease in London busmen. *Lancet* 2:553–559, 1966.
9. Mann, G. V. Medical intelligence: Current Concepts: Diet-heart: End of an era. *N. Engl. J. Med.* 297:644–650, 1977.
10. Bricklin, M. Trade yourself in for a new model. *Prevention* 29(2):32–42, 1977.
11. Cureton, T. K., Jr. *Physical Fitness and Dynamic Health,* Second Ed. New York: Dial Press, 1973.
12. Cooper, K. H. *The Aerobics Way.* New York: M. Evans and Co., Inc., 1977.
13. Editorial. Vitamin C, HDL and a healthier heart. *Prevention* 30(2):86–90, 1978.
14. Editorial. Before they ski, stress cardiography. *Phys. Sportsmed.* 2(1):22, 1974.
15. Barney, V. S., Hirst, C. C. and Jensen, C. R. *Conditioning Exercises: Exercises to Improve Body Form and Function,* Second Ed. St. Louis: C. V. Mosby Co., 1969.

16. Editorial. Exercise after 30. *Exec. Fitness Newletter,* Sample Issue 2, 1977.
17. Editorial. Relaxation formula: Jogger, si! jigger, no! *Phys. Sportsmed.* 3(10):16, 1975.
18. Anderson, J. L. and Cohen, M. *The West Point Fitness and Diet Book.* New York: Rawson Associates, 1977.
19. Bassler, T. J. Marathon running and immunity to heart disease. *Phys. Sportsmed.* 3(4):77–80, 1975.
20. Runner's World Editors. *The Complete Runner,* Second Ed. Mountain View, Calif.: World Pubns., 1975.
21. Fixx, J. F. *The Complete Book of Running.* New York: Random House, 1977.
22. Sheehan, G. *Running and Being.* New York: Simon and Schuster, 1978.
23. Higdon, H. Can running cure mental illness? *Runner's World* 13(1):36–43, 1978.
24. Nevins, M. A., Levy, A. and Lyon, L. J. When a pro athlete's ECG mimics heart disease. *Phys. Sportsmed.* 2(1):27–30, 1974.
25. Henderson, J. Our normal "abnormalities." *Runner's World* 9(2):26–27, 1974.
26. Rose, K. D. Which cardiovascular "problems" should disqualify athletes? *Phys. Sportsmed.* 3(6):62–68, 1975.
27. Kirk, C. Loosen up your tight, aching shoulders. *Prevention* 29(4):70–76, 1977.
28. Lear, L. Here's help for your aching back. *Prevention* 29(2):103–109, 1977.
29. Norris, C. Is your back biting back? *Dent. Manag.* 17(9):57–60, 1977.
30. Gottlieb, B. Release your tension with massage. *Prevention* 29(2):134–142, 1977.
31. Reibstein, L. Foot rubs a cure for ills? *Philadelphia Sunday Bull.* NxC:3, Aug. 6, 1978.
32. Foley, W. J. Stress from many sources affects your health and well being. *Dent. Stud.* 55(8):34–35, 1977.
33. Editorial. Heat is on saunas as possible teratogens. *Med. World News* 19(6):37, Mar. 20, 1978.

12

Sleeping, Napping and Relaxing

To sleep: perchance to dream; ay there's the rub.*

THE HAPPY SLEEPER**

Some people have difficulty in falling asleep. Their problem is known as insomnia. They may resort to sleeping pills, psychotherapy, hypnosis or even shock therapy. There are other people who can get to sleep but only under certain conditions. The typical example is the person who sleeps well only in his own bed. Some individuals can only sleep on one side of a bed. Many people have difficulty in sleeping on trains and buses but have no problem on planes and vice versa. And, of course, there are students who are wide awake all the time except when they attend lectures.

Sleeping for some people is a means whereby they avoid or evade stressors. One of us (DM), who is an endodontist (a root canal

* Shakespeare, *Hamlet,* Act III, Scene I.
** Any relationship to *The Happy Hooker,* by Xavier Hollander, is purely coincidental.

specialist), had such an individual as a patient. People fear many things in dentistry, but the one procedure that seems to be the most fear-provoking is having a "nerve" removed from a tooth. Root canal therapy is often a completely painless procedure, but the general public doesn't know this. Hence, it is not unusual for a root canal specialist to see many apprehensive patients each day. Until trained to relax (see Chapter 17), the average person sits in the chair and holds on to the arm rests for dear life. But not Fred Morris (whose name we have changed for purposes of anonymity).

Fred Morris was seen ten times (he needed root canal therapy on four teeth). From the very first visit, as soon as he got his "Novocaine" injection, he fell asleep. However, he was very cooperative—he would sleep with his mouth open.

Mr. Morris was a great patient, but on occasion he would disturb the other patients with his loud snoring. A gentle tap on the shoulder usually broke the snoring pattern, but he would still sleep on. It was really a shame to end each visit, as Mr. Morris was so relaxed. Finally, at the last session, Mr. Morris was asked about his ability to sleep throughout the procedures. His response was classic: "This is the only place that I can go to where I can *really* relax. Your chair is more comfortable than my own bed. And the sound of the drill and saliva ejector is so soothing, that it puts me 'right out.' "

Well, all you fearful patients, if Mr. Morris could do it, so can you!

INTRODUCTION

This is a short chapter for two reasons. The first is that not too much is known about the role of sleeping and napping in stress control. The second reason is that we do not want to put our readers to sleep by talking too much about sleep. Sleeping, napping and relaxing are all means to counteract the stress response. The best way to do this is by initiating the relaxation response, which is covered in the next chapter. We begin this discussion with sleeping.

SLEEPING

Without adequate sleep, people do not function normally. Deprived of sleep, they tend to experience hallucinations and may become psychotic.

Definition

The definition of adequate sleep varies with individuals; but as discussed previously, Nedra Belloc's study showed an average of eight hours per night to be associated with the best results.[1] That is, she found that eight-hours-per-night sleepers had the lowest mortality of the three groups that were compared. Those who slept either six hours or less, or nine hours or more, had higher mortality as compared to the eight-hour sleepers. Probably less than six hours per night is not sufficient for most people for adequate body renewal. Sleeping more than nine hours nightly often results from some concurrent disease, and that could affect mortality.

Functions of Sleep

As was illustrated in the introductory story, one role of sleep is to cut off stressors that are potential causes of distress. Sleep also provides the opportunity for the body to prepare itself for the next day's stressors.

One reason why sleep may not be as effective as meditation (a deep relaxation method) is that during sleep, periods of deep relaxation alternate with periods of vigorous mental activity. That may be what Shakespeare's Hamlet meant when he spoke about the "rub" in sleeping.

Dreaming occurs during sleep, and apparently it has both beneficial and deleterious aspects. Dreaming has been shown to be accompanied by electroencephalographic (EEG) changes and rapid eye movements (REM).[2] The EEG patterns of deep sleep show slow delta waves, while dreaming shows the beta rhythms that generally occur during wide-awake alert thinking (see Fig. 12.1 for examples of these patterns). On one hand, dreaming may serve to relieve the stresses of the day; while on the other, nightmares may trigger stresses of their own. It is for these reasons that an early morning meditation is recommended (discussed in Chapter 15).

Sleep Induction Methods

There are various ways to help induce sleep.[3-6] As preparation, it is important to empty the bladder; for, as one gets older, weak bladder

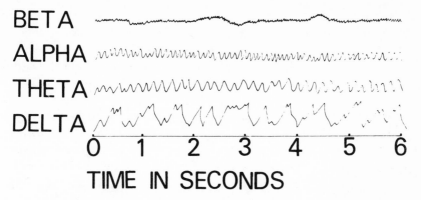

Fig. 12.1 The brain wave patterns. Beta rhythms (14–60 cycles per second) occur during the wide-awake, alert state and during dreaming periods. Alpha rhythms (8–13 cycles per second) occur during meditation and relaxation-hypnosis. Theta rhythms (4–7 cycles per second) occur during deep meditation and in the hypnagogic period (time between awake and sleep when hallucinations can occur). Delta rhythms (1–3 cycles per second) occur during restful sleep.

and prostate problems (in men) may develop, which make for frequent nocturnal bathroom visits.

The room should be well ventilated and quiet. One should never go to bed with a grudge, since it preys on the mind, making it difficult to get to sleep.

Taking a few deep breaths and focusing on them may relieve anxiety and bring on sleep. "Counting sheep"—a device along the lines of self-hypnosis and meditation (see Chapters 14 and 15)—may also help. Self-hypnosis itself is an excellent way to relax the body and allow for sleep.

A good time for meditation is generally before dinner, but it can also be practiced about two hours after dinner. However, meditating too late at night can alert an individual to the extent that sleep becomes difficult. On the other hand, meditation in an inclined position seems to be an effective way to induce sleep. After one has been awakened, meditation may help him get back to sleep. (For further discussion on meditation, see Chapter 15.)

Eating moderately during the day and not heavily right before bedtime permits restful sleep. Still, if a person is hungry, then a light snack will relieve the hunger pangs and help induce sleep. Late night coffee drinking keeps many people awake. There are drinks that are soothing and relaxing, such as herbal teas. The warm glass of milk with its calcium and tryptophan content may be the best one of them all. However, drinking too much of anything at night can result in mid-night interruptions for a trip to the bathroom.

Exercise during the day tends to induce relaxation and permit a good night's sleep. However, it is not advisable to take a strenuous workout at night, since it may make the individual overly wakeful. Light exercise such as taking a stroll may be a good practice.

For many people, sex at bedtime is a precursor of sleep. The combination of mild exercise, sexual release and mental peace seems to be a good formula. Another good practice to help induce sleep is to take a warm bath.

The kind of bed one sleeps in may affect the ease with which one falls asleep. A mattress that is either too soft or too hard—remember the story of, "Goldilocks and the Three Bears"?—may not be just right for sleeping purposes. The new water beds are reported to be quite comfortable and conducive to relaxation.

If all of these tried and true ways for inducing sleep do not work, then sleeping pills may be used as a last resort. They should be used sparingly because of the potential for addiction and dangerous interaction with other drugs (e.g., alcohol). These various sleeping aids are summarized in Table 12.1.

It may be worth considering that insomnia is not truly an inability to get to sleep as much as a device to escape from troubles by sleeping more than the body requires. That is, the individual may perceive that he is not getting enough sleep, but actually he may be oversleeping. Those people who really do not get enough sleep at night may be

TABLE 12.1   Sleeping Aids

1. Eat moderately.
2. Do not drink late-night coffee.
3. Drink a warm glass of milk.
4. Drink a cup of herbal tea.
5. Empty the bladder before going to bed.
6. Arrange the bedroom for quiet and comfort.
7. Resolve the grudge before retiring.
8. Take a few deep breaths.
9. Exercise moderately.
10. Try self-hypnosis, meditation or "counting sheep."
11. Take a warm bath.
12. Pick a comfortable bed—one that is not too soft.
13. Take a sleeping pill as a last resort.

able to compensate by taking daytime naps, the topic of the next section.

NAPPING

Daytime sleeping is known as napping, whereas daydreaming is really a form of self-hypnosis (discussed in Chapter 14). An interesting study on napping was undertaken by Fred Evans and his coworkers.[7]

The attitudes toward napping and patterns of napping were determined in a survey of 430 college students. Sixty percent of the students napped either sometimes, usually or always; 40% never or rarely napped. Those who did not nap reported that the aftermath of the naps was so unpleasant that napping was actively avoided. Many of those who did nap found that it had a restorative effect, which was in excess of the time spent. The nap helped them get through the day better.

It was determined that there were basically two types of nappers. The first was replacement nappers, who napped to make up for lost sleep or anticipated lost sleep. The second type was appetitive nappers, who tended to nap for psychological reasons. A psychological and physiological evaluation was undertaken of the two subgroups of nappers and the nonnappers. The nappers were able to fall asleep easily under various conditions in contrast to the nonnappers. Nappers felt better afterwards as compared to the nonnappers. Also, several minutes after the conclusion of the nap, the nappers had decreased fatigue, which was not the case with the nonnappers. There were also EEG differences among the restorative nappers, appetitive nappers and nonnappers.

The results of this study reinforce the idea that napping for some people is a means of overcoming fatigue and helping to meet the stressful challenges of the day. Then there are some people who can meet the day's challenges merely by having a period of relaxation, the next topic.

RELAXING

"Now just relax." How many times have you heard that phrase? Can't you just see that needle take its ominous path toward your mouth as the dentist reassuringly tells you to—"relax!"

And don't you feel the pulsations building up inside your arm and head as the nurse inflates the blood pressure cuff while urging you to —"relax!"

And as your best forehand shots go soaring over the baseline, don't you listen with "deaf ears" to the repeated suggestions of the tennis pro to—"relax!"

And how about the traffic jam, and you with that important early morning appointment? You tell yourself to—"relax!"

And what about that first presentation before a live audience when you know the material "cold," but your heart is pounding and your mind goes blank? And you repeat to yourself—"relax!"

It is often the case that these self-imposed pleas to relax are usually not much more effective than the admonitions of others. The fact is that most people do not know how to relax—especially in a doctor's office. (This topic is covered in Chapter 18.)

Studies

In the two studies at Temple University that were discussed previously, no physiological differences were found among self-hypnosis, meditation and relaxation.[8,9]

This finding of no difference could have been related to the fact that the subjects volunteered for the study. That is, many of the subjects were students who took the opportunity to get out of class. As a result of the preliminary interviews, they anticipated a pleasant experience having to do with hypnosis, meditation and relaxation. Also, the mere suggestion to relax might have had an interactive effect, since the person giving the suggestion was also the hypnotist.

On the other hand, significant subjective differences were found.* When the subjects were questioned about the perceptions of the various states, most of them found that relaxation didn't begin to compare with self-hypnosis or meditation. In the first study, all 48 of the subjects reported that meditation and self-hypnosis were better on the measures of best dissociation (i.e., to mentally transport one's self somewhere else), best euphoria (i.e., feelings of intense

---

* The differences between the mental and physical phenomena may be more in the means of measurement; physiological differences are measured behaviorally, as through pulse rate and skin resistance, whereas mental differences are determined in terms of subjective reports.

pleasure), greatest depth and most effortless induction.[8] In the second study, only six of the 48 subjects preferred relaxation to meditation.[9] Those few subjects who did prefer relaxation stated that mentally repeating a sound (as is done in meditation) interfered with their ability to get into a deep state. Conversely, the great majority of subjects in the two studies (90 of 96) found that the use of meditation or self-hypnosis was a far easier, more predictable and more pleasurable method of becoming deeply tranquilized.

Relaxation Aids

A variety of things may help to induce relaxation. Among them are the following: a quiet room with few distractions; sitting or lying in a comfortable position; listening to light semiclassical music; and taking a few deep breaths.[6]

SUMMARY

Sleeping, napping and relaxing are stress-relieving methods. Sleep is a period for both physical and mental restoration that gives one the capability of coping with the stressors of the following day. However, disturbed sleep can be stressful.

Napping is a good practice for some people and not beneficial for others. Where sleep at night has not been sufficient, napping may "carry" the individual for the remainder of the day. By the same token, relaxation can be of benefit to many individuals. Nevertheless, it has been found that most people need additional methods to counteract the stress response. For instance, they need to initiate the relaxation response, which is the subject of the next chapter.

REFERENCES

1. Belloc, N. B. Relationship of health practices and mortality. *Prev. Med.* 2:67–81, 1973.
2. Kratochvil, S. and MacDonald, H. Sleep in hypnosis: A pilot EEG study. *Am. J. Clin. Hyp.* 15:29–37, 1972.
3. Wiley, D. B. Sleep: Too much or too little, it's a problem. *Philadelphia Eve. Bull.* BK: 37, Aug. 17, 1978.
4. Wheeler, A. C. Try a tisane for tranquility. *Prevention* 24(6):142–146, 1972.
5. Sharpe, R. and Lewis, D. *Thrive on Stress.* New York: Warner Books Inc., 1977.

6. Editorial. Deep breathing: More than a sigh of relief. *Prevention* 30(6): 58–62, 1978.
7. Evans, F. J., Cook, M. R., Cohen, H. D., Orne, E. C. and Orne, M. T. Appetitive and replacement naps: EEG and behavior. *Science* 197:687–688, 1977.
8. Morse, D. R., Martin, J. S., Furst, M. L. and Dubin, L. L. A physiological and subjective evaluation of meditation, hypnosis, and relaxation. *Psychosom. Med.* 39:304–324, 1977.
9. Morse, D. R., Martin, J. S., Furst, M. L. and Dubin, L. L. A physiological and subjective evaluation of neutral and emotionally-charged words for meditation. *J. Am. Soc. Psychosom. Med. Dent.* 26(1–4):(1979), in press.

13

The Relaxation Response

When angry, count four; when very angry, swear.*

A LITTLE BIT OF HISTORY

As mentioned in Chapter 7, the best way to counteract the results of stress is to initiate the opposite reaction, the relaxation response. Mark Twain knew something about this when he said to count to four when angry. That is, silent counting (e.g., "counting sheep") is a means of inducing a hypnotic state, which is a form of the relaxation response. Mark Twain's other suggestion was to use a vocal venting method of stress release if the first method failed (the shouting method was discussed in Chapter 8).

In a similar vein, we have a tennis acquaintance who tries to induce the relaxation response when he makes an unforced error. He says, "Borg, Borg, Borg, Borg, Borg, Borg" (i.e., the unforced

* Mark Twain, *Pudd'n head Wilson's Calendar.*

error in the given situation may have a value of a "6-Borg'er"), in the hopes that the repetition of that great tennis player's name will calm him down in the same way that Bjorn Borg "keeps his cool."

In order to understand the relaxation response, we go back about 20 years to the experiments of Walter Hess with cats.[1] Hess stimulated various parts of the cat hypothalamus and found that he could elicit two opposite reactions. The first reaction was one aspect of the previously described stress response. This response Hess called the "ergotropic reaction," and it corresponds to the "fight or flight" sympathetic nervous system response of Cannon, in which catecholamines are released and blood pressure and heart rate increase.[2] (You may want to refresh your memory about this aspect of the stress response by reviewing Chapter 3.) The second reaction, which Hess obtained from stimulating a different part of the cat hypothalamus, he called the "trophotropic response." In this response, there was increased activity of the parasympathetic division of the autonomic nervous system and a decreased activity of the sympathetic division. In other words, the response was diametrically opposite to the ergotropic reaction. For example, blood pressure and heart rate decreased.

Herbert Benson recently examined the human counterpart of the cat trophotropic response and concluded that a similar response can be achieved by deep relaxation.[3] He called the psychological and physiological changes of deep relaxation the "relaxation response."

As was done with stress, let us now consider the three components of deep relaxation: the relaxors; the individual makeup; and the relaxation response. The interrelationships are shown in the following equation:

RELAXORS + INDIVIDUAL MAKEUP = RELAXATION RESPONSE

RELAXORS

Just as the stress response is brought on by stressors, the stimuli that elicit the relaxation response can be called "relaxors." The definition of a relaxor is similar to the one previously given for a stressor except that the opposite response is elicited. A simple definition is: A relaxor is any stimulus or technique that is capable of inducing deep relaxation. In the same way that stressors were subdivided, relaxors can also be considered as of three types: physical, social and psychological. However, the types are often combined. For example, T'ai Chi is a physical form of meditation; but it is also social, as it is an expression of the Taoist religion. It involves a serious of slow, fluid movements and postures. T'ai Chi is a physical method to induce relaxation that is practiced regularly in China and recently has attracted a strong following in the United States. Akido is one of the Japanese martial arts and contains elements of meditation and visualization along with physical activity.

Nichiren Shoshu is a form of physical meditation in which active chanting is used to induce deep relaxation. It is also social in the sense that it is a branch of Buddhism. Zen meditation is psychological and social in the sense that it is a highly ritualized Buddhist practice. The same is true for Sufi meditation, which combines psychological with social practice (an Islamic technique). In many other religious practices, silent meditation combines psychological and social aspects. Examples are found in Judaism, Christianity, Confucianism and Shintoism. Yoga is physical (Hatha Yoga), psychological (Raja Yoga) and social (it is an expression of Hinduism).

A current controversy is over whether Transcendental Meditation (TM) is simply psychological or is social as well. TM has recently been banned in New Jersey's public schools as it has been judged to be an expression of the Hindu religion.*

Some purely psychological relaxors are Progressive Relaxation (Jacobson's method), Autogenic Training (Schultz-Luthe technique), Sentic cycles (Clynes method), self-hypnosis (various techniques), simple-word meditation (Benson's method; Morse's method), Clinical Standardized Meditation (CSM; Carrington's method) and meditation-hypnosis (Morse's method). Meditation (psychological) is also a part of various group encounters (social) such as Esalen, est, Silva Mind Control and Alpha Meditation and Mind Control.

The type and duration of the specific relaxor (i.e., the amount of time spent in practice per day) and the individual's makeup (i.e., categorized as normal, neurotic or psychotic) determine how the person will react to the specific relaxor. In other words, there should be

* Editorial. Judge bans Transcendental Meditation in N.J. schools. *Philadelphia Eve. Bull.* NA9, Oct. 21, 1977.

different relaxors for different people. As with stress, relaxation responses can be neutral, favorable or unfavorable. A neutral response is the rested feeling following an average morning meditation. A favorable response is the euphoric feeling following a "good" late afternoon meditation. A negative response is the feeling of loss of control that could lead to mental breakdown in susceptible individuals. These descriptions are summarized in the following equation:

RELAXORS +	INDIVIDUAL MAKEUP	= RELAXATION RESPONSE	
Physical	Heredity	Unfavorable	Mental Breakdown
Social	Environment	Neutral	Rested
Psychological		Favorable	Euphoria

INDIVIDUAL MAKEUP

Whereas the genetic and environmental factors in relationship to stress have been adequately investigated, very little study has been undertaken with respect to the relationship between relaxors and different types of individuals. As discussed in Chapter 2, people have different personalities (e.g., introverts or extroverts; internals or externals), and individuals vary in their autonomic nervous system responses to stressors (e.g., sympathicotonics, vagotonics, normal responders).

These individual variations could modify the type of relaxor that should be used. Other factors that could affect the choice of relaxor are age, sex, diet, disease, drug intake, conditioning (physical and mental), biorhythm, brain laterality, occupation and family situation. In other words, the same things that can affect stress can affect relaxation. Unfortunately, these factors are rarely considered when people are instructed in relaxation methods.

A technique that relaxes one person can act as a stressor for another person and vice versa. This turned out to be the case in the two previously discussed studies performed at Temple University.[4,5] It was found that most subjects preferred meditation and self-hypnosis to instructed relaxation (the subjects were told to simply close their eyes and try to relax). However, about 13% of the subjects in one study found that the repetition of the word in meditation actually interfered with relaxation. They reported that they felt more relaxed when they simply closed their eyes and did not repeat anything.

Physiologically—i.e., using measures such as heart rate, blood pressure, breathing rate, muscle activity, skin resistance (to measure sweat gland activity) and alpha brain wave patterns—no significant differences were found among meditation, relaxation-self-hypnosis and instructed relaxation (see Figs. 13.1 and 13.2). This may mean that there are no real differences among the methods, or that the physical measures are not sensitive enough to detect the differences that the subjects reported. At any rate, an individual should not practice a method that he does not find satisfying.

Another finding in the Temple studies was that silently repeating a series of numbers with eyes closed, was a stressful procedure, both physiologically and subjectively, for most people (see Fig. 13.3). That is, even though they were physically relaxed, the active mind interfered with their relaxation. However, a few subjects actually enjoyed the mental task of repeating numbers, and for them the mental activity actually induced physiological relaxation (as indicated by the physical measures). Probably for those individuals, the repetition acted as a monotonous hypnotic-like device, somewhat like counting sheep.

There is other evidence that people vary in their need for relaxors. The following two studies seem to show that the effectiveness of certain words and sounds for meditation is related to personality. In a study at Temple University, subjects were tested using emotionally charged words ("love" and "hate") as compared to a neutral word ("one") and instructed relaxation.[5] Physiologically, no significant differences were found between any of the words for meditation and instructed relaxation. Subjectively, most subjects preferred "love" (25 of 48). But surprisingly, more preferred "hate" to the neutral "one" (11 to 6). Six of the subjects preferred instructed relaxation to any type of meditation. The majority of subjects who preferred "love" had comments such as: "saying 'love' makes me feel so good, so relaxed, so peaceful"; and " 'love' brings forth such pleasant feelings." Their comments about "hate" included: "saying 'hate' makes me dizzy"; "I see knives, blades and swords when I say 'hate' "; " 'hate' brings forth terrible thoughts"; and "the 'tuh' sound of 'hate' bothers me when I say it." On the other hand, those who preferred "hate" had different comments such as: "I don't

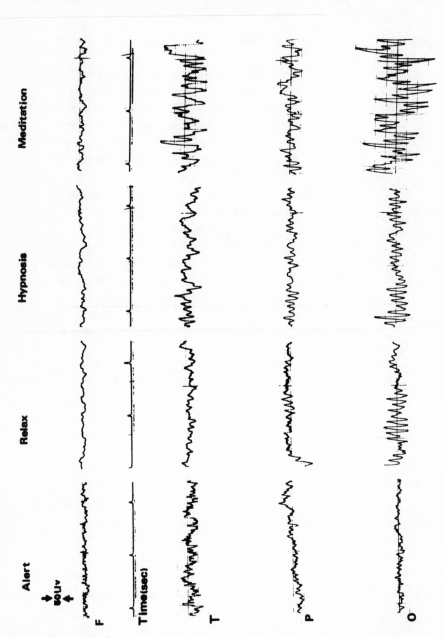

Fig. 13.1 Brain wave comparison of three relaxation states and the alert state. Abbreviations: uv = microvolts; F, T, P and O are four scalp areas in which the electrodes are placed (F = frontal; T = temporal; P = parietal; O = occipital). For this subject, who is in the partly stressful alert state, beta waves are found in all four areas. Similar patterns are seen in each of the three relaxation states (Relax, Hypnosis, Meditation), with predominantly beta waves in the frontal area and alpha rhythms in the

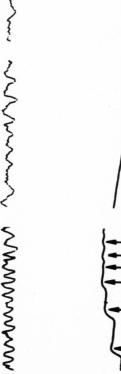

Fig. 13.2 Physiological comparison of three relaxation states and the alert state. P = pulse (heart) rate; R = respiratory rate; B = skin resistance; ↑ = skin resistance nonspecific fluctuations (indicative of a stressful reaction); and ↓ = direction of increased skin resistance (less stress). For this subject, during the partly stressful alert state, there is a slightly faster pulse and respiratory rate than during the relaxation states. The principal difference is for skin resistance with decreased levels and increased fluctuations (known as the galvanic skin response or GSR) found during the alert state. The physiological responses for the three relaxation states (Relax; Meditation; Hypnosis) are seen to be similar.

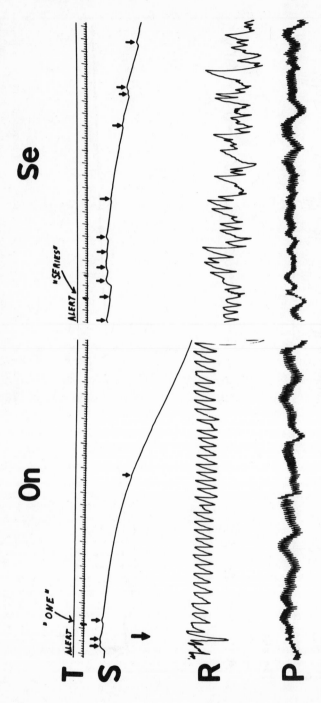

Fig. 13.3 Stressful response to silent repetition of a number series. On = meditation with the word "one"; Se = silent repetition of a series of numbers; T = time in seconds; S = skin resistance; ↓ = skin resistance, nonspecific fluctuations (indicative of a stressful reaction); ↓ = direction of increased skin resistance (less stress); R = respiratory rate; and P = pulse rate. In this subject, the silent repetition of a series of numbers induced a stressful response as shown primarily by increased fluctuations and faster and more irregular breathing. (From Morse, D. R. et al., 1979. A physiological and subjective evaluation of neutral and emotionally-charged words for meditation. Reprinted from *The Journal of the American Society of Psychosomatic Dentistry and Medicine*, Volume 26, 1979.)

hate anyone, so the word has no bad meaning for me"; " 'hate' is easy to say." Their comments about "love" were interesting. For instance, "When I say 'love,' I get so emotionally involved that I can't relax"; and "The 'vuh' sound of 'love' really bothers me." Most subjects reported that "one" didn't do anything for them subjectively, but it was easy to say.

At Princeton University, Patricia Carrington performed a similar experiment.[6] Meditation was compared with pleasant- and unpleasant-sounding nonsense words. Most subjects felt better and did better with the pleasant-sounding words (e.g., "lohm"). However, a few had better results with the unpleasant-sounding words (e.g., "grik"). Carrington found some evidence that depressed individuals had beneficial results from using the unpleasant-sounding "grik." It may be that this sound helps those individuals get rid of their negative feelings.* Hence, it certainly appears that the variability of people should be taken into consideration before any type of relaxor is used.**

Transcendental Meditation (TM)

In the indoctrination program, the TM teachers state that personality and other factors are considered in the assignment of individual mantras (sounds for meditation). Yet, a former TM teacher has just released a sworn affidavit in which he stated that there are only 16 mantras, and they are assigned solely on the basis of age.[7] Some examples he gave are: up to the age of 11, "eng"; age 16–17, "ema"; age 30–34, "shiring"; and age 45–49, "hirim." A recent report by Carrington corroborated the age basis of TM mantras.[6] The members of the Junior Class at Princeton University who were TM practitioners were invited to write their individualized mantras on a slip of paper. Then the folded papers were placed in the center of the room. It was found that practically all the students reported the

---

* Bernard Glueck from The Institute of Living (Hartford, Conn.) and Patricia Carrington are currently collaborating in the analysis of brain wave patterns with respect to personalities and meditation word preferences. The hope is that certain definite relationships will emerge.

** The authors are currently conducting a study in which personality and moods are being correlated with words used for meditation. Each individual answers a personality-mood questionnaire and then selects a word for meditation from a carefully prepared list of 52 different words. An interesting preliminary result is that about one-third of the subjects preferred a word with an m or n ending (e.g., "lum"; "om"; "woman"; "shirim").

same mantra—and just about all the students fell in the same age range.

With TM, it is also stated that meditation should be performed before breakfast and before dinner for 20 minutes per session. Other than testimonials, there does not seem to be any evidence to show that this is essential or even beneficial for everyone. From speaking to a number of meditators, and from the results of the physiological studies undertaken at Temple University, the authors have found that some people get maximum benefit from 10 minutes of meditation, while others require at least 30 minutes. The time period also seems to vary with the day, the weather, the location and other factors. When people are sick in bed, they appear to do better with longer periods of meditation. Conversely, when these same people are feeling well, long periods of meditation can be upsetting to them. Religious people may do better with meditation associated with prayer than with TM or self-hypnosis. On the other hand, an avowed atheist attempting religious meditation might find it to be quite stressful.

Finally, it seems that certain people should not use any type of relaxor. For instance, people who dislike being alone or who fear loss of control can become extremely anxious during meditation or self-hypnosis. Individuals who suffer from migraine may get an attack during the deep relaxation phase of meditation or self-hypnosis.[8] Also, it is not recommended for people who do not believe in the method's effectiveness. It may be that the effectiveness of the method lies in the positive attitude of the practitioner (see Chapter 16, Biofeedback). For those individuals who should not use a relaxor, employment of the other stress-relieving methods previously discussed should prove beneficial (e.g., exercise, positive attitudes, diversions, consultations).

Now that the relaxors and the individual makeup have been discussed, let us examine the changes of the relaxation response.

THE RELAXATION RESPONSE

Physiological Changes

As was the case with the stress response, the relaxation response is initiated in the hypothalamus. It is believed that an unknown signal causes activation of the parasympathetic division of the autonomic nervous system and deactivation of the sympathetic division of the autonomic nervous system.[9] It is not definitely known if the hypothalamus–anterior pituitary–adrenal cortex (H-AP-AC) axis is involved. However, considering the close relationship of the autonomic nervous system and the H-AP-AC axis in stress (see Chapter 3), it would appear that activation of the relaxation response would cause a deactivation of the H-AP-AC axis. This should result in a curtailing of the release of cortisone, vasopressin and thyroid hormones. These relationships are shown in Fig. 13.4.

The activation of the parasympathetic nervous system and the deactivation of the other systems causes reactions to occur that are generally opposite to those seen with stress. There have been several studies on the physiological changes of the relaxation response, including investigations by Wallace, Benson and our group at Temple University.[3-5,9,10] These studies have examined meditation (TM and simple-word type), relaxation-hypnosis and instructed relaxation. Although differences in the magnitude of the changes are reported, there was agreement about the nature of the changes. The major findings are as follows:

1. Decrease in both intake of oxygen and removal of carbon dioxide.

2. Decrease in the breathing rate. As the body and all its tissues are in a state of rest, there is less need for oxygen and gaseous exchange; hence, the decreased intake and breathing rate.

3. Increase in skin resistance. There is less sweating from the palms and the soles. An individual who is calm tends not to sweat. This is related to the decreased activity of the sympathetic nervous system.

4. Blood changes showing a decrease in blood cholesterol and

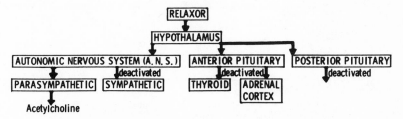

Fig. 13.4 A preliminary view of the relaxation response.

blood lactate.[3,9,11] The decreased amount of cholesterol is added to the lowered cholesterol level that may result from aerobic exercise (see Chapter 11). Together, these changes may prove beneficial in preventing heart disease. The decreased blood lactate results from the muscles' inactivity, which is associated with a decreased energy expenditure.

5. Decreased blood flow to the skeletal muscles, since it is no longer needed for activity.

6. Skeletal muscle activity also diminished, for the same reasons as above.

7. An increase in alpha and theta rhythms, shown by examination of the brain wave patterns. These changes are indicative of deep relaxation, but there is disagreement over the importance of these patterns. For instance, in one of the studies at Temple University, it was found that most subjects had increased alpha rhythms with deep relaxation.[4] Yet, there were some subjects who were deeply relaxed

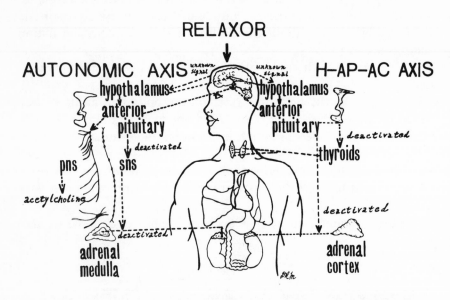

Fig. 13.5 Major physiological changes of the relaxation response. pns = parasympathetic nervous system; sns = sympathetic nervous system. An unknown signal from the hypothalamus activates the pns, deactivates the sns, and probably also deactivates the H–AP–AC (hypothalamus–anterior pituitary–adrenal cortex) axis. As a result of pns activation, acetylcholine is released. (The resultant physiological changes are described in the text.)

and produced no discernible alpha. Other subjects were wide awake, and a high level of alpha was indicated.

8. Constriction of the pupils of the eye, possibly because visual acuity is not needed under relaxation as it is under stress.

9. In contrast to stress, saliva increased in flow, probably to aid in the digestive process.

10. Observations by Benson, Patel, Datey, Stone and others that meditation, hypnosis and biofeedback used over a period of months cause definitive decreases in blood pressure for patients who had high blood pressure (hypertensives).[12-16] Thus, this is another important reason for practicing the relaxation response in one form or another.

11. Evidence presented by Benson that regular practice of meditation can decrease the incidence of heart arrhythmias (irregular heart activity).[12,17]

12. Some reports that asthma attacks can be reduced and muscle "tension" decreased by the use of regular meditation or self-hypnosis.[18,19]

The major physiological changes of the relaxation response are shown in Fig. 13.5. The potential benefits resulting from regular practice of the relaxation response are shown in Fig. 13.6.

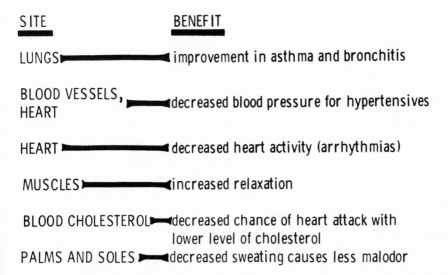

SITE   BENEFIT

LUNGS ━━━━━◀ improvement in asthma and bronchitis

BLOOD VESSELS, ━━◀ decreased blood pressure for hypertensives
HEART

HEART ▶━━━━━◀ decreased heart activity (arrhythmias)

MUSCLES ▶━━━━◀ increased relaxation

BLOOD CHOLESTEROL ▶━◀ decreased chance of heart attack with
                     lower level of cholesterol
PALMS AND SOLES ▶━◀ decreased sweating causes less malodor

Fig. 13.6 Potential physiological benefits of the relaxation response.

Psychological Responses, Objective Signs and Social Benefits

Subjective reports for the relaxation response vary with the individual, the time of day, the technique that is practiced and the type of technique employed. Still, certain common feelings are often described.[4] These include warmth, tingling, numbness, floating, out-of-body sensation, dissociation (feeling as if one were in two places at once), euphoria (extreme pleasure) and various mental images. The subjects often report that they do not hear their heartbeats and are unaware of their breathing. They generally verbalize feelings of peace and tranquility.

The individuals often look relaxed; their arms and legs hang loosely, and the skin of the face and scalp appears unwrinkled. If their eyes are open—e.g., during a phase of hypnosis and some forms of meditation—they may have a "spaced-out" appearance.

There is some evidence that regular practice of the relaxation response results in improved psychological health. People report better study and work habits, decreased aggression, less anxiety and overall improvement in interpersonal relationships.[3,18,19]

SUMMARY

Relaxation is an important and effective way to counteract the stress of today's life style. Although relaxation may result from simply relaxing, napping or sleeping, a far better and more predictable method is to elicit the relaxation response.

The physiological and subjective changes seen with the relaxation response are opposite to those seen with stress. Although the relaxation response is beneficial for most people, there are variations in techniques that should be considered. These variations should be based on personality and physical differences among individuals. However, particular people may experience detrimental results from the practice of the relaxation response. For these individuals, alternative methods of stress reduction should be considered. (Review Chapters 8–12.)

In the next two chapters, we consider two major methods of inducing the relaxation response, hypnosis and meditation.

REFERENCES

1. Hess, W. R. *The Functional Organization of the Diencephalon.* New York: Grune & Stratton, 1957.
2. Cannon, W. B. The emergency function of the adrenal medulla in pain and the major emotions. *Am. J. Physiol.* 33:356-372, 1914.
3. Benson, H. *The Relaxation Response.* New York: William Morrow, 1975.
4. Morse, D. R., Martin, J. S., Furst, M. L. and Dubin, L. L. A physiological and subjective evaluation of meditation, hypnosis and relaxation. *Psychosom. Med.* 39:304-324, 1977.
5. Morse, D. R., Martin, J. S., Furst, M. L. and Dubin, L. L. A physiological and subjective evaluation of neutral and emotionally-charged words for meditation. *J. Am. Soc. Psychosom. Dent. Med.* 26(1-4):1979, in press.
6. Carrington, P. New directions in meditation research. Read before the Symposium on Meditation Related Therapies, St. Louis, Oct. 28-29, 1977.
7. Randolph, G. J. Declaration on TM. Paper presented at the Symposium on Meditation Related Therapies, St. Louis, Oct. 28-29, 1977.
8. Dudley, D. L. and Welke, E. *How to Survive Being Alive.* Garden City: Doubleday and Co. Inc., 1977.
9. Benson, H. Your innate asset for combatting stress. *Harvard Bus. Rev.* 52(4):49-60, 1974.
10. Wallace, R. K. Physiological effects of transcendental meditation. *Science* 167:1751-1754, 1970.
11. Editorial. Just relax—Transcendental Meditation reduces cholesterol level. *Jewish Press* 27(40):53, Oct. 7, 1977.
12. Benson, H. Systemic hypertension and the relaxation response. *N. Engl. J. Med.* 296:1152-1156, 1977.
13. Patel, C. H. Yoga and bio-feedback in the management of hypertension. *Lancet* 2:1053-1055, 1973.
14. Stone, R. A. and DeLeo, J. Psychotherapeutic control of hypertension. *N. Engl. J. Med.* 294:80-84, 1976.
15. Friedman, H. and Taub, H. A. The use of hypnosis and biofeedback procedures for essential hypertension. *Int. J. Clin. Exp. Hypn.* 25:335-347, 1977.
16. Frumkin, K., Nathan, R. J., Prout, M. F. and Cohen, M. C. Nonpharmacologic control of essential hypertension in man: A critical review of the experimental literature. *Psychosom. Med.* 40:294-320, 1978.
17. Benson, H. The relaxation response: An innate capacity for dealing with stress. Read before the Symposium on Stress and Behavioral Medicine, New York, Dec. 3-4, 1977.
18. Bloomfield, H. H., Cain, M. P. and Jaffe, D. T. *TM* Discovering Inner Energy and Overcoming Stress.* New York: Delacorte, 1975.
19. Kroger, W. S. and Fezler, W. D. *Hypnosis and Behavior Modification: Imagery Conditioning.* Philadelphia: J. B. Lippincott, 1976.

14

Hypnosis:
The Deep Down Dive

And the Lord God caused a deep sleep to fall upon Adam, and he slept: and he took one of his ribs, and closed up the flesh instead thereof.*

"TRIPPING"

Your eyelids begin to flutter, and as they close, you feel yourself slowly sinking into the stuffed chair. The muscles of your body relax, and soon you are surrounded by quiet. Yet within you, the feelings are intense.

First, there is a slight tingling of the toes, and then the fingertips react with their own mini-pulsations. Soon these pleasant vibrations spread throughout your body, and a sensation of chilling warmth permeates your very being.

* Genesis 2:21.

"So, this is hypnosis!" Other changes are now superimposed—a calf muscle twitches; an arm feels numb; a foot feels light.

"I can't even hear myself breathe." And your heart beats slower, and your mouth gets moist.

"Where is my nose? Do I still have my toes?" Your body feels suspended in space, relieved of weight, relieved of tension. The mind begins to unfurl its treasure trove of images, and the "trip" begins.

It starts with a yellow haze that gradually dissipates. As the view unfolds, a typical beach scene is evident. It is a sun-drenched afternoon. The sea is calm, the sand glistens, and *you* are there.

You don't ask how you got there or why you chose this place. You accept the reality of the moment, and are part of it.

"The sun is really intense today and that water looks so inviting. I think I'll take a swim." You let the lukewarm waves caress your body, and sensation is more than pleasant.

Still, there is the body-mind dichotomy: Part of you is back in that quiet, dark room, comfortably relaxed and dozing off; and part of you is squinting from the sun while basking in nature's water bed. But it doesn't matter—it is perfectly natural, nothing to ponder over. So you continue the trip.

And then the day changes, and the water is colder. Now you are swimming steadily and smoothly toward an isolated island. "When I get there I'll just lie in the sand and sleep." Your pulse rate quickens, your breathing is rapid, and your muscles contract. You make it to dry land and flop on the sand, where the warmth pervades your body. Your pulse rate slackens, your breathing is slow, and your muscles relax. You look up at the sun, and close your eyes; and your mind takes over for another trip.

Soon you become part of a pastoral scene. You turn and see a field of flowers with daisies in bloom. You reach out toward the flowers, and they entwine you, engulf you, enrapture you. You feel your presence in the field at the same time that you sense your being in the stuffed chair. The fragrance seems to come from both places so that the wonderful aroma becomes part of you.

You feel such inner tranquility, but know it is time—and time takes precedence. So you begin to move, and the mist returns. You stretch, and darkness supervenes. Finally, you sigh and open your eyes.

"So that was hypnosis!"

THE NATURE OF HYPNOSIS[1-4]

But what is hypnosis really? Although many articles and books have been written on the subject, we still know very little about its true nature. What do we know?

Well, it is known that hypnosis is related to suggestibility, the ability to readily accept and act upon suggestions. Generally speaking, the more easily an individual will uncritically accept ideas and concepts, the more easily will he be hypnotized. But hypnosis is much more than just suggestibility.

Hypnosis is also related to an individual's ability to focus or concentrate his attention on something. The object of the concentration may be a fixed point, an outside noise, a specific smell, a mental image or even a silently repeated sound. But mere concentration does not denote hypnosis.

The act of concentrating upon something allows the field of awareness to become narrowed. Other external or internal stimuli tend to become blocked out. It then becomes easier for suggestions to enter the individual's secondary consciousness.*

It is also known that monotony is important in inducing hypnosis. It can be the constant pitter-patter of falling raindrops, a speaker's boring, repetitive tone, a candle's flickering flame or the constant internal repetition of a word.

To be hypnotized, we must desire it. Contrary to public belief, it is usually not possible to hypnotize someone against his will. This knowledge lets us know something else about hypnosis. The more an individual desires it, the easier it is for him to be hypnotized. Motivation is a key factor. People in extreme pain or fear often are the best hypnotic subjects. The reason is related to their great need for outside assistance.

It has also been observed that children often are more easily hypotized than adults. It may be that they usually have more vivid imaginations and do not have the "hang-ups" of their elders.

THE HYPNOTIC TRANCE

We now have established that hypnosis is more easily induced in motivated and suggestible people, and that concentration and

---

* There is controversy over whether we can talk logically about concepts such as the mind, the unconscious or the subconscious because these "areas" have never been pinpointed in the human nervous system. Hence, we use the term "secondary consciousness" to designate that part of a person's mental functioning that he is not aware of in the alert state.

monotony are important in reaching the hypnotic state. But what is this state? What is a hypnotic trance? Can it be measured?

We do know that there are two basic phases of hypnosis, the induction procedure and the trance itself. The methods that facilitate hypnotic induction (e.g., fixation, monotony) have already been covered. In a subsequent section the various means of induction are discussed. Hence, let us now focus on the trance.

The trance is the component of the hypnotic state that follows the induction phase. At times it is difficult to determine the exact point where induction ends and trance begins. With the eye-fixation method, trance is usually considered to begin when the eyes close.

The hypnotic trance has been the subject of many research projects. Studies have been made of blood pressure, pulse rate, breathing rate, brain wave patterns, body temperature, eye movements, muscle changes and skin responses. To date, no changes have been found that would clearly differentiate the hypnotic state from the awake state[1,5]—partly because different types and stages of hypnosis were studied.

When a subject is under hypnosis, he may be able to do various things. Some individuals can only achieve a light trance. In a light trance, a person often feels relaxed, both mentally and physically, but he is completely aware of his surroundings. In a medium trance, an individual is often able to take a mental "trip" and achieve an even deeper state of relaxation. A deep trance is called the somnambulist stage.* In this state, a person can generally realize the more distinctive phenomena of hypnosis, which include the following:

1. Hand levitation; a hand or an arm rises, apparently of its own free will.
2. Eyelid catalepsy—an inability to open the eyes.
3. Limb rigidity; an arm or a leg locks in a straightened position.
4. Automatic writing; a hand appears to write of its own free will.
5. Automatic movements; a hand or a leg moves continuously.
6. Dream induction; vivid dreams occur easily.
7. Dissociation—an ability to feel either as if one is in two places at the same time or that one can separate the mental from the physical state.

* Related to the term somnambulism; the ability to walk while in a deep state of sleep. However, in hypnosis, the subject is presumed not to be asleep.

8. Hallucination—to be able to see, smell, hear or feel objects that are not present (known as positive hallucination) or not to see, smell, hear or feel objects that are present (known as negative hallucination).
9. Age regression and progression; the former is the ability to go back in time, while the latter is the belief that one can go ahead into the future.
10. Amnesia—to be able to forget that which has occurred during the hypnotic state.
11. Posthypnotic suggestibility—to act out at a later time, a suggestion given by the hypnotist.
12. Analgesia—the ability not to perceive pain (perhaps, more appropriately, an example of a negative hallucination).

Not all of these phenomena are seen in the people who can achieve a deep trance. On the other hand, these phenomena may be seen in some individuals who are in medium and even light stages. But generally, the deeper the state a person can reach, the more probable it is that these things will occur.

The lack of consistency found in objective measurements taken with respect to hypnosis may be due to the stage a subject is in and the task being performed while he is being monitored. For example, if one were in a light state and relaxing, the pulse and breathing rates would probably decrease. However, if one were in a deep state and engaged in automatic writing (i.e., doing work), the pulse and breathing rates would likely increase.

These opposite results were obtained in the first of the studies previously reported on at Temple University.[6] Hypnosis, meditation and simple relaxation were compared in this study. As part of the investigation, relaxation-hypnosis was compared with task-hypnosis. The task the subjects were asked to work at while under hypnosis was to obtain numbness of the right hand. The subjects were continually monitored during the two types of hypnosis for blood pressure, pulse rate, breathing rate, slow alpha brain wave patterns and skin resistance levels.

An alteration in skin resistance level is indicative of minute changes in sweating. When an individual is relaxed, sweating decreases, and skin resistance goes up.

Under the condition of relaxation-hypnosis, it was found that blood pressure, pulse rate and breathing rate decreased, while skin resistance and slow alpha brain waves increased. Under the condition of task-hypnosis, the opposite results were found. Hence, the mixed results seem to show that the objective measurements, in and of themselves, do not indicate when one is under hypnosis.

Can the hypnotic state be inferred from subjective feelings? Even these subjective reports are difficult to evaluate. Some people report that all they feel is relaxation. These individuals tend to achieve only a light state of hypnosis. Probably about 90% of the population can achieve this stage. In this phase, the body sensations have been described as tingling, numbness, heaviness, warmth, floating, lightness and chills. Outside sounds tend to become distant and distorted. There is a slight air of unreality, and yet the individual knows where he is and why he's there.

About 70% of the population can get into a medium trance. At this stage, an individual begins to feel even more relaxed, almost as if his body were weightless. It becomes easier for him mentally to leave his present surroundings. Various scenes can be visualized, and the subject begins to become part of them (as in the introductory story). Reality is still present at this stage, and the individual is aware of his identity and environment. Often in this phase, people may achieve some degree of control over pain (analgesia).

About 20% of the population are capable of entering a deep trance. This stage is believed by some hypnotists to be the only true state of hypnosis. The other stages are considered just forms of deep relaxation. However, most authorities designate somnambulism as the deepest stage in hypnosis. In this phase, the person is usually the most relaxed, both mentally and physically.

The mental images are most intense in this state, and the person may recall memories better than in the awake state. The subject may actually believe that he is somewhere else. For instance, he may believe that he has left his body in the place where the session was taking place and taken himself to another place and even another time. Sensations can become intense, including sight, sound, smell and touch. Many subjects report pleasurable feelings that are almost ecstatic in nature.

In this deepest stage, it is often possible not to feel pain and to control autonomic nervous system functions such as breathing, heart beat, blood pressure and salivation. With all this, this person is not a "zombie." Although it is difficult to substantiate, many authorities believe that even in this deep state most subjects are still aware of reality.[1-4] They still know that they are back in the place of the hypnotic session even though they are somewhere else in their imagination. The explanation for this "double life" may lie in the fact that the deeply hypnotized subject takes everything literally. The individual simply does not initiate thinking or attempt to reason. For instance, he does not consider it illogical that he is back home on his fortieth birthday and in an office simultaneously—the incongruity is merely accepted.

THE HYPNOTIC STATE

Now that the factors in induction, the stages, and the subjective feelings of hypnosis have been described, let us try to arrive at some definition of the state. Hypnosis may be considered as an altered state of awareness in which an individual achieves varying degrees of relaxation, subjective changes in body image, certain distortions of reality, and the ability to exert some control over autonomic nervous system functions.[7] Since some people can achieve many of these various things while alert under proper motivation, there are authorities who state that hypnosis does not exist as a separate state, but is merely role playing.[8] However, most investigators consider hypnosis to be separate and distinct from the awake or relaxed states.[1-4,6,7]

As part of the Temple University study, each subject was asked to compare his subjective feelings of relaxation and hypnosis.[6] It has been shown that people who participate in a study in which a well-known technique is compared with a control expect that they would do better with the popular technique[9] Thus, most subjects would expect to do better with hypnosis or meditation than with simple relaxation.

It also has been shown that since it is possible voluntarily to control autonomic functions (e.g., heart beat, breathing rate), some subjects may actually do better under hypnosis or meditation. This can occur even if the experimenter says nothing to the subjects about the expectations of the experiment. Ideally, the subjects should not be told that they are even using hypnosis or meditation. However, because of the regulations of the Temple University Commission of Human Experimentation, all subjects had to told of the nature of the experiment.

In order to offset the bias of the subjects, they were told prior to the sessions that the results to date had shown no significant differences among hypnosis, meditation and simple relaxation with respect to the various parameters being tested (pulse rate, breathing rate, skin resistance levels, blood pressure, slow alpha waves and muscle activity). It was felt that this precaution would dissuade the subjects from deliberately trying to do better under hypnosis or meditation.

In the next chapter, the physiological findings of this study are discussed in detail. As far as the subjective feelings were concerned, over 95% of the 48 subjects reported that they were completely alert and aware of everything that was occurring during the relaxation condition. However, a great difference was felt both mentally and physically between hypnosis and the alert state. This even held true for those people who had physiological changes with relaxation similar to or larger than those with hypnosis. For instance, some subjects showed a greater decrease in breathing rate, heart rate and blood pressure with simple relaxation than with hypnosis. Yet they felt subjectively that relaxation was similar to the awake state and hypnosis was completely different. Hence, it may be inferred that either there is a real difference, or that the result is due to the subjects' expectations that they would feel differently under hypnosis as compared to simple relaxation.

COMMON HYPNOTIC PHENOMENA

Even though it is generally thought that about 10% of the population are not capable of being hypnotized, this is probably not true. Given strong motivation and appropriate hypnotic conditions, almost anyone can enter at least a light trance.

To support this position, let's look at three common occurrences. There is a phenomenon called "highway hypnosis," which most superhighway drivers have experienced. The fixed hypnotic point is often the sun's reflections on the road, which produce a water mirage. This "wet" area is sustained for long periods of time and tends to fatigue the eyes. The roads themselves are usually straight with few distractions, thus tending to increase the monotony, which helps in the hypnotic induction. These factors probably contribute to highway accidents and to drivers' missing their exits.

Daydreaming is a second example of a hypnotic phenomenon. It frequently occurs when one reads a book, watches TV, listens to a speaker or runs. The attention of the individual may not be fully engaged in the ongoing activity, and it may be that the repetitive or boring aspects tend to divide his attention and promote daydreaming.

Another well-known instance of a hypnotic phenomenon may occur when one looks for a familiar object that has been misplaced. For example, a person places a pen on his desk but not in its usual place. As much as he tries, he cannot find it. Someone else comes into the room, asks about the problem and immediately locates the pen. What has occurred is known as a negative hallucination. This phenomenon tends to occur when someone is overly tired and, thus, amenable to self-hypnosis.

MISCONCEPTIONS AND FALLACIES

Now that we know something about what hypnosis is presumed to be, let us examine what it seems not to be. Let us also consider the misconceptions and the fallacies about hypnosis First of all, hypnosis is not sleep. The brain wave patterns are different, and the subjective perceptions are not the same.[10] However, if an individual is tired, hypnosis can easily lead to sleep. Hypnosis is also not dreaming, although dreamlike images can be visualized during hypnosis.

Hypnosis is not a form of meditation, although relaxation-hypnosis is related to meditation (see next chapter). Hypnosis is not a state of amnesia, although in a deep stage it is possible to forget some of the occurrences. Usually, a hypnotized subject can recall most of what has happened.

Hypnosis is not merely a conditioned reflex, although some of the reactions by subjects who are in a deep trance appear to be automatic. This assumption may be easily tested by instructing the hypnotized subject to cease the given activity. If it were a reflex not under one's control, it would continue.

Hypnosis is not an electrical or magnetic phenomenon in which a hypnotist transfers or extracts energy from another person. The contemporary belief is that all hypnosis is really self-hypnosis. The hypnotist serves as a guide to the subject, who achieves the deep state of relaxation and who gains control over certain functions and feelings.

The poorly understood phenomena of extrasensory perception (ESP), thought transference and medium seánce activity appear to be enhanced during a hypnotic trance. But nobody knows if there is any actual transfer of energy or if in fact any abnormal or unusual changes do occur.

During hypnosis, a person does not lose control to the hypnotist. As we have said, the individual is still aware of his surroundings. A person does not do anything against his moral, ethical or personal code. Hypnosis does not alter a person's way of behavior. However, a person under hypnosis may act differently than he would if he were completely awake. It is somewhat similar to the unloosening effect of a couple of drinks. It also could be compared to the wearing of a mask at a masquerade party. In that disguise, the person might feel free to alter his behavior. Nevertheless, the individual is still aware of his principles and—unless he really wanted to—would not deliberately violate them.

A person is not and does not become weak-willed if he can be hypnotized. Just the opposite seems to be true. If an individual can achieve a deep enough state so that he can relax completely and alter some of his autonomic responses (e.g., breathing rate, heart rate), this indicates good control. In the usual case, long-range effects of hypnosis are beneficial rather than damaging.

If a person is hypnotized by a trained physician, dentist or psychologist, he does not have to fear that he will be made to perform stupid acts. Many people have seen stage demonstrations of hypnosis in which people bark like a dog, lie still as a board while supporting a weight or do other theatrical tricks. The ethics of their profession prohibits doctors from engaging in such conduct.

Another worry is the fear of not being able to come out of the trance. Even if the hypnotist should die, the person would shortly come back to the normal state, or else the trance would convert into normal sleep. Frequently, people do not want to awaken because they are enjoying the state too much. A little gentle prodding usually brings them around rapidly.

DANGERS OF HYPNOSIS

Having dispelled some commonly held misconceptions, we now examine the possible dangers in the use of hypnosis. If a person is psychotic or pre-psychotic, it is possible for hypnosis to induce a bizarre reaction. Hence, only those doctors trained to deal with such individuals should employ hypnosis.

There is danger in employing hypnosis to remove an unwanted habit. For instance, a posthypnotic suggestion can inhibit smoking, but it may also remove that which serves to keep the individual functional.

Prolonged, continual use of hypnosis could lead to habituation, idling and withdrawal. If a person spent most of the day in a trance, it is easy to see that very little of a useful nature would be accomplished.

In the recent mass suicide in Jonestown, Guyana, hypnosis may have been a factor (although this has not been verified). Individuals with strong "personalities," such as the Reverend Jim Jones and Adolph Hitler, markedly influenced people's behavior. Some authorities believe that the subsequent negative group activities such as suicide and murder resulted from mass hypnosis. However, people can be influenced to perform antisocial and immoral activities without being hypnotized.

Aside from these hazards, hypnosis can be used on anyone provided that it is employed by a qualified practitioner.

HISTORY OF HYPNOSIS[1-4,9]

Now that we have some idea of what is meant by hypnosis, let us briefly consider how it began. It may be that God was the first hypnotist. According to the Bible, Adam was put in a momentary sleep (hypnotic trance?) so that a rib could be removed for the creation of Eve.

Apparently, hypnosis has been employed since the dawn of history. Primitive man seems to have used trances for healing purposes. The "laying-on of hands" has been used in many religions to effect divinely inspired cures. It is possible that many of the cures effected by the biblical prophets were based on suggestibility, trance induction and control of autonomic functions. In the Middle Ages, the kings of England and France were also believed to have miraculous powers of curing. It is probable that the positive results were based on suggestion.

The modern origins of hypnosis can be traced to the work of Franz Mesmer in the late 1700s. He came to believe that there was a transfer of magnetic energy from himself to his patients. There is a description of him dressed in a silken robe and effecting his cures with the help of an iron wand. Mesmer believed that the planets influenced human health by their effect on an invisible magnetic fluid that all people possessed. It was his willpower that caused change in this fluid and thereby resulted in cures of various disorders. By making "passes" over the patient's body, Mesmer believed that magnetic fluid was transferred from his fingertips to the patient. This would allow for redistribution and eventual restoration of health.

Although Mesmer's basic premises are erroneous, he did actually get his patients into deep trances and must have had some effect on their many diseases (probably primarily psychosomatic). At the time, the medical fraternity considered him a charlatan. He had some followers though, and his work was kept alive for many years. The term describing the state was mesmerism. Up to the mid-1800s, the phenomenon was used primarily for stage appearances and rarely was used by physicians.

Around 1850, the physician James Braid saw a stage demonstration and was impressed; he soon began using the technique for medical and surgical purposes. He realized that magnetic energy was not involved, but that suggestibility was a key component. Braid then coined the term hypnosis* to describe the phenomenon. Other physicians began to use hypnosis, including Liebeault, Bernheim and Breuer. Joseph Breuer, in the 1880s, was the first practitioner to employ hypnosis for analysis.

Sigmund Freud also employed hypnosis early in his career, but apparently Freud was not a very effective hypnotist. He soon abandoned hypnosis, once he discovered the free association method. Hypnosis was again on the wane for many years as a result of the disapproval of Freud and other physicians.

However, during World War I a rapid form of psychotherapy was needed for symptom removal and treatment of war neurosis. Hypnotherapy then came back into more general use.

---

* Hypnosis is derived from "Hypnos," the name for the Greek god of sleep.

Within the last 20 years, both the American and the British medical societies have recognized hypnosis as an effective means of therapy in the hands of qualified doctors. Hence, at the present time hypnosis is used in medical, dental and psychologic practices. To the continued disapproval of organized professional hypnosis societies,* stage demonstrations of hypnosis are still given in a carnival atmosphere. It is hoped that the future will see licensing and regulation of the practice of hypnosis.

USES OF HYPNOSIS

Having examined hypnosis and explored its origins, we shall now look into its current uses. In medicine and dentistry, hypnosis is employed for fear removal, pain elimination, bleeding control and distraction[7,11] (see Fig. 14.1). In dentistry, hypnosis has been used successfully for patients allergic to "novocaine," to prevent gagging and to cause a diminution in the flow of saliva. Hypnosis is also effective for the elimination of deleterious dental habits such as thumbsucking, nailbiting, tongue thrusting and teeth grinding.

In medicine, hypnosis is employed for childbirth delivery, wart removal and treatment of drug abuse, smoking, alcoholism, high blood pressure, asthma and sleeplessness. It is used as a preventive measure for people who are susceptible to stress-related conditions such as stroke, heart diseases and headaches. An important medical use of hypnosis is for the determination and removal of deep-seated psychological conflicts. (These dental and medical uses are more fully covered in Chapters 16 and 17.)

Hypnosis can be useful in areas other than the health field. For instance, it is effective in helping many people develop better study habits. As a result of hypnosis, people seem to improve their memories, overcome the fear of taking exams, reduce "stage fright," become more aware of their surroundings, develop better interpersonal relationships and perform better in various sports. Most of these effects result from learning to relax through hypnosis, which is discussed in the latter part of this chapter.

* Society for Clinical and Experimental Hypnosis; American Society of Clinical Hypnosis; American Society of Psychosomatic Dentistry and Medicine.

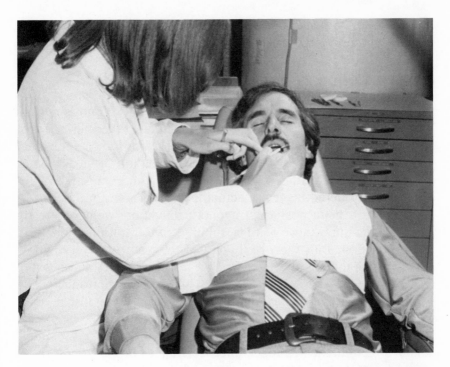

Fig. 14.1 Dental treatment under hypnosis. The author (DM) is having dental treatment performed on himself while under meditation-hypnosis. The dentist performing the treatment is
Carole N. Hildebrand. (From Morse, D. R. and Hildebrand, C. N., Case report: Use of TM in
periodontal therapy, *Dental Survey,* 52(11):36, 1976. Copyright© 1977 by Harcourt Brace
Jovanovich, Inc.)

Hypnosis is used in the legal field for the purpose of recalling
details of criminal incidents. The subject is placed under hypnosis
and asked to recall things that he might not remember in the awake
state (e.g., the license plate number of a car).

A more exotic use of hypnosis is in espionage. For instance, under
hypnosis a subject might be told a secret that he could only recall
when rehypnotized by another designated individual.

"Brainwashing" has been used in military situations. A "good"
hypnotic subject could become so disoriented that he would do
things that normally he would not do. For instance, a person might
be told under hypnosis that his fellow soldier was a traitor. The subject believing this might then shoot his "enemy." This would not be
against his moral code because he would be acting according to what

he believes to be the true situation.* The latter two uses of hypnosis are not ordinarily encountered.

FACTORS CONDUCIVE TO HYPNOSIS

Now that we are somewhat knowledgeable about hypnosis and its uses, it is appropriate to consider how it actually takes place. There are various techniques to induce and deepen hypnosis. An individual should learn hypnosis for treatment and prevention of medical conditions only from a trained doctor. Hence, the mechanisms of hypnosis are considered here, but actual techniques are not described.

In terms of the mechanics of hypnotic induction, we have already discussed the importance of suggestibility, concentration, monotony and motivation. But, this is only part of the picture. A very important consideration is the interpersonal relationship established between hypnotist and subject. Trust is of primary importance. The would-be subject must have implicit faith in the hypnotist because without this motivation, concentration is not possible.

How a hypnotist generates trust depends upon his personality, ability to communicate, appearance, tolerance and perseverance. A good hypnotist should be able to match his approach and technique to each subject. For instance, the hypnotist would assume a dominant role in the case where the person is used to following orders. The suggestion might be as follows: "Mr. Jones, I want you to listen to every word that I say and do exactly as I tell you."

For the individual who is more self-assured, the approach should be one of equal footing. The hypnotist might say the following: "Mr. Brown, I want you to be able to control your mind and body so that you will be more successful."

To the subject who has a fear of losing control, the hypnotist might say the following: "Mr. Smith, I will merely guide you. It is you yourself who is in control."

For the subject who says he cannot be hypnotized, but nevertheless wants it attempted, the hypnotist might resort to guile. For instance, he might talk about the weather or the details of a painting.

---

* Some people consider that the recent mass suicide in Jonestown, Guyana, resulted from Jim Jones's "brainwashing" of the entire "People's Temple" cult. The concept was that his followers were led to believe a "heavenly" future with Jones was preferable to their dismal present life on earth.

The idea is for the hypnotist to get the subject involved in something innocuous and then, when the subject's resistance is down, to make suggestions about deep relaxation that would not be perceived on a conscious level.

Some subjects require constant talking to for reinforcement; others find the hypnotist's chatter to be intrusive. Some individuals have vivid imaginations; for them, only vague descriptions are necessary. Others cannot visualize so readily; for them, a detailed word picture may be necessary.

Since the hypnotist is often the health practitioner as well, the subject must have complete trust in the capabilities of his doctor. Once under hypnosis, he is in the "hands of his doctor," much as in surgery.

Although it is not mandatory, hypnotic induction is facilitated in a quiet, darkened, pleasant environment. The reason is that distractions such as noise and bright lights tend to interfere with the induction and maintenance of the hypnotic state. However, this is not always the case. There are individuals who can effectively block out all distractions and can even be hypnotized with their eyes open.

Instead of having complete quiet, listening to soothing music can have a hypnotic effect. Another helpful factor is comfort. A soft, reclining chair is conducive to deep relaxation. This is also not mandatory, since some people can relax even in a hard, straight-backed chair.

Although drugs are definitely not recommended, it has been observed that hypnosis is often more readily induced in subjects who have taken tranquilizers or sedatives or who are given nitrous oxide and oxygen simultaneously.[12]

HYPNOTIC INDUCTION AND DEEPENING METHODS

Now that the factors conducive to hypnosis have been examined, let us consider a few of the induction methods.

The most popular method of hypnotic induction is the eye-fixation technique. The subject stares at an object while keeping his head motionless. Objects frequently used are fixed points, a moving pendulum, a flame, a finger, a pencil, a coin or even the hypnotist's eyes. As the subject concentrates, suggestions are given of progressive relaxation.

Another induction method is for an individual to concentrate on his arm and watch it rise as the hypnotist gives suggestions of arm elevation and progressive relaxation.

Rapid methods of hypnotic induction are often achieved when the subject closes his eyes immediately and silently counts backward, counts his breaths or repeats a word while the hypnotist gives suggestions of progressive relaxation.[7,13]

Once hypnosis is initiated, the state may be deepened by various means. In one popular method, the hypnotist describes a descending elevator or escalator ride that is associated with the subject's getting deeper into the trance. Another well-known method of enhancing the deepening is to describe a pleasant scene; e.g., walking down to the shore, taking a boat ride and cruising downstream. The authors have found that the silent repetition of a word is an effective means of deepening hypnosis.[7,13]

The subject comes out of the hypnotic state as the result of the hypnotist's suggestions. One popular method is to have the subject count backward from ten to one, with awakening occurring at the count of one. Also, like describing the deepening scene, the hypnotist can ask the subject to cruise upstream, get out of the boat, walk back from the shore and so on.

It must be reemphasized that the novice should not attempt to hypnotize someone, even though this superficial discussion makes it seem simple. The techniques are more complex than this presentation shows, but of even greater importance, untoward reactions can occur with some people. Therefore, only a trained doctor should employ hypnosis where the human body and mental activities are involved. As far as self-hypnosis is concerned, that is the next topic to be considered.

SELF-HYPNOSIS

Self-hypnosis (auto-hypnosis) is a technique whereby an individual brings himself into a state of hypnosis. Just as was said with regard to induced hypnosis, we believe that an individual should not hypnotize himself for medical, dental or psychological reasons unless he has been so trained by a doctor.

However, for purposes of relaxation, self-learned self-hypnosis is permissible. There are two reasons for this. First, as has been described, in the early stage of hypnosis physical and mental relaxation occurs. Therefore, there is no need to go any deeper. Second, with only a superficial depth of hypnosis, untoward reactions are held to a minimum. Also, it is difficult for an individual to get himself into a deep enough state through auto-suggestion. While hetero-hypnosis* is more effective for most people, the primary purpose of self-hypnosis is for relaxation, and for this, great depths are not necessary.

Techniques of self-hypnosis are similar to those for hetero-hypnosis. A popular method is for an individual to stare at a fixed object while suggesting to himself muscular relaxation beginning with the tips of the toes and going all the way to the top of the head. When the eyes begin to tire, they tend to close. The subject then programs himself to take a mental trip to a pleasant place. A more detailed description of a self-hypnosis–meditation combined technique is given in the next chapter.

Other techniques, which are variations of self-hypnosis are progressive relaxation and autogenic training.

PROGRESSIVE RELAXATION

In 1938, progessive relaxation was devised by Edmund Jacobson in the United States.[14] In this technique the subject closes his eyes and concentrates on different parts of the body in order to relax them in turn. It is practiced in six stages, starting with the arms, followed by the legs, breathing, the forehead and the eyes and ending with the muscles of larynx. Pain and anxiety often decrease when progressive relaxation is employed. This method is often used in conjunction with the eye-fixation method of hypnosis.

AUTOGENIC TRAINING

In 1932, autogenic training was introduced by J. H. Schultz in Germany and popularized by Wolfgang Luthe.[15] Individuals are taught to gain self-initiated control over feelings of anxiety. The subject closes his eyes and passively concentrates on a brief set of mental exercises. Training takes place over a period of several weeks.

* Hetero-hypnosis is hypnosis induced by another person, as opposed to self- or auto-hypnosis.

The trainee makes mental contact with different parts of his body while responding to verbal cues. These include the following: "My right arm is heavy; my right arm is warm"; "My heart is beating calmly and regularly"; "My breathing is calm and regular"; "My abdomen is warm"; and "My forehead is cool."

As is the case with relaxation-hypnosis, subjects report sensations of warmth, heaviness, coolness and a slowing of the heart and breathing rate. In the method of autogenic training, these responses are noted and reinforced. However, it can be seen that both progressive relaxation and autogenic training are still methods of self-hypnosis.

SUMMARY

Hypnosis is neither a magical nor a mystical state. It is rather an altered state of awareness in which, among other things, an individual can control certain autonomic nervous system functions. Of direct concern to us here is the ability to relax and block out psychological stressors. Not everyone is a good hypnotic subject, but those who can be hypnotized and learn self-hypnosis usually find it to be an excellent relaxation method.

In the next chapter, another excellent relaxation method, meditation, is considered, and its relationship to hypnosis is examined.

REFERENCES

1. Crasilneck, H. B. and Hall, J. A. *Clinical Hypnosis: Principles and Applications.* New York: Grune & Stratton, 1975.
2. Frankel, F. H. *Trance as a Coping Mechanism.* New York: Plenum Medical, 1976.
3. Bowers, K. S. *Hypnosis for the Seriously Curious.* Monterey, Calif.: Brooks/Cole, 1976.
4. Erickson, M. H., Rossi, E. L. and Rossi, S. I. *Hypnotic Realities: The Introduction of Clinical Hypnosis and forms of Indirect Suggestion.* New York: Irvington Publ. Inc., 1976.
5. Crasilneck, H. S. and Hall, J. A. Physiological changes associated with hypnosis: A review of the literature since 1948. *Int. J. Clin. Exp. Hypn.* 7:9–49, 1959.
6. Morse, D. R., Martin, J. S., Furst, M. L. and Dubin, L. L. A physiological and subjective evaluation of meditation, hypnosis and relaxation. *Psychosom. Med.* 39:304–324, 1977.

7. Morse, D. R. Hypnosis in the practice of endodontics. *J. Am. Soc. Psychosom. Dent. Med.* 22:17–22, 1975.
8. Barber, T. X. *Hypnosis: A Scientific Approach.* New York: Van Nostrand Reinhold, 1969.
9. Shor, R. E. and Orne, M. T. *The Nature of Hypnosis.* New York: Holt, Rinehart and Winston, Inc., 1965.
10. Diamant, J., Dufek, M., Hoskovec, J., Kristof, M., Perárek, V., Roth, B. and Velek, M. An electroencephalographic study of the waking state and hypnosis with particular reference to subclinical manifestations of sleep activity. *Int. J. Clin. Exp. Hypn.* 8:199–212, 1960.
11. Hilgard, E. R. and Hilgard, J. R. *Hypnosis in the Relief of Pain.* Los Altos, Calif.: William Kaufman, 1975.
12. Carnow, R. Hypnosis and N_2O-O_2 sedation *J. Nat. Anal. Soc.* 3(3):47–61, 1974.
13. Morse, D. R. Use of a meditative state for hypnotic induction in the practice of endodontics. *Oral. Surg.* 41:664–672, 1976.
14. Jacobson, E. *Anxiety and Tension Control.* Philadelphia: J. B. Lippincott, 1964.
15. Luthe, W. *Autogenic Training.* New York: Grune & Stratton, 1969.

15

Meditation: The Silent Word Game

In the beginning was the Word, and the Word was with God, and the Word was God.*

THE MYSTICAL SOUND OF SILENCE**

With poetic license, impressions and reflections of a first mantra-type meditation are presented.

> A sound is heard
> An eerie word
> I close my eyes
> I hear its vibes
>
> I speak it softly
> I feel it gently

---

* The Gospel According to St. John 1:1.
** By D. R. Morse. From Morse, D. R. and Furst, M. L., *Stress and Relaxation: Application to Dentistry,* 1978. Courtesy of Charles C Thomas, Publisher, Springfield, Illinois.

And my limbs lighten
As my thoughts quicken

Then the sound repeats
In rhythmic beats
And my mind retreats
From its daily feats

Thoughts come and go
My breathing's slow
And the sound repeats
With leisure beats

And my toes tingle
As new thoughts mingle
And the sound repeats
With lulling beats

My mind is still
Without a will
Then the sound repeats
With quiet beats

And then no mind
No thoughts to find
And the sound repeats
In silent beats

A yawn, a sigh
A stretch, a cry
Then the sound retreats
And my mind's at peace

THE NATURE OF MEDITATION

Definition

Many people have heard of meditation, but few know what it is really like. Therefore, let us first define meditation and then give some examples.

Meditation may be considered an altered state of awareness in which an individual achieves varying degrees of relaxation, subjective changes in body image, certain distortions of reality and the ability to decrease autonomic nervous system functions. As may be seen, this definition is similar to the one that was given for hypnosis. Without further amplification, the reader might assume that the two states are identical. However, there are some critical differences.

One difference is related to concentration or control. In self-hypnotic induction, an individual deliberately concentrates on something—an object, a speaker's voice, a mental picture, a mental task (e.g., counting backward) or a part of the body.

Types of Meditation

There are several types of meditation.[1-5] Some are identical to self-hypnosis in the induction phase. In these, concentration is also used (i.e., active techniques). Meditation can take place with the eyes either open or closed.

Contemplative. When the eyes are open, the individual concentrates on an external object. This has been called contemplative (external) meditation. In Yoga, the object of concentration is called a Yantra. If the object is a drawing or painting with a typical multicolored square within a circle design (symbolizing unity of micro-and macro-cosmos), it is called a mandala. Other forms that have been used for external concentration are statues, crucifixes, pictures, flowers, colors, inscriptions, the sun, the moon, stars and planets, the sea and candle flames. With partially closed eyes, one can concentrate on the tip of the nose (nasal gaze).

Concentrative. With the eyes closed, concentration is on a mental picture (internal). It can be part of the body as in Zen (Buddhism) and Yoga (Hinduism) meditations. In one technique, concentration is on the navel. In another, one mentally fixates on a spot inside the center of the forehead. This is the frontal or "third eye gaze." With Kundalini meditation, concentration is on specific parts of the body.

With other closed-eye concentration techniques, a mental image is used. In Hindu and Buddhist methods, the thousand-petal lotus flower can be employed. In Christianity, a crucifix or a sacred rose may be the internal object. With Judaism, it can be a Star of David. In Islam, the crescent moon is a favorite mental picture. Concentration can also be on the sound of one's breathing. In one Zen practice, a meditator mentally examines a koan, which is an apparently unsolvable riddle. A favorite illustration is, "What is the sound of one hand clapping?" In some techniques, one observes thoughts without clinging to them.

Physical. With certain aborigines, chants, drum beating (and other music) and dancing are used to induce hypnoticlike trances. These practices can also bring on meditative states. Shamanism is a mystical practice that is common with tribes in Africa, the Americas, Indonesia, Japan and Siberia. Singing, chanting and drum-beating are used to induce trancelike states. In Sufism, a mystical Islamic practice, constant repetition of God's name is used along with rhythmic breathing, music and dance for meditation. A Buddhist method is Nichiren Shoshu practice. A specific chant, "Nam-Myoko-Renge-Kyo," is constantly repeated in this meditative method. Quaker meetings with their vocal chants can result in hypnotic or meditativelike states. In T'ai Chi, a Taoist practice, graceful body movements are used to bring on a state of meditation.

The use of "worry beads" could also be considered as a form of physical meditation. The author (DM) had a Hare Krishna practitioner as a patient. All during the dental procedure, the patient fondled the worry beads while placing himself into a deep meditative state.

Thus, it may be seen that with contemplative (external), concentrative (internal), and physical (chants, music, dance) meditative methods, the beginning phases are practically identical to self-hypnotic inductions.

Mantra Meditation. The most popular meditation is mantra* meditation. A strict definition of a mantra is a Sanskrit syllable, word or phrase derived from one of the ancient Hindu texts that is used to induce a state of meditation. However, we shall use the term for any word or phrase that is used in a repetitive manner to bring on a meditative state. The sound is generally repeated silently with the eyes closed.

Depending upon the viewpoint, mantra meditation involves concentration or nonconcentration. With many Hindu practices, mantras are holy and meaningful words. They are believed to have great

* The correct Sanskrit term is mántra, although in common English usage the acute accent has been dropped.[5]

power, possibly even supernatural powers. The most sacred mantra is the syllable "om" ("aum"). It is the highest symbol of Brahman and is related to the creation. Other mantras are symbols of various deities. From this standpoint, the power of a mantra is related to its mystical meaning and an individual's attention to that meaning. Attention requires definite concentration. Use of mantra meditation in this way is similar to self-hypnotic induction.

Maharishi Mahesh Yogi, the founder of Transcendental Meditation (TM), has derived a number of mantras from the ancient Vedic Hindu tradition for use in the TM technique. These mantras are not primarily used for their mystical meanings. In fact, they are supposed to have no real meanings, but are employed for their vibrating or soothing effects on the mind and body. The Maharishi personally trains the TM instructors to select one of these mantras for an individual who is being initiated into the TM technique.* The selection is supposedly based on the personality and behavioral characteristics of each subject.

However, as mentioned in Chapter 13, it now appears that there are only a few TM mantras, and age is the only basis for assignment.[6,7] An individual being inducted into the TM program receives his mantra from a TM teacher during a semireligious ceremony. The inductee brings fruit and flowers into an incense-filled room and emerges with his own gift—a mantra that he is told never to disclose to anyone. He is further warned not to speak the sound aloud or even think it when he is not meditating. Should he not follow this advice, the power of the mantra would be lost. However, there is no evidence that the disclosure of one's mantra makes any difference whatsoever.[7]

The most important apparent difference in types of meditation lies between the active meditative techniques and the passive TM technique in which the mantra is supposed to be used effortlessly.[8] That is, no conscious effort is made to concentrate, and the sound (mantra) is repeated at any pace. If thoughts intrude, they are allowed to be completed; i.e., when realization occurs, then the mantra is repeated. Although TM teachers emphasize that concentration is not

---

* Formerly all TM teachers were personally instructed in Switzerland by the Maharishi. Presently, a few experienced TM teachers have also taken the role of instructing new teachers.

used, investigators point out that the mental effort required to return to the repetition of the mantra is a form of concentration.

Still, it is apparent that intense concentration is not used with TM. This was verified in the first study undertaken by the authors at Temple University.[9] As part of that study, mantra meditation and hypnosis were compared with respect to the activity of scalp muscles. When a person concentrates, there is a good possibility that those muscles of the head will contract. It was found that muscle activity was twice as frequent during hypnosis as it was during mantra meditation. (See Fig. 15.1.)

However, muscle contraction usually occurred during the induction of hypnosis, when the subject was concentrating on an object. Once the eyes closed, the muscle activity stopped. Therefore, comparing just the actual trance with meditation, it was found that there was practically no muscle contraction discernible during either technique.

Thus, it can be stated that one difference between eye-fixation self-hypnotic inductions and TM is the lack of concentration in the latter. Yet, the induction methods may still be similar.

One of the bases of hypnotic induction is the use of a repetitive stimulus to the central nervous system. This can be in the form of a constant monotonous voice or a flickering flame. Both are externally-originating methods that permit suggestions easily to enter the secondary consciousness, resulting in a hypnotic trance.

On the other hand, the constant repetition of a mantra is an internally-originating method of repetitive stimulation to the central nervous system. This also allows for the subsequent development of a hypnotic trance.[10] In the early part of this century, Emile Coué developed techniques of self-hypnosis.[11] A popular phrase that he had individuals repeat was: "Every day in every way I am getting better and better." At the time, it was considered a pseudoscientific approach. However, it is now reminiscent of current meditative techniques. Another well-known technique for inducing self-hypnosis is based on the constant repetition of the word "relax."

Is it essential to use a Sanskrit mantra to meditate effectively? There is a difference of opinion on this point. TM teachers state that it is necessary that the mantra be personally assigned by a trained instructor as part of a specific initiating process.[2,8] Benson has shown

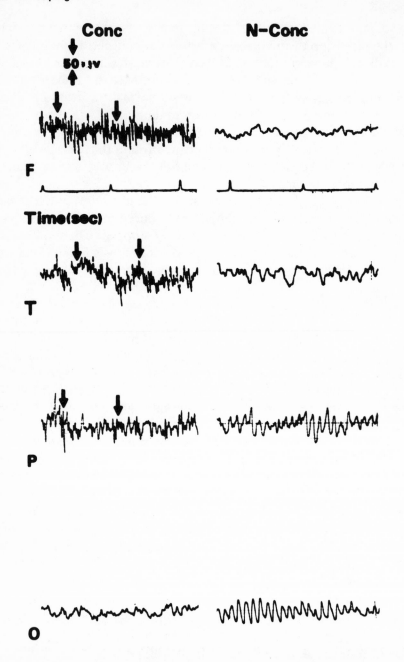

Fig. 15.1 Muscle activity during hypnosis and meditation. Conc = the concentration involved during the inductive phase of eye-fixation hypnosis; N-Conc = the absence of concentration

in his studies that the use of the word "one" coordinated with each out-breath is just as effective.[3] Carrington permits trainees to choose their own mantras from a list of 16, and she reported obtaining results similar to TM.*[5] Since Benson did not examine brainwave patterns, it is claimed by some that he did not prove that the use of the word "one" coupled with breathing out is comparable to the TM and CSM methods.

Research now in progress by Bernard Glueck at the Institute of Living in Hartford, Connecticut, suggests that brainwave patterns for TM and CSM do differ from the brainwave patterns found in Benson's technique. In both TM and CSM the mantras are repeated at any pace. With Benson's method, the mantra is repeated only on exhalation. Carrington has suggested that the difference in brainwave patterns is apparently related to the extra concentration required to link a mantra with every out-breath.**

As part of the aforementioned study at Temple University, TM meditators were compared with subjects assigned a simple word for meditation.[9] As was the case with the TM subjects, the subjects who were assigned a simple word repeated the word at any pace. They had no previous training in meditation. Words that were offered included the following: "one," "om," "flower," "garden," "sail," "ocean," "fishing" and "rock." Each subject chose his own word. During the meditation, both groups (TM and simple-word subjects) were monitored for breathing rate, pulse rate, blood pressure, skin resistance levels, slow alpha brain waves and muscle activity. The results were similar for both groups of meditators. Hence, at least with respect to physiological measures, these findings seem to negate the proposition that TM mantras are unique. (Criteria for selection of mantras are discussed later.)

In the previously mentioned clinical study in which the author

---

* Carrington's technique is known as Clinically Standardized Meditation (CSM). It involves no religious initiating ceremony and is a simple nonconcentrative form of meditation.
** P. Carrington, Personal communication, 1978.

---

during meditation; uv = microvolts; F, T, P, and O are four scalp areas in which the electrodes are placed (F = frontal; T = temporal; P = parietal; and O = occipital). Large arrows point to areas of muscle concentration. With respect to this subject, there is intense muscle activity during hypnotic induction in the frontal, temporal and parietal scalp areas. (From Morse et al., 1977. *Psychosom. Med.* 39:305–324. Reprinted with permission of Elsevier North-Holland, Inc.)

(DM) used meditation for hypnotic induction, it was found that TM meditators using their own mantras got into a hypnotic trance a few minutes sooner than subjects who were assigned a word.[10] Some of the following possibilities could account for this finding:

1. The Sanskrit word has no meaning to most individuals. Hence, no subjective impressions would interfere with its monotonous effect.

2. The mantra is chosen specifically for the subject, and it is not supposed to be disclosed. Because of this, it may more likely command his attention and be used regularly. It might be considered a gift, and as such would probably have a facilitating effect. It may also act as a signal to the meditator that he should feel relaxed and as such might have the effect of a conditioned reflex.[12]

3. The TM meditators all had been practicing longer than the subjects who were assigned a word. Hence, the effect would make it easier for them to get deeper more rapidly.

4. Finally, there may be specific effects from the Sanskrit words. There is some research to show that sounds that resonate and rise slowly may decrease heart rate and help induce relaxation.[12] However, Benson's, Carrington's and our findings seem to show that the effect, if it occurs, is not limited to Sanskrit words.

So far in our clinical and research studies we have taught simple-word meditation to about 200 subjects.[9,10,13-16] The various words used for meditation included the following: "one," "aum," "flower," "garden," "sail," "fishing," "rock," "love" and "hate." Physiologically, it was found that it didn't really matter what word was repeated—the effects were similar. Subjectively, most of the subjects reported that the word—regardless of which one it was—lost its meaning, usually by the halfway point of the meditation. This reinforces the idea mentioned in Chapter 14, that the repetitive sounds of a mantra is similar to the repetitive stimulus that induces hypnosis. For instance, the constant, monotonous voice of the hypnotist and staring at the flame of a candle, both send repetitive stimuli to the central nervous system which tend to make the person languid and receptive to suggestions. The repetitive mantra appears to do practically the same thing.

In the clinical study undertaken by the author (DM), meditation was used to induce hypnosis for patients undergoing dental treatment.[10] As part of that study, the subjects were given a choice of words for meditation (see above). They were asked to pick out one of the words, to repeat it out loud and then silently, and see how it felt to them. They were told that if none of the words appealed to them, then they could choose their own word. Most subjects chose one of the profferred words, but some used their own. A couple of subjects even used their own names. Some words were of one syllable, others were two-syllable words, and a few were three-syllable words. Analysis of the words used showed that the two-syllable words were most popular. The most frequently used word was "flower."*

In Chapter 13, it was reported that there are people who actually prefer and do better with negatively charged words such as "hate" and "grik." At present, it is not clear what are the best words or sounds to use for mantra meditation. The ancient Sanskrit mantras have a long history of use, but even those sounds are not necessarily effective for everyone. It also may be that the gurus are very knowledgeable about people and thus are able to match the proper mantra with the individual. Nevertheless, it does appear that the effectiveness of a word for meditation is related to something like personality or attitudes.

Hence, at this point it can be stated that the inductions of self-hypnosis and meditation are similar with the possible exception of TM and TM-like methods such as CSM where concentration is not used.

Control

A second possible difference between hypnosis and meditation has to do with control. With hypnosis, one generally tries to control certain body actions or functions (e.g., relax muscles, slow breathing, obtain pain control). With passive meditation, one does not try to control or concentrate on anything. The things that do occur are apparently spontaneous. Without deliberately trying, one can obtain results such as relaxed muscles and quiet breathing. This is related to the relaxation that usually accompanies meditation.

* We are currently correlating various words for mantras with personalities and moods. To date (32 subjects), the most popular mantras are "om," "love" and "shirim."

Subjective Differences

Are subjective feelings different for meditation and self-hypnosis? In the above-mentioned study comparing hypnosis and meditation, there were four groups of subjects: (1) those who were trained in TM and untrained in self-hypnosis; (2) those who were trained in self-hypnosis and untrained in meditation; (3) those who were trained in both TM and self-hypnosis; and (4) those who were trained in neither meditation nor self-hypnosis.[9] All subjects were monitored for various physiological changes as they went through the states of hypnosis, meditation, relaxation and alertness. Also, the subjects were asked to report on their subjective feelings in the various states.

In the previous chapter, it was mentioned that the subjects felt that hypnosis was subjectively different from relaxation. As for their impression of hypnosis versus meditation, that depended upon their orientation. These were the usual results: (1) subjects trained in TM experienced greater mental relaxation and more intense sensations during the meditation condition; (2) subjects trained in self-hypnosis experienced better results during the hypnosis condition; and (3) subjects trained in both techniques or in neither technique had variable subjective impressions—some found meditation more effective and others found hypnosis better.

Subjective reports by individuals included feelings of tingling, numbness, warmth, chilling, floating, spinning, being "suspended in space" and being "somewhere else." For some subjects, sensations were intense, and there were feelings of euphoria. At times, they felt as if their minds were completely blank. At other times, subjects had altered body images. Some reported that their bodies felt large and swollen; others stated that they felt small and shrunken. Still others felt as if they had no body at all but were just a floating mind. Time was also distorted. For some, minutes felt like hours; others felt as if only a few seconds had passed. These feelings were reported with both self-hypnosis and meditation.

Let us now summarize: Hypnosis and meditation are similar in method of induction—with the possible exception of nonconcentrative forms of meditation such as TM and CSM—and in subjective feelings. They differ in the matter of control of body functions. Are there any other differences? This depends upon whether one can believe in unverifiable concepts such as the various stages of consciousness.

The Stages of Consciousness

During Transcendental Meditation, one is supposed to expand his consciousness and to achieve higher states of consciousness.[2,8] Through TM, a person attempts to understand himself, his thoughts and his mental images. Progression is then supposed to occur so that self-understanding merges with understanding of others, and then unification of consciousness. Finally, one reaches cosmic consciousness or unity with nature, the universe and God. In other forms of meditation, this is called "Satori" (Zen) and "Samadhi" (Yoga); TM calls it "Unity Consciousness."

The traditional forms of meditation are purported to purify consciousness, to give mental peace, to allow one to attain the highest form of self-realization and enlightenment and ultimately to be one with the cosmos. Modern forms of meditation such as Benson's technique and CSM make no such claims. Self-hypnosis also lays no claim to the achievement of any higher states of consciousness. Thus, we can state that hypnosis and the traditional forms of meditation apparently differ in this respect.

Association with Religion

One other difference between hypnosis and the traditional forms of meditation is that unlike hypnosis, these kinds of meditation are often linked with religious ceremonies.[3] Yoga is part of Hinduistic tradition; Zen is derived from Buddhism; Sufism is a mystical Islamic practice; and there are meditative techniques involved with various forms of Judaism, Christiantiy, Taoism, Confusianism and Shintoism. Even though TM is purported not to have religious significance, it is derived from Yoga, and the initiating ceremony uses Sanskrit dialogue.[2]

With respect to religion and meditation, the authors have done some preliminary investigation into meditation during prayer. It appears that silent religious meditation may be just as effective as other kinds of meditation in inducing the relaxation response. If further investigation corroborates this finding, it may help spur a return to religion.

Extrasensory Perception (ESP)

Another kind of behavior that has been reported to be common to both hypnosis and meditation is extrasensory perception (ESP).[8] As a result of continued practice of both disciplines, some individuals seem to enhance their mental telepathy, clairvoyance and precognition abilities. (This is a highly controversial subject; we leave it to others to evaluate the evidence.)

Revised Definition of Meditation

We can now give a revised definition of meditation. Meditation is an altered state of awareness that is induced by the repetitive action of some constant stimulation. The stimulation may be external, internal or physical. As a result of repeated constant stimulation, an individual, without trying, achieves varying degrees of relaxation, subjective changes in body image, certain distortions of reality and the ability to decrease autonomic nervous system functions. In addition, the subject appears to gain a better understanding of himself and sometimes believes that he expands his consciousness and achieves higher states of consciousness. As a result of the process, the individual may feel closer to his God or a oneness with the universe.

MEDITATION STUDIES

Now that we have some understanding of the meaning of meditation, let us look at a few of the studies that have investigated this phenomenon. First, the physiological studies of meditation will be examined.

Various Responses

In these physiological studies, various responses were monitored, including the following: blood pressure; heart rate; breathing rate; oxygen consumption; carbon dioxide elimination; blood lactate concentration; muscle contraction; skin resistance levels; brain wave patterns. When an individual is relaxed, all of these responses normally decrease with the exception of GSR and alpha brain wave rhythms, which generally increase.

The accumulation of blood lactate seems to be related to stress. People who have anxiety and high blood pressure tend to have higher resting blood lactate levels than controls.[17] As mentioned in the previous chapter, skin resistance levels are related to sweating and increase with relaxation. Skin resistance is also one of the most important measurements in the lie detector test. When a person lies, the skin resistance often decreases and becomes irregular. This response is related to the sweating that usually occurs when a person is confronted with his fabrication.

Brain Wave Patterns

The brain wave patterns are interpreted from the electroencephalograph (EEG) record. The EEG is recorded by the placement of electrodes over different areas of the scalp. Many sites can be used, but the general areas are the occipital (back of the head), temporal and parietal (side of the head) and frontal (front of the head).[18] The patterns that are recorded apparently reflect activity from within the brain, although no one is certain of this.

There are four basic types of brain waves: beta, alpha, theta and delta. They are differentiated by their frequency and amplitude. Beta, 14–60 cycles per second, occurs when an individual is alert and is concentrating. It can also occur when one is actively thinking during dreaming. Alpha, 8–13 cycles per second, appears to be related to a deeply relaxed, but awake state. Theta, 4–7 cycles per second, occurs just prior to falling asleep. Hallucinations may be associated with the production of these waves. Delta, 1–3 cycles per second, the slowest of all, is found in a sleeping individual. (See above, Fig. 12.1, for diagrams of these various brain wave patterns.) These wave activities are not an all-or-none phenomenon. For instance, an alert person can produce alpha, but beta activity predominates. On the other hand, when one is deeply relaxed, alpha and beta are both produced, but alpha is usually more prevalent.

Alpha State.   In terms of alpha activity, the so-called alpha state is not a true state. Alpha is not produced solely throughout all areas of the brain—there is always some beta activity as well. And no one has shown conclusively that it is beneficial to produce a large amount of alpha. In fact, recent research by Orne indicates that alpha control cannot be learned, and alpha production is not related to decrease of anxiety.[19]

A somewhat similar finding was reported by Chisholm and his associates.[20] It was found that subjects who were trained to produce alpha could maintain alpha even in the face of an electric shock (a physical stressor). However, their heart rates did not decrease, and subjectively the individuals felt anxious. Hence, in this study the increased alpha apparently did not help in the reduction of anxiety that accompanied an electric shock.

Nevertheless, other studies do indicate that increased relaxation is often accompanied by an increase in alpha production.[1-3,21] Thus, right now alpha remains an enigma. Theta waves may be more indicative of deep relaxation, since some studies have shown that they are produced during deep meditation.[22-24]

Synchronization. Synchronization of alpha production is also observed. The alpha rhythms begin in the occipital area and sweep forward to the parietal, temporal and frontal areas and then to the opposite hemisphere.[22,23] This synchronization is supposed to be associated with a deep state of relaxation. However, critics suggest that the synchronization may be just an artifact created by the placement of the ground electrode.[25] That is, the apparent production in all areas of the brain may be due to the superimposition of occipital alpha—which often occurs just from closing the eyes or rolling the eyes upward when they are closed—on other areas. Still, most investigators believe that the spread of alpha forward does occur and is related to deep relaxation.[2,22,23]

Problems of the Studies

First of all, variables such as hypnosis, meditation and relaxation do not easily lend themselves to measurement as others do (e.g., drugs). Also, factors other than the variables of interest tend to affect the measurements taken (e.g., pulse rate, breathing rate and skin resistance). For instance, as was discussed in the previous chapter, subjects may expect to do better with a technique such as meditation than with a control condition, simple relaxation. Thus, possible conscious and unconscious control of autonomic functions may affect the results.

In addition, the two main strategies used to control extraneous variables* are not particularly effective where the techniques interact with each other and the subjects. For example, if one were comparing meditation and relaxation and started a subject with 20 minutes of relaxation, by the time the meditation condition was being tested the subject would be more relaxed than when he began. One way to control for this effect is to balance or reverse the order of the conditions; i.e., start an equal number of subjects in the meditation and relaxation conditions and subsequently switch to the opposite condition.

Also, there are serious design limitations where both the experimenter and the subjects know which group they are in. The technique of not letting subjects know which group they are in—the single-blind technique—is not appropriate, since the cooperation of the subject is needed for hypnosis, meditation or relaxation. Moreover, it is not possible to keep the experimenter in the dark about which subjects are in which group—e.g., he either is the hypnotist or is promoting meditation. Obviously, it would be best to disguise group membership from both the experimenter and the subjects (a method known as the double-blind technique).

Beyond these design limitations, a common problem with many studies of this kind is that the data are not analyzed independently. That is, the principal investigators generally are the ones who analyze the results, a fact that could prejudice the findings. However in meditation studies, a blind technique of having independent analysis of the data by unbiased judges is possible and indicated.

Various Studies

Let us now proceed with the studies. In 1935, Brosse monitored cardiac activity in Indian Yogis. Based on the results of an electrocardiograph (EKG), it was concluded that one of the subjects was able to stop his heartbeat.[26] However, since the equipment was not very sensitive and relied on peripheral phenomena, those results are not

---

* One strategy uses control groups; the other strategy has each subject serve as his own control.

considered conclusive. In 1957, Bagchi and Wenger also monitored meditating Yogis.[27] It was found that these individuals had a decreased heart rate (but no complete stoppage), increased alpha brain wave activity and a 70% increase in galvanic skin resistance.

In 1961, Anand, Chhina and Singh examined other Yoga meditators and found markedly reduced oxygen consumption and carbon dioxide elimination.[28] Examination of Zen meditators by Suzi and Akutsi showed similar results.[29] Increased alpha and theta waves were found in meditating Yogis and Zen practitioners by other investigators in the 1950s and 1960s.[30,31]

In 1970, Wallace and Benson performed the first investigation of TM meditators.[26,32] Marked decreases in oxygen consumption, carbon dioxide elimination and blood lactate were found. Respiration rate and heart rate also slowed from the resting state. There were marked increases in skin resistance levels and alpha waves, and some subjects had theta wave production. Blood pressure did not significantly decrease. Wallace considered the findings to be so unique that the TM state was proposed as a fourth state of consciousness—distinct from the alert state, sleep, dreaming and hypnosis.

All the studies prior to Wallace and Benson's were not well controlled and are difficult to evaluate. In the Wallace and Benson study, the subjects acted as their own controls. The monitoring began with relaxation, which was then followed by meditation. The reverse order was not done.

Several other studies have reinforced Wallace and Benson's findings about the uniqueness of the TM state. Banquet compared a group of meditators with a control group who just relaxed.[22] He found that the meditators had a large increase in alpha even with the eyes open as compared to the controls. The meditators also showed theta activity and synchronous activity of alpha, which the controls did not show. Glueck and Stroebel also found increased alpha and synchronized activity during the use of Transcendental Meditation.[23] However, their results were clinical observations and not a controlled study.

Orme-Johnson, in a controlled study of meditators and nonmeditators, found that meditators had fewer fluctuations in skin resistance than the nonmeditators had.[33] This is indicative of better ability to handle stress. Goleman and Schwartz also found that meditators recovered more rapidly from a stressful stimulus than did nonmeditators.[34]

So at this point, the studies had been uniformly favorable for the TM technique. However, recently some discordant elements have begun to emerge. Beary and Benson, using subjects as their own controls, compared meditation using the word "one" (linked with each out-breath) with alert states (eyes open and eyes closed).[35] They alternated the order with various subjects to try to control for interactive effects. Oxygen consumption, carbon dioxide elimination and respiratory rate were measured, and all three were found to be markedly decreased during meditation as compared to results for controls. These results then became the basis for Benson's subsequent best-selling book, *The Relaxation Response*.[3] As mentioned previously, TM teachers dispute Benson's contention that the use of the word "one" linked with breathing, is as effective as TM techniques in inducing the meditative response.

In 1975, an important study was undertaken by Walrath and Hamilton.[36] Three groups of subjects were involved: TM meditators; self-hypnosis (relaxation-type) practitioners; and individuals taught instructed relaxation. The latter group was given meditationlike instructions to "view both thoughts and external events non-evaluatively." Heart rate, respiratory rate and skin resistance levels were monitored, and the results showed decreases that were similar for all three groups. In other words, contrary to previous findings, the physiologic responses that were examined showed that TM was not unique.

All the original EEG findings showed that TM was not related to sleep.[2,22,23,26,32,37] However, a recent study of well-experienced TM meditators (minimum of 2.5 years training) showed that they spent 40% of their meditation time in sleep.[38] Based on this limited study, one might conjecture that the so-called cosmic consciousness is no more than sleep.

Recent reports from Great Britain have challenged the claimed uniqueness of TM.[5,25] One study showed that if long periods of rest preceded testing of TM meditators, there was practically no decrease in oxygen consumption. Only when they started with a relatively alert state was there a pronounced drop in oxygen consumption.

Another study showed that people lying still while listening to soothing music had a drop in oxygen consumption comparable to that found with TM meditators.

A recent study by Bennett and Trinder showed that TM and relaxation control subjects did not differ on brain laterality.[39] (In Chapter 2, it was mentioned that the right hemisphere is supposed to be important in gestalt, holistic and spacial types of thinking, while the left brain is concerned with cognitive-type thinking.) Neither the TM subjects nor the controls showed any preference for right brain activity. Meditation had previously been considered to be characterized by right brain activity. Bennett and Trinder also found that both the TM subjects and the relaxation controls had a symmetrical distribution of alpha activity, and TM was not any better in this respect.

A recent study by Cauthen and Prymak (University of Calgary, Alberta, Canada) showed no significant differences between TM subjects and relaxation controls on skin conductance (the inverse of skin resistance) and respiration rate.[40]

One other recent study, by Kanas and Horowitz at the University of California, showed that meditators and nonmeditators did not differ significantly in their reactions to stress films.[41] The films shown are well known in the stress field. The first, "Woodshop," depicts accidents occurring because of carelessness with power tools. The second film, "John," shows the life of an abandoned child. Since TM practitioners are supposed to manage stress well (suggested by the previous studies of Orme-Johnson and Goleman and Schwartz), it was assumed that they would react well to the films. But on all measures taken they did no better than the controls.

In short, these last three studies do not support the claim that TM is unique.

In the first study undertaken by the authors at Temple University, an attempt was made to overcome some of the inherent problems that plagued many of the previous studies.*[9] For instance, in a preliminary survey it was found that there was a marked difference between individuals in the skin resistance level response and in the production of slow alpha waves (8–10 cycles per second). This

---

* Studies are quoted in many articles and books, but the reader has no idea about the design, validity or reliability of those studies. To help overcome this shortcoming, the authors describe the first study at Temple University in some detail.

occurred with both trained and nontrained individuals even if all they did was sit and close their eyes.

Some subjects produced less that 1% slow alpha, whereas others had over 50% slow alpha. With respect to skin resistance, the authors found, as did others, that there were two diametrically opposite kinds of subjects: underresponders and overresponders.[42] The underresponders showed approximately no change in skin resistance as compared to the base level alert state. The overresponders had almost a 100% increase over the baseline. And remember that was without meditation or hypnosis, merely with the eyes closed.

Hence, it was surmised that if different groups were used in the study, it would be possible for a majority of underresponders to be in one group (e.g., meditation group) and a majority of overresponders to be in a second group (e.g., relaxation group). If this had occurred, it would have been erroneously concluded that relaxation causes more alpha and greater skin resistance increases than does meditation. It may be that an individual's normal production of alpha rhythms and tendency to show skin resistance changes may not be related only to the ability to relax. Because of the drastic differences we found in individuals, it may be that the levels produced are partly due to genetic and hormonal differences between people. As a result of these great individual differences, it was decided not to rely on random assignment but to use subjects as their own controls.

The techniques compared were Transcendental Meditation, simple word meditation, hetero-hypnosis-relaxation type, hetero-hypnosis-task type, self-hypnosis-relaxation type and simple relaxation—with the awake state as the control. As previously stated, there were 48 subjects: 12 trained in TM, 12 trained in self-hypnosis, 12 trained in both and 12 trained in neither. All subjects were monitored for respiratory rate, heart rate, blood pressure, skin resistance, muscle activity and the production of slow alpha waves. Sites selected for the EEG were in the frontal, temporal, parietal and occipital areas.

There were four different orders of condition used for each group:

1. Relaxation, meditation, hypnosis; (and in reverse) hypnosis, meditation, relaxation.
2. Relaxation, hypnosis, meditation; (and in reverse) meditation, hypnosis, relaxation.

3. Hypnosis, meditation, relaxation; (and in reverse) relaxation, meditation, hypnosis.
4. Meditation, hypnosis, relaxation; (and in reverse) relaxation, hypnosis, meditation.

The subjects were in each state for about six to seven minutes, with a three-minute alert break between each state, which helped to control for the interactive effects. As mentioned before, in order to control for the bias against relaxation, the subjects were told prior to being tested that no significant differences had been found to date among relaxation, relaxation-hypnosis and meditative states. Thus, if there was a real difference between the techniques, the confounding with expectations would be minimized.

Also, subjects were not told how they were doing during the experiment. The testing was done in a relatively quiet, semidark room, at the same time of the day, on the same day of the week, in the same place for all subjects. The same investigator (Morse) met with all the subjects.

A psychological test was administered, and all subjects were found to be within psychologically acceptable limits. All subjects were in good medical health, except two who had slightly elevated blood pressure. It was determined from some preliminary work that only six to seven minutes in each experimental state was a good compromise. It had been found that if a subject was monitored for 20 minutes in each state, the entire experiment took several hours, and the subjects might get extremely restless and irritable. It was felt that the shorter period would be sufficient because previous studies had shown that most of the changes in meditation occur within the first few minutes. [22,23,26,35]

All the subjects had been tested for hypnotic susceptibility, and they were all considered to be of moderate to high susceptibility according to the Spiegel Eye-Roll Susceptibility Test. [43] As a result, no difficulty was experienced in hypnotizing the subjects rapidly. Also, since they all were volunteers for the experiment, they were highly motivated. As we have discussed, motivation is important for the induction of hypnosis.

The results were reviewed by members of the physiology department who were not involved in the study. They did not know the subjects, which groups they were in or the states that were being monitored. The results were as follows:

There were no statistically significant changes in blood pressure through all the states, but there were some trends; there was a slight decrease during simple relaxation, meditation and relaxation-hypnosis as compared to the alert state, and there was a slight increase during task-hypnosis.

There was a significant but small decrease in pulse rate (about 4–5 beats per minute) for all the relaxation states as compared to the alert state and task-hypnosis. The same was true for respiratory rate. There was a decrease of about 2.5–3.5 respirations per minute in all the relaxation states as compared to the alert state and task-hypnosis. In muscle contraction, which was discussed previously, meditation showed the best results.

In slow alpha production, there was a significant increase from the alert state to all the other states. Synchronization of alpha was found in several areas of the brain, but this property was more related to the individual himself than to the relaxation state he was in. If a person manifested this phenomenon it was seen in all of the relaxation states; and if he didn't show it, none of it was seen in any of the states. (See Fig. 15.2.)

The greatest significant differences were found with skin resistance. All relaxation states showed increased and more stable skin resistance as compared to the alert and task-hypnosis states. The lower skin resistance finding during task-hypnosis is the result of mental work that was being done to concentrate on numbing of the hand. That is, mental work as well as physical work can cause an increase in sweating.

What can be concluded from these findings? It appears that TM is an effective means of achieving a deep state of physical and mental relaxation. But TM did not show itself to be unique. Similar results can be achieved with the use of simple word meditation, relaxation-type self-hypnosis and just sitting comfortably in a chair and relaxing.

However, a few points need to be made. One reason why subjects did so well in simple relaxation may have been that they were in a laboratory experiment and wanted to try to impress the investigators with their ability to do as well as prior subjects. Also, the laboratory

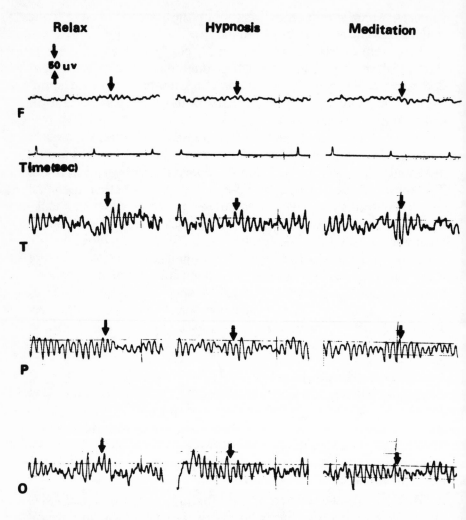

Fig. 15.2 Synchronization of alpha rhythms. Abbreviations: uv = microvolts; F, T, P and O are four scalp areas in which the electrodes are placed (F = frontal; T = temporal; P = parietal; O = occipital). The arrows point to areas of synchronous alpha activity. With respect to this subject, there is similar synchronous activity in the four areas during the three relaxation states. (From Morse et al., 1977. *Psychosom. Med.* 39:305-324. Reprinted with permission of Elsevier North-Holland, Inc.)

is different from the home situation. With the investigators present for reassurance and with no interruption, it may have been much easier for the subjects to relax in the laboratory than it would have been at home. Conversely, when they were by themselves at home—with the possibility of distractions—they might have performed much better with methods that aid in relaxation such as meditation and hypnosis.

Also, oxygen consumption, carbon dioxide elimination and blood lactate concentration were not monitored.* As a result, it is possible that meditation would show better results for these measurements than would be found for hypnosis or relaxation, although other recent experiments have not shown this to be the case.[3-5,25,35]

In no way can it be assumed from these results that relaxation, hypnosis or simple word meditation can cause the elevation or expansion of consciousness that may accrue from the practice of Transcendental Meditation.[44] Even though at this time consciousness expansion is not measurable, this does not mean that it does not occur or that the individual does not feel as if it occurred. (The field of mind expansion is left to more intrepid investigators.)

Psychological and Sociological Benefits

Apart from physiological studies, there have been some investigations of psychological and sociological benefits of meditation. Shaw and Kolb found that TM practitioners had faster reaction times than nonmeditators.[45] Graham compared auditory discrimination (ability to detect different sounds) in TM meditators after meditation for 20 minutes and after reading a book for 20 minutes (the TM Ss were used as their own controls); better results were found following meditation.[46] Another group found that meditators had better psychological health than nonmeditators.[47] Shelly found that meditators as compared to controls developed greater self-sufficiency, stability and happiness.[48]

As previously mentioned, the confounding variable with studies of this kind is that practitioners of TM are much more highly motivated than people who just relax or are practicing a method for control purposes. But the consequences of the studies are not necessarily

* It was felt that there might be adverse effects due to the invasive procedures (e.g., drawing blood from the arm) required for these measures.

bad—not if people can be motivated to do something that is good for them. The problem is that one cannot definitely attribute to TM alone the cause of the results described.

Contrary Findings

White has reported on two interesting studies conducted by Jonathan Smith of Roosevelt University in Chicago.[4] In the first study, one group was trained in TM; the second group was trained in relaxation with eyes closed, but with simulated TM-like indoctrination. In the second study, one group was taught a TM-like exercise; the second group was taught an "anti-meditation" exercise. The latter group was taught to sit with eyes closed and think as many positive thoughts as possible.

After a few months, the results from both studies showed a greater effect in reducing anxiety from all groups as compared to no treatment at all. But the mere act of sitting with eyes closed regardless of what was done mentally was equally effective for the TM group, the eyes-closed group, the TM-like group and the anti-meditation group.

An interesting paper was written recently by Lewis Thomas on "Transcendental Metaworry" with "tongue-in-cheek."[49] Thomas suggested that individuals spend two 20-minute periods a day (as in TM) sitting quietly with their eyes closed, concentrating all their worries into those two periods. Thus they would not have to worry the rest of the day. Although this suggestion was presented in jest, Smith's findings about the "anti-meditation" group may show that Thomas's technique has merit. Could it be, then, that sitting quietly for a certain period each day is the most important aspect of TM—at least as far as stress release is concerned? Even if this is true, the motivation that is generated by such organized approaches as TM makes them very useful techniques.

DANGERS OF MEDITATION

Are there dangers in meditation? For the normal individual, probably not. For the highly neurotic or psychotic person, meditation might be hazardous. When one is in this deep state of relaxation, stresses are released, and repressed problems and emotions could surface, which could cause psychosomatic symptoms or bizarre behavior. Harmful results of this kind were reported by Otis.[50] This danger is similar to the possible dangers of hypnosis, as discussed in the last chapter.

For instance, the deep relaxation during meditation could bring on a migraine attack in a susceptible individual, since it is during quiet periods that migraines can occur.[51] During meditation, some subjects experience dizziness or a sense of loss of control. This sensation is disturbing to some. Overprolonged periods of meditation can lead to hallucinations, "nervous breakdown," insomnia, depression and schizophrenia.[4,5,52,53]

Akers and his group found that personality variables can affect an individual's response to meditation.[54] Williams and his co-workers found that TM practitioners were more introverted and neurotic than normal nonmeditating subjects.[55] Considering these findings, we believe that before anyone begins using any of the relaxation response methods, he should have a complete examination by his physician and approval by his therapist (if he is in treatment).

HISTORY OF MEDITATION

Now that we are somewhat knowledgeable about meditation, let us briefly consider the history of this practice. Meditation was probably first used in the Eastern religions. In the Indian scriptures of the sixth century B.C., the use of meditation is discussed.[56] Yoga developed as part of the Hindu religion. Zen, an important component of Buddhism, evolved from Yoga techniques. Meditative practices spread from India to China, Japan and other Far Eastern countries. Other Eastern religions in which meditative techniques developed are Shintoism, Taoism and Confucianism. In the Kabbalistic tradition, mantra meditation was practiced using the Hebrew letters of God's name.[52]

In Christianity, meditative techniques were also common. A fourteenth-century practice was to say repetitively "Lord Jesus Christ have mercy on me."[52] Distractive thoughts were supposed to be put aside.

In Islam, the mystic practice of Sufism used meditative techniques. During the twelfth century its followers included exercises, breath control and repetition of a secret holy word.[57]

The so-called nature mystics included Wordsworth, Thoreau,

Tennyson and William James. They achieved meditation by the quiet contemplation of nature.[52]

Within the last few years, many other meditative techniques or religious practices have been introduced into the Western world. These include the following: Arica, Nichiren Shoshu, T'ai Chi, Gurdjieffian technique, Sabud, Sufi, Kundalini, Vipásyána, Esalen, Hare Krishna, Meher Baba, Scientology, Sentic Cycles, Cotention and Ditention, Sensory Awareness Methods, Black Muslimism, Ananda Marga Meditation, The Divine Light Sect and various other offshoots of Yoga and Zen. The most popular movement, Transcendental Meditation (TM), was introduced into the United States in 1959 by Maharishi Mahesh Yogi;[2] TM is based on a Yoga meditative technique.

Recently, an effective new program was introduced by Patricia Carrington, called Clinically Standardized Meditation (CSM).[5,7] Like TM, it is relatively effortless and easy to learn. Unlike TM, it emphasizes individual adjustment of the technique to suit the trainee. CSM has no secret mantras or mystical overtones. It is usually taught by a set of recordings plus a programmed instruction text.*

Other techniques that include meditation have recently been developed in the United States. These are Silva Mind Control, Alpha Meditation and Mind Control, and est (Erhard Seminar Training).

USES OF MEDITATION

Now that we have examined meditation and traced its origins, let us consider its uses. The foremost uses of meditation are for coping with stress and reducing anxiety.

In a recent report, Schwartz and his co-workers found that meditation reduced cognitive anxiety, while exercise reduced somatic anxiety.[58] Cognitive anxiety is conscious awareness of negative feelings about oneself or outside stimuli. Some examples are as follows: "I worry a lot about unimportant things"; "I have thoughts that crop up, and I can't control them." Somatic anxiety is conscious awareness of body changes related to the negative thoughts. Some

---

* Those interested in obtaining information on CSM can write to: Pace Systems, P.O. Box 113, Kendall Park, N.J. 08824.

examples are as follows: "I sweat a lot", "I often have diarrhea"; "I feel a pounding in my chest."

Meditation also allows for deep muscular relaxation. Other reported uses of meditation—especially TM—are as follows: increased well-being; better intuition; more energy; improved emotional stability; improved interpersonal relationships; better perceptiveness; more creativity; decreased use of drugs, alcohol and cigarettes; improved grades in school; increased productivity; improved athletic performance.[2]

As far as health is concerned, studies have shown that meditation can do the following: reduce blood pressure in hypertensives;[3,59,60] help in the treatment of heart rhythm irregularities (cardiac arrhythmias); act as an aid in the treatment of mental diseases;[61] help in the control of tension headaches and asthma;[62] help control fear, pain, muscle contractions and salivation in dentistry.[13] (In Chapter 18, further details are given with respect to the medical and dental benefits of meditation.)

However, not everyone benefits from meditation. In our studies at Temple University, it was found that there were no physiological differences between meditation and simple relaxation in responses to physical stressors (e.g., the taking of blood pressure) and psychological stressors (e.g., hearing the word "needle").[9,16] As mentioned earlier, a study by Jonathan Smith showed that there were no significant differences in reduction of anxiety levels between meditating subjects and subjects sitting quietly with active thoughts.[4] William Morgan reported on a study conducted at the University of Wisconsin.[63] There were three groups involved: (1) an exercise group; (2) a meditating group (used Benson's relaxation response); and (3) a seated relaxation control group. All three groups showed similar reductions in anxiety. As was discussed in Chapter 9, Diversions, it may be that meditation, relaxation and exercise are all forms of diversion, and this is part of the reason for the anxiety reduction.

WORDS FOR MEDITATION

In Chapter 13, the results of a study at Temple University on the use of various words for meditation was discussed.[16] Also mentioned were Carrington's findings with respect to pleasant- and unpleasant-sounding words.[7] Although no significant physiological differences were found with any of the words by the authors, there were subjective preferences (Carrington also found subjective preferences). The investigations are being continued with a focus on personality and mantra selection. Let us now consider what the authors believe is important in mantra selection.

Although there is a long-standing tradition with mantra meditation, at present, words and sounds for mantras are being assigned with few or no criteria. It is important to establish criteria for mantra selection, especially since meditation is being used for medical and psychological purposes. In selecting a word or sound for meditation, certain factors should be considered.

Meaning and Meaningfulness

First to be considered are the "meaning" and "meaningfulness" of the word. Words with "meaning" tend to generate a large number of associations.[64] Should a meditation word have meaning? As has been mentioned, the TM mantras have no significance to Western meditators. However, words without direct meaning can still be "meaningful." That is, they can bring forth some related or unrelated associations (e.g., "bzzz" has no meaning that is denotative or connotative and yet may elicit thoughts of insects).[65] Hence, even to Westerners, mantras can still be "meaningful."

Benson picked "one" presumably because it was basically a neutral word, low in association value.[66] Yet, "one" does have "meaning," and many Sanskrit mantras have deep "meaning" (e.g., "aum"—a mantra that purportedly gives cosmic power).[4] With religious meditation in Judaism, Christianity and Islam, the repetition of the deity's name has great "meaning."[52]

Emotionality

A second factor to consider with mantra selection is the emotional impact of the word. Single encounters with emotionally charged words, especially taboo words, cause more severe stress reactions than do neutral words.[67] As was mentioned in Chapter 13, it was found that, physiologically, silent repetition of emotionally charged words did not cause stress reactions.[16] However, subjectively most people reported "hate" to be stressful.

Familiarity

A third important factor in mantra selection is the "familiarity" of the word.[65] A word may be low in "meaning" or "meaningfulness" and yet be "familiar." For instance, "quark" is becoming "familiar", but aside from physicists and astronomers, few people know what it denotes.* With repetition, words become "familiar."

Repetition

A fourth consideration is the effect of repetition. Does the word retain its "meaning" throughout the meditation period, or does it tend to lose its "meaning"? In our study, the subjects reported that the words lost their meaning, usually by about the midpoint of the meditation period.[16] Words may also change in their significance. For example, with repetition, "Constantinople" can change to "can't stand an apple." Many meditators have reported that their mantra changes with repetition. Does this matter?

Miscellaneous Considerations

Other unanswered questions are as follows:
1. Is there a difference between using simple words (i.e., those recalled easily) and using complicated words (i.e., those recalled with difficulty)?
2. Are multisyllabic words better than single-syllable words? According to one TM teacher's disclosure, people below the age of 13 were given a one-syllable TM mantra and those over the age of 14 were given a two-syllable word.[6] As discussed before, in his three clinical studies using meditation, the author (DM) found that most subjects preferred a two-syllable word for meditation (e.g., "flower")[10,13-15]**
3. Does the "pronounceability" of the word have anything to do with its effectiveness?[65] For instance, is there a difference between

---

* A recent definition of quark is: "Any particle of fractional charge $\pm e/3$, $\pm 2e/3$, $\pm 4e/3$ . . . where e is the electron charge" (Zweig, G., Quark catalysis of exothermal nuclear reactions, *Science* 201:973-979, 1978). The term was originally "coined" by James Joyce in *Finnegan's Wake*.
** However, in our ongoing study correlating personalities and moods with words for meditation, to date, 20 of 32 subjects have selected a one-syllable word.

using harsh-sounding syllabic words as contrasted to soft-sounding syllabic words? Is this related to the rhythm imparted by the word repetition?

TM mantras purportedly have a soothing effect on the central nervous system.[2,12] Glueck and Stroebel sought the relationship between the relaxing effectiveness of TM mantras and resonance frequencies.[23] They stated: "The mantra represents a rather powerful input stimulus to the central nervous system, most likely the limbic circuitry. We have been informed that analysis of the resonance frequencies of a number of mantras gives a value of 6–7 Hz, which is in the high-theta EEG range and also approximates the optimal processing of the basic language unit, a phoneme, by the auditory system."* Unfortunately, no significant relationship has ever been found between mantras and resonance frequencies, although this remains a possibility.

In the study at Temple University, it was found that the pronounceability of the word did affect the subjects' feelings about it.[16] As discussed in Chapter 13, some people had difficulty with the "vuh" sound in love, while others disliked the "tuh" sound in hate.

At the present time there are many unanswered questions, but it may eventually be discovered that specific words are effective for particular people in overcoming anxiety and helping in the treatment of medical conditions. The authors contend that education in the proper use of meditation and self-hypnosis is a public health responsibility. Moreover, these techniques should be practiced not only for relaxation and to instill pleasurable feelings but to prevent diseases and help in the attainment of health.

MEDITATION TECHNIQUES

Now that we have considered meditation, its history, its uses and the various words, let us examine a few of the more popular techniques. As we have said, there are three basic methods: physical, external and internal. An example of each will be given.

T'ai Chi is a well-known physical form of meditation, which is derived from the Chinese religion Taoism. It involves difficult

---

* Glueck, B. C. and Stroebel, C. F., Biofeedback and meditation in the treatment of psychiatric illnesses, *Compr. Psychiat.* 16:303–321, 1975. Reprinted by permission of Grune & Stratton, Inc., a subsidiary of Harcourt Brace Jovanovich, Publishers.

postures and the performing of exacting exercises together with sitting meditation, walking meditation and breathing exercises. It takes years to perfect the postures and exercises in order to relax various areas of the body, but it is said to be an extremely rewarding way to achieve deep physical and mental relaxation. The physical exercises are used not only to improve physical strength and health but to help clear and calm the mind.

In Yoga or Zen meditation, one can concentrate on an external object or on a mental image. Traditional postures are used, which tend to decrease body activity and allow the subject to concentrate his attention on mental activities. The spine, neck and head must be kept in a straight line. The legs are crossed in the typical lotus position. This posture is a stable position in that it helps prevent one from tipping over. Besides concentration, breathing exercises are also very important. These meditative practices also take years to perfect, but apparently the results are worthwhile.

From their experience with hypnosis and meditation, the authors have devised a combination method which is believed to provide the advantages of both techniques.[68-70] Called meditation-hypnosis, it is described in the next section.

TIME AND SPACE TRAVEL

The only requisites for meditation-hypnosis are time and patience. If you seriously want to learn a method to counteract stress, it is yours for the asking. But it has to be practiced regularly and does require self-discipline. However, with repetition it gets easier, as one improves. And after a while, it becomes a habit. If you should happen to skip a session, you may feel a letdown just as with exercise.

If you are a person who only does something when there is constant reinforcement, then perhaps you should learn meditation (e.g., TM) at a meditation center. On the other hand, if you tend toward self-help, them you might look into the CSM tape-program. Whichever way you go, the chances are good that you will continue once you start experiencing the benefits.

Meditation-hypnosis is generally practiced twice a day for 20–30 minutes per session. Before breakfast and before dinner are the usual times, but it has been found that it can be practiced at other periods. It can be done after dinner if you wait about two hours.

And there is no rule that says you can't meditate during the day. In fact, if you anticipate stressful periods or if you have just come out of a stressful situation, you can spend 3–10 minutes in a "quickie" meditation (called a "mini-meditation" by Carrington).[7]

If you happen to be very thirsty or hungry, then have a quick drink and small snack and wait an hour before beginning. Experience has shown that either an empty or a full stomach interferes with proper meditation-hypnosis. Also, alcoholic and caffeinated beverages and drugs (e.g., Valium, marijuana) can interfere with effective meditation-hypnosis.

Before beginning the technique, it is important to relieve yourself, since fullness of the bladder or rectum interferes with relaxation. When you are all set, then go to a quiet, darkened room away from distractions such as the TV, radio and telephone. The room should be attractive and well-ventilated with a moderate temperature. Cold, warmth, drafts and dust all impede relaxation. Pick a comfortable chair, and you are ready to start. However, don't let these restrictions faze you. It is best to follow these suggestions, but "good" meditations may take place in uncomfortable seats in bouncy, noisy buses. Once your body gets accustomed to the technique, you can "turn on" even under adverse conditions.

When you get in the chair, sit partially inclined. If you lie all the way back and begin to meditate, you can easily fall asleep. That may be fine if you suffer from insomnia, but if you want to use meditation for stress-relief, then be sure to sit up. In the seated position, keep your feet on the ground, uncrossed. Next, loosen your clothes and remove your shoes, watch, rings, glasses and anything else that might be clinging tightly to your body. Place your hands, uncrossed, on your lap or on the sides of the chair. The idea is to decrease the outside pressure on your body. Again, don't worry if you can't follow everything that has been suggested; but the easier you make it for yourself, the better.

Now close your eyes, inhale, exhale and remain quiet for about a minute. Then begin to repeat your word silently. As was discussed before, it is not known what is the best word for each person. But experience has shown that people do prefer words that are pleasant to them. So try out a few words and pick one that is easy to say and brings forth either pleasant or neutral associations. Personal experience in teaching over 800 people this technique has disclosed that most people prefer a two-syllable word, and for many "flower" is the favorite.*

The word should be repeated at any pace; that doesn't seem to matter as long as it feels comfortable. You can say it to your heartbeat, to the sound of your breathing, to some melody or any way you choose. After a while, thoughts may intrude. As you have the thoughts, complete them, and then return to the silent repetition of the word.** In time, the word will probably appear distorted or devoid of meaning. But don't concern yourself. The word may even appear to come and go by itself. That also is not unusual.

While meditating, mentally concentrate on your toes. Think about them and then relax them. Do this same sequence with your ankles and calves. Then gradually continue up your body to your thighs, fingers, wrist, forearm, upper arm, shoulders, stomach, chest and neck. Always begin by concentrating on the particular area and then relaxing it completely. It should relax so completely that the part appears to have separated from the rest of the body.

When you get to your jaw, let your mouth muscles relax. Your mouth should then hang loose; you may even have some saliva drooling. If this should happen, then wear a towel or napkin over your chest to make you feel comfortable. You can either wipe your mouth or, if you are completely relaxed, just "drool on."

The next place to really "let go" is your scalp. Many headaches are caused by contracted scalp muscles, so try to "tense" your scalp and then relax it completely. You should now be relaxed from the tip of your toes to the top of your head. All the while you are contracting and relaxing the various muscles of your body, you should still effortlessly return to the repetition of the word. It may sound difficult when we talk about it in this way, but in actual practice it is easy.

Now you should proceed internally with the concentration-relaxation. Consider your lungs, your intestines, your heart and

---

* In our ongoing study correlating personality types and moods with words for meditation, to date, 20 subjects have chosen meaningful words (e.g., "love"; "smooth"); while 12 subjects have chosen neutral or meaningless words (e.g., "lum"; "shirim").

** However, if an important thought occurs to you that you do not want to forget, it is preferable gradually to come out of the meditation, write the thought down on a piece of paper and then return to the meditation. If you don't do this, the thought itself, if it is important enough to you, can act as a psychological stressor, creating anxiety and making for an unrewarding meditation.

blood vessels, and then work your way down to smaller things like nerve fibers and individual cells. After a while, you may feel a warm, tingling, floating, heavy sensation throughout various parts of your body.

You are now ready to take a mental trip. Think about a lovely, quiet place. It could be a lake, a stream, a mountaintop or the shore. But it should be a place where *you* want to go. The more engrossed you become with the trip, the easier it is for you to forget your word. But don't be concerned. However, if you feel that you are becoming alert, then return to your word. In time, you may forget your word and your trip. Your mind may be a complete blank. In this case, you have either achieved cosmic consciousness or you have fallen asleep. According to a recent study, the two events may be similar[38]—but nobody can really scientifically investigate the mystical states of deep consciousness. Whatever you call it, for most people this is a very pleasant state. It is the natural "high" that you hear about. You don't always feel this euphoric sensation, but even without it most meditations are very pleasant.

You should keep a watch nearby, to glance at occasionally. But don't use an alarm clock or a kitchen timer because you don't want to be jolted out of meditation. After about 20 minutes, you should begin to arouse yourself. Take about one to two minutes to gradually come back to the present. As you awaken, stretch and slowly open your eyes. You should feel alert and refreshed. If you feel a little light-headed, then close your eyes again, and take another minute to awaken.

The regular practice of this technique will go a long way in helping you counteract the stressors of everyday life. You may also find that meditation-hypnosis will really help control your anxieties in the medical or dental office or before a major surgical operation (discussed further in Chapter 18).

CHOOSING A TECHNIQUE

According to Benson's, Carrington's and our Temple University studies, it can be seen that the use of a simple word is an effective means of inducing a state of meditation. The question that is often asked is, "Is it advantageous to learn meditation at a meditation center from a trained teacher?"

The answer depends upon one's belief and the kind of individual involved. If one believes that the Sanskrit mantra is one that is personally suited to the individual involved and can only be given by a trained teacher, then he should learn meditation at a regular center. However, there is no evidence to show that physiological benefits are superior with the use of a Sanskrit sound. At this time, studies are not able to show that simple word meditation is better than TM for prolonged use. This is so because the techniques of TM have been practiced much longer than simple word meditation.

As far as the achievement of higher states of consciousness is concerned, that does not lend itself to scientific testing.

There is a more important reason to learn meditation at a regular center, related to the fact that most people do not do things unless they are strongly motivated. Merely telling someone that he should sit, close his eyes and repeat a word silently twice a day does not ensure that it will be done. With TM, there is a well-organized program. There are interesting lectures, impressive visual handouts and a charismatic figure, the Maharishi. There are also fellow meditators who share their experiences in group sessions. This is almost like group therapy. There is an intriguing ceremony, and the reception of the mantra is almost like a gift to be cherished. There are regular checkups by seemingly interested teachers. Also, there are periodic lectures, weekend retreats and regular mailings directly to the individual. So even though there is a costly initiation fee (about $165, but it may vary), many people willingly pay it.

Similarly, the tape presentation given in Carrington's Clinically Standardized Meditation is a superb program that one can easily follow and listen to repeatedly for reinforcement. However, a highly motivated person can definitely learn meditation by following the instructions given above.

Let us now consider the combination of two stress-control methods, exercise and meditation.

RUNNING MEDITATION

Earl Solomon recently reported on the running meditation response.[71] It is a combination of slow, long distance running with TM. Solomon observed the following:

1. The runner usually becomes addicted to the combination in between two and four months.

2. The benefits are physical as well as emotional.

3. Even though he is meditating, the runner remains vigilant and attentive to traffic and other possible dangers (such as ferocious dogs) and his eyes stay open most of the time.

4. When it is carried out for an hour or more, there is vigorous and rhythmic contraction and relaxation of the large muscles of the trunk and legs.

5. The meditating runner uses a special breathing technique.

The author (DM) has devised a similar method. He meditates for about one-third of the time during a typical six-mile run. The meditation is done during periods when he feels either bored or "achy." This technique, using simple words for mantras, has been taught to several joggers and "run-of-the-mill" runners who find it to be very effective in helping to overcome simple running problems.

However, recent studies have shown that world class marathoners keep in touch with their bodies for signs of distress rather than dissociating as is done with meditation.[72] During dissociation one can block pain and possibly cause bodily damage. On the other hand, Benson found that subjects who meditated while exercising consumed less oxygen than when they exercised without meditation.[73] This could be of benefit.

Dyreke Spino advocates another method to reduce energy expenditure during running.[74] Since keeping the eyes fully open requires energy expenditure, Spino used semi–eye closure during the running to induce enhanced relaxation. With this method, the eyelids are relaxed until the eyes are almost closed. The individual still is able to see, but the view is one of softness and restfulness.

Bill Gordon reported on running with the eyes completely closed.[74] He stated that at the start it was "eerie" and frightening, but the feeling soon changed to exhilaration. He perceived a heightened awareness of his whole body.

With both semi– and total eye-closure methods, one must make sure that no obstacles are in the running path. There was a report on one runner who did not heed this warning and ran smack into a tree.

SUMMARY

Meditation is an excellent means to bring forth the relaxation response. If one needs constant reinforcement and encouragement, it is best to learn meditation from a center (e.g., TM), a personal instructor (e.g., Yoga; Zen; Sufi; Silva Mind Control; various other groups) or carefully programmed tapes such as those offered by CSM. However, if a person can motivate himself, he can read a book such as Benson's *The Relaxation Response* or Carrington's *Freedom in Meditation* and learn an effective technique that way. We believe that the technique presented in this chapter is an easily learned, easily applied combination of meditation and hypnosis. Meditation can also be used to complement exercise, and, as is discussed in the next chapter, it can be used with biofeedback.

REFERENCES

1. Woolfolk, R. L. Psychophysiological correlates of meditation. *Arch. Gen. Psychiat.* 32:1326–1333, 1975.
2. Bloomfield, H. H., Cain, M. P. and Jaffe, D. T. *TM* Discovering Inner Energy and Overcoming Stress.* New York: Delacorte Press, 1975.
3. Benson, H. *The Relaxation Response.* New York: William Morrow, 1975.
4. White, J. *Everything You Want to Know About TM Including How to Do It.* New York: Pocket Books, 1976.
5. Carrington, P. *Freedom in Meditation.* Garden City: Doubleday Co., Inc., 1977.
6. Randolph, G. J. Declaration on TM. Paper presented at the Symposium on Meditation Related Therapies, St. Louis, Oct. 28–29, 1977.
7. Carrington, P. New directions in meditation research. Read before the Symposium on Meditation Related Therapies, St. Louis, Oct. 28–29, 1977.
8. Green, E. and Green, A. *Beyond Biofeedback.* New York: Delacorte Press/ Seymour Lawrence, 1977.
9. Morse, D. R., Martin, J. M., Furst, M. L. and Dubin, L. L. A physiological and subjective evaluation of meditation, hypnosis and relaxation. *Psychosom. Med.* 39:304–324, 1977.
10. Morse, D. R. Use of meditative state for hypnotic induction in the practice of endodontics. *Oral Surg.* 41:664–672, 1976.
11. Coué, E. *My Method Including American Impressions.* Garden City: Doubleday, Page & Co., 1923.
12. Schwartz, G. TM relaxes some people and makes them feel better. *Psychol. Today* 7(4):39–44, 1974.
13. Morse, D. R. and Hildebrand, C. N. Case report: Use of TM in periodontal therapy. *Dent. Surv.* 52(1):36–39, 1976.
14. Morse, D. R. An exploratory study of the use of meditation alone and in combination with hypnosis in clinical dentistry. *J. Am. Soc. Psychosom. Dent. Med.* 24(4):113–120, 1977.
15. Morse, D. R. Nonsurgical endodontic therapy for a vital tooth with meditation-hypnosis as the sole anesthetic: A case report. *Am. J. Clin. Hypn.* (1979), in press.

16. Morse, D. R., Martin, J. M., Furst, M. L. and Dubin, L. L. A physiological and subjective evaluation of neutral and emotionally-charged words for meditation. *J. Am. Soc. Psychosom. Dent. Med.* 26(1-4): (1979), in press.

17. Pitts, F. N., Jr. The biochemistry of anxiety. *Sci. Am.* 220(2):69-75, 1969.

18. Brazier, M. A. B. The analysis of brain waves. *Sci. Am.* 206(6):142-153, 1962.

19. Editorial. Alpha rhythms: Back to baselines. *Science News.* 109:148, Mar. 6, 1976.

20. Chisholm, R. C., DeGood, D. E. and Hartz, M. A. Effect of alpha feedback training on occipital EEG, heart rate, and experimental reactivity to a laboratory stressor. *Psychophysiol.* 14(2):157-163, 1977.

21. Brown, B. B. *Stress and the Art of Biofeedback.* New York: Harper & Row, 1977.

22. Banquet, J. P. Spectral analysis of the EEG in meditation. *Electroenceph. Clin. Neurophysiol.* 35:143-151, 1973.

23. Glueck, B. C. and Stroebel, C. F. Biofeedback and meditation in the treatment of psychiatric illness. *Compr. Psychiat.* 16:303-321, 1975.

24. Herbert, R. and Lehmann, D. Theta bursts: An EEG pattern in normal subjects practicing the Transcendental Meditation technique. *Electroenceph. Clin. Neurophysiol.* 42:397-405, 1977.

25. Nova. "Meditation." Presented on the Public Education Television Network, Channel 12, Philadelphia, 1976.

26. Wallace, R. K. and Benson, H. The physiology of meditation. *Sci. Am.* 226: 84-90, 1972.

27. Bagchi, B. K. and Wenger, M. A. Electrophysiological correlations of some yoga exercises. *Electroenceph. Clin. Neurophysiol. Suppl.* 7:132-149, 1957.

28. Anand, B. K., Chhina, G. G. and Singh, B. B. Some aspects of EEG studies in yogis. *Electroenceph. Clin. Neurophysiol.* 13:452-456, 1961.

29. Suzi, Y. and Akutsu, K. Studies on respiration and energy-metabolism during sitting in Zazen. *Res. J. Phys. Ed.* 12:190-206, 1968.

30. Das, N. N. and Gastaut, H. Variations de l'activité electrique du cerveau, du coeur et des muscles squelettiques au cours de la meditation et de l'extase yogique. *Electroenceph. Clin. Neurophysiol. Suppl.* 6:211-219, 1957.

31. Kasamatou, A. and Hirai, T. An electroencephalographic study on Zen meditation (Zazen). *Folia Psychiat. Neurolog., Japan* 20:315-316, 1966.

32. Wallace, R. K. Physiological effects of Transcendental Meditation. *Science* 167:1751-1754, 1970.

33. Orme-Johnson, D. W. Autonomic stability and Transcendental Meditation. *Psychosom. Med.* 35:341-349, 1973.

34. Goleman, D. J. and Schwartz, G. E. Meditation as an intervention in stress reactivity. *J. Consult. Clin. Psychol.* 44:456-466, 1976.

35. Beary, J. F. and Benson, H. A simple psychophysiologic technique which elicits the hypometabolic changes of the relaxation response. *Psychosom. Med.* 36:115-120, 1974.

36. Walrath, L. C. and Hamilton, D. W. Autonomic correlates of meditation and hypnosis. *Am. J. Clin. Hypn.* 17:190-196, 1975.

37. Wallace, R. K. TM: Meditation or sleep? *Science* 193:719, 1978.
38. Pagano, R. P., Rose, R. M., Stivers, R. M. and Warrenburg, S. Sleep during Transcendental Meditation. *Science* 191:308–309, 1976.
39. Bennett, J. E. and Trinder, J. Hemispheric laterality and cognitive style associated with Transcendental Meditation. *Psychophysiol.* 14:293–296, 1977.
40. Cauthen, N. R. and Prymak, C. A. Meditation versus relaxation: An examination of the physiological effects of relaxation training and of different levels of experience with Transcendental Meditation. *J. Cons. Clin. Psychol.* 45:496–497, 1977.
41. Kanas, N. and Horowitz, M. J. Reactions of Transcendental Meditators and nonmeditators to stress films. *Arch. Gen. Psychiat.* 34:1431–1436, 1977.
42. Toomin, M. K. and Toomin, H. GSR biofeedback in psychotherapy: Some clinical observations. *Psychother. Theory Res. Practice* 12:33–38, 1975.
43. Spiegel, H. An eye-roll test for hypnotizability. *Am. J. Clin. Hypn.* 15:25–28, 1972.
44. Ornstein, R. E. *The Psychology of Consciousness.* San Francisco: W. H. Freeman, 1972.
45. Shaw, R. and Kolb, D. One-point reaction time involving meditators and nonmeditators. Cited in *The Psychobiology of Transcendental Meditation,* Los Angeles: Maharishi International University, 1973.
46. Graham, J. Auditory discrimination in meditators. Cited in *The Psychobiology of Transcendental Meditation,* Los Angeles: Maharishi International University, 1973.
47. Nidich, S., Seeman, W. and Dreskin, T. Influence of Transcendental Meditation: A replication. *J. Counsel. Psychol.* 20:565–566, 1973.
48. Shelly, M. W. The theory of happiness as it relates to Transcendental Meditation. Cited in *The Psychobiology of Transcendental Meditation,* Los Angeles: Maharishi International University, 1973.
49. Thomas, L. Notes of a biology-watcher: On Transcendental Metaworry (TMW). *N. Engl. J. Med.* 291:779–780, 1974.
50. Otis, L. S. If well-integrated but anxious, try TM. *Psychol. Today* 7(4):45–46, 1974.
51. Dudley, D. L. and Welke, E. *How to Survive Being Alive.* Garden City: Doubleday & Co., Inc., 1977.
52. Benson, H., Beary, J. F. and Carol, M. P. The relaxation response. *Psychiatry* 37(2):37–46, 1974.
53. Lazarus, A. A. Psychiatric problems precipitated by Transcendental Meditation *Psychol. Rep.* 39:601–602, 1976.
54. Akers, T. K., Tucker, D. M., Roth, R. S. and Vidiloff, J. S. Personality correlates of EEG change during meditation. *Psychol. Rep.* 40:439–442, 1977.
55. Williams, P., Francis, A. and Durham, R. Personality and meditation. *Percept. Motor Skills* 43:787–792, 1976.
56. Organ, T. W. *The Hindu Quest for the Perfection of Man.* Athens, Ohio: Ohio University Press, 1970.
57. Trimmingham, J. S. *Sufi Orders in Islam.* Oxford: Clarendon Press, 1971.

58. Schwartz, G. E., Davidson, R. J. and Goleman, D. J. Patterning of cognitive and somatic processes in the self-regulation of anxiety: Effects of meditation versus exercise. *Psychosom. Med.* 40:321–328, 1978.

59. Benson, H. Systemic hypertension and the relaxation response. *N. Engl. J. Med.* 296:1152–1156, 1977.

60. Cohen, M. C. Nonpharmacologic control of essential hypertension in man: A critical review of the experimental literature. *Psychosom. Med.* 40:294–320, 1978.

61. Daniels, L. K. The treatment of psychophysiological disorders and severe anxiety by behavior therapy, hypnosis and Transcendental Meditation. *Am. J. Clin. Hypn.* 17:267–269, 1975.

62. Honsberger, R. and Wilson, A. T. Transcendental Meditation in treating asthma. *Resp. Ther. J. Inhal. Techn.* 3:79–81, 1973.

63. Higdon, H. Can running cure mental illness? *Runner's World* 13(1):36–43, 1978.

64. Underwood, B. J. and Schulz, R. W. *Meaningfulness and Verbal Learning.* Philadelphia: J. B. Lippincott, 1960.

65. Hall, J. F. *Verbal Learning and Retention.* Philadelphia: J. B. Lippincott, 1971.

66. Benson, H. The relaxation response: physiology and applications. Read before the Symposium on Meditation Related Therapies, St. Louis, Oct. 28–29, 1977.

67. Eriksen, C. W. Perception and personality. *In* Wepman, J. M. and Heine, R. W., *Concepts of Personality.* Chicago: Aldine, 1963.

68. Morse, D. R. Overcoming "practice stress" via meditation and hypnosis. *Dent. Surv.* 53(7):32–36, 1977.

69. Morse, D. R. Variety, exercise, meditation can relieve practice stress. *Dent. Stud.* 56(3):26–29, 1977.

70. Morse, D. R. and Furst, M. L. *Stress and Relaxation: Application to Dentistry.* Springfield, Ill., Charles C. Thomas Publ., 1978.

71. Solomon, E. Running and meditation. Read before the Symposium on Meditation Related Therapies, St. Louis, Oct. 28–29, 1977.

72. Morgan, W. P. The mind of the marathoner. *Psychol. Today* 11(11):38–49, 1978.

73. Benson, H., Dryer, T. and Hartley, L. H. Decreased VO_2 consumption during exercise with elicitation of the relaxation response. *J. Human Stress* 4(2):38–42, 1978.

74. Bricklin, M. This year make time for fun. *Prevention* 30(1):32–42, 1978.

16

Biofeedback: The Art of Self-Control

They can because they think they can.*

EMOTIONAL TALK

It's "eating me up alive."
You make me "sick to my stomach."
I can't "stomach it."
I've got a "gut feeling" about that.
Oh! That "turns me inside out."
That "nauseates" me.
I don't "swallow" that line.
You're a "pain in the neck."
You give me a "headache."
Boy, that sent "chills up-and-down my spine!"
That gave me "goose bumps."
"Cold hands, warm heart."
That really "turns me on."
He is a real "warm-hearted" person.

* Vergil (70–19 B.C.).

He is cruel and "cold-blooded."
I get a "sinking feeling in the pit of my stomach."
I was "flushed with excitement."
When I saw what happened, "my heart stood still."
That gives me a "cold sweat."
He was "swollen with pride."
The mere sight of it "makes my mouth water."
I was "sweating bullets."
I was so excited, I "could hardly catch my breath."
"My nerves are frayed" from all that happened.
I was "scared stiff."

In these commonplace sayings, people talk about controlling their autonomic nervous system responses. For example, they activate the acidity in the stomach; they contract the throat muscles; they increase the sensitivity of pain receptors; they constrict their blood vessels; they release adrenaline (sympathetic response); they release acetylcholine (parasympathetic response); they slow down the heart rate; they increase the blood flow to the heart; they activate the salivary and sweat glands; they increase the respiratory rate; and they make nerve endings more receptive.

However, most often people don't take the blame themselves for doing these things. Rather they state that he/she/they/it caused it to happen to them (i.e., projection takes place). But, in reality, all these reactions are produced by ourselves and to ourselves as a result of the effect of psychological stressors upon us. For instance, the sight and smell of a particular savory food (e.g., a steak) activates the parotid, submaxillary and sublingual salivary glands in the mouth. This, in turn, causes the "drooling" reaction. After a while, merely the thought of that "mouth-watering" steak is sufficient to set the saliva in motion. All of these examples show that we can really affect our autonomic nervous system. The relationship of all this to biofeedback is now described.

THE NATURE OF BIOFEEDBACK

It was formerly believed, in the United States, that autonomic nervous system responses could not be brought under voluntary control. However, recent experiments performed in the Soviet Union[1] and later ones done in the United States by Neal Miller with rats[2] showed that autonomic nervous system responses could be brought under voluntary control. Furthermore, it was shown that this control could be selective. For example, one could slow down pulse rate while simultaneously increasing blood pressure. In light of these findings, the technique of biofeedback came into prominence.

Biofeedback is a technique that uses various procedures and instruments to teach people how to voluntarily control "involuntary" activities such as blood pressure, heart rate, brain wave production, certain muscle activity, body temperature, vasodilation (opening up of blood vessels), vasoconstriction (closing down of blood vessels) and skin resistance levels and fluctuations (control of sweat gland activity).

When one uses the relaxation response (e.g., relaxation-type self-hypnosis; meditation; progressive relaxation), there is no selectivity in the changes in the autonomic nervous system. There are usually decreases in breathing rate, pulse rate, blood pressure, muscle activity and fluctuations in skin resistance (less sweating). However, with the use of biofeedback, it is possible selectively to alter each one of these physiological responses.

As discussed in Chapter 2, reaction to stress is a function of individual makeup. Individuals may have selected areas of their body affected by stress and, therefore, come down with specific symptoms and diseases. Theoretically, then, one could selectively control different parts of his autonomic nervous system with biofeedback, so that for instance, one could reduce blood pressure, control stomach acidity or induce muscle relaxation in the scalp muscles to help control hypertension, ulcers and tension headaches, respectively.

As mentioned in Chapter 5, placebos (harmless sugar pills) may also work, as a result of the individual's belief in the purported power of the pills. For instance, if a patient received a pill that he believed to be an analgesic (pain reliever), he could in some (unknown) way affect the autonomic nervous system. He could cause an activation of the anterior pituitary gland. The activated gland could then release the morphinelike substances endorphins and enkephalins, which, in turn, could block the perception of and/or reaction to pain (see Chapter 3).* Acupuncture and hypnosis conceivably may work similarly to block pain.

Now let us return to biofeedback. There are three major features

---

* A recent study showed that placebos could actually cause the body to release endorphins and thus control pain (Fields, H. L., The brain: Secrets of the placebo, *Psychol. Today* 12(6):172, 1978).

of biofeedback control.[3] First, the physiological activity must be one that can be monitored and amplified by electronic instrumentation so that the subject can be made aware of it. The usual methods are visual (seeing a moving signal) or auditory (hearing a specific sound). Second, physiological changes must send off appropriate messages to the individual to let him know that something is occurring in his internal environment; e.g., the "sinking feeling in the gut" with stomach neurochemical activity. The third feature is that knowing a change is occurring and becoming aware of its direction by the appropriate signal, the person then tries to change the activity in the desired direction (i.e., alter the "sinking feeling" to one of calmness).

In order to change the activity, the individual employs his own particular method. For instance, he could use self-hypnosis, meditation, autogenic training or some visualization technique, or work by trial and error. The person is made aware of the alteration in physiological activity by a change in the signal. For example, one way is to attach electrodes from the biofeedback monitor to the fingertips in order to detect skin resistance levels and changes. A second connection is made to an FM radio: When the electrodes are first connected, there is only a slight hum coming from the radio. When the person is asked to increase skin resistance level (a decrease in sympathetic nervous system activity would do this), he might do so by using self-hypnosis or meditation. Without being fully aware of what was happening physiologically (i.e., no "vibes" come from the skin to tell him when he was or was not beginning to sweat), he would know that he was successful when he heard music coming from the radio. The louder the music sounded, the greater the increase in skin resistance would be. Should the music stop, then the individual would have a way of knowing—i.e., the feedback or information aspect—that he was not changing the skin resistance in the desired direction.

USES OF BIOFEEDBACK

In psychology and medicine, there are several types of biofeedback instruments, which are adapted for use with the following: heart rate and blood pressure; skin resistance (galvanic skin resistance or GSR); brain wave patterns (specifically trying to attain high levels of alpha or theta waves for deep relaxation); blood flow (to try to reduce tension or migraine headaches); and muscle activity (to attempt to decrease microvoltage output from muscles; known as electromyographic activity or EMG).[4]

In dentistry, the most popular technique is the use of EMG biofeedback.[5] The electrodes are put in a band that is placed over the patient's forehead to measure the frontalis muscle activity (see Fig. 16.1).[6] As the muscles relax, the EMG activity lessens, whereas the

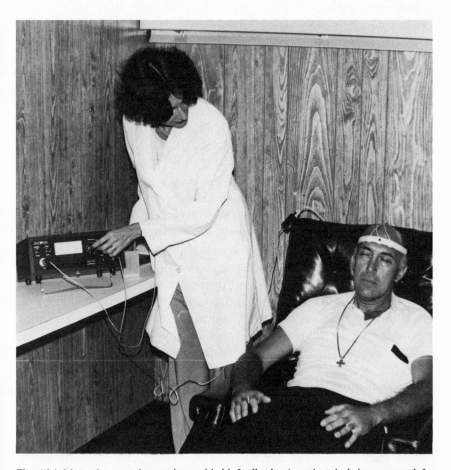

Fig. 16.1 Measuring muscle reactions with biofeedback. A patient is being prepared for biofeedback-assisted relaxation by biofeedback trainer Judith Proctor. The EMG biofeedback unit is the EMG P433, manufactured by Cyborg Corporation. The electrodes are placed in a band that is fitted over the patient's frontalis muscle. (Courtesy of Dr. Andrew Cannistraci, New York, New York).

reverse occurs with muscle contraction. Associated with these changes in muscle activity are changes that may be seen on the machine dial, and the patient hears or fails to hear an auditory beeper tone. When the patient hears the tone, he knows his muscles are contracting, and he initiates a technique to relax the muscles (e.g., meditation). If the patient hears a reduction in the tone, he knows he is relaxing the muscles, and he continues to use his particular relaxation method.

Since biofeedback is expensive and its use takes time and training, one may wonder why we use this method when meditation and self-hypnosis require no machinery and are relatively rapid. One reason is that some people cannot get as deeply relaxed with meditation and hypnosis as they can with the use of biofeedback. This was shown in a clinical study comparing biofeedback with relaxation techniques.[7] It was found that subjects using EMG biofeedback were able to attain lower levels of muscle activity than those who used relaxation methods without feedback. It may be that when subjects become aware of their level of relaxation by a direct signal, they can achieve a deeper state of relaxation than when they relax without knowing specifically how "deep" they really are.

Another possible reason to employ biofeedback is that certain people cannot or will not use meditation or hypnosis. For them, the "scientific" appearance of the biofeedback technique might be appealing so that they would attempt to use this method.

Once people become proficient in the use of biofeedback, they can respond directly to the associated body cues they receive when they are achieving deep relaxation. They can then transfer to a relaxation method without the aid of the machine.

Although it is not a form of biofeedback, there is an interesting topic that is related to biofeedback. Considering that one of the ways to manage stress is through diversion, this may be a good time for a diversion—the fascinating subject of voodoo.

There is some evidence that the damaging results from voodoo are related to control of the autonomic nervous system. That is, voodoo deaths may result from overstimulation of the parasympathetic nervous system, causing the heart rate to slow down, the body temperature to drop drastically and breathing to stop.[8] Exactly how this can be effected by sticking pins in a doll or by having one person impose his will on another is not known. But let us think about a couple of examples anyway.

If a tribal taboo is broken among the Australian aborigines, then the native committing the infraction is "cursed" by having a bone pointed at him.[9] The "boned" man apparently gets "glassy-eyed" and white with terror, his face becoming distorted. He becomes mute and may froth at the mouth. He trembles, moans and writhes piteously. In time, he crawls home, doesn't eat, gets very sick and dies. However, if a medicine man reverses the curse before death occurs, the victim returns to normal within hours.

James L. Mathis reported on a case of a contemporary "voodoo" death.[10] The involved person, as a young man, had been married twice. Each time he got married, his mother said it wouldn't last. Whether or not she influenced the outcome, both marriages ended up in divorce. With the financial help of his mother, he bought a nightclub. After 10 successful years, the man decided to sell the business. His mother was distraught and said, "Do this and something dire will happen to you."

Although the son had never previously had asthma, he soon developed a severe attack, from which he had to be hospitalized. He subsequently had many more asthmatic attacks and was constantly in and out of hospitals. After psychiatric help, in which the connection of asthma to his mother was elucidated, the man's health improved. In fact, he decided to begin another business venture, this time without his mother's aid. He called her to let her know of his decision. She was angry and repeated her threat of dire results. Within the hour, he was dead from a fatal asthma attack.

It is hoped that none of our readers will choose to learn the techniques of voodoo, but rather will stick to biofeedback.

SUMMARY

For the person who has difficulty in relaxing and doesn't know specifically how well he is doing, biofeedback is an excellent method to use. By the use of a direct signal from a machine, the individual is informed of his level of relaxation; then, with practice, he can eventually learn to reach this level without the use of the machine. Biofeedback is also effective in selective control of different aspects of the autonomic nervous system (e.g., lower heart rate at the same time that skin temperature is increased). The latter aspect is helpful in the control of various diseases such as high blood pressure, jaw disturbances and migraine and tension headaches.

Finally, for those who are influenced by "scientific" apparatus, biofeedback may be a better choice than either meditation or hypnosis. The use of biofeedback in medicine and dental treatment is covered in the next chapter.

REFERENCES

1. Ivanov-Smolensky, A. G. *Essays on the Pathophysiology of the Higher Nervous Activity According to Pavlov and His School.* Moscow: Foreign Language Publishing House, 1954.
2. Miller, N. E. and Dworkin, B. R. Effects of learning on visceral functions—Biofeedback. *N. Engl. J. Med.* 296:1274–1278, 1977.
3. Pelletier, K. R. *Mind as Healer Mind as Slayer: A Holistic Approach to Preventing Stress Disorders.* New York: Dell Publ. Co. Inc., 1977.
4. Brown, B. *Stress and the Art of Biofeedback.* New York: Harper & Row, 1977.
5. Morse, D. R. and Furst, M. L. *Stress and Relaxation: Application to Dentistry.* Springfield, Ill.: Charles C. Thomas Publ., 1978.
6. Cannistraci, A. J. A method to control bruxism: Biofeedback-assisted relaxation therapy. *J. Am. Soc. Prev. Dent.* 6(12):12–15, 1976.
7. Budyznski, T. and Stoyva, J. An electromyographic feedback technique for teaching voluntary relaxation of the masseter muscle. *J. Dent. Res.* 52:116–119, 1973.
8. Richter, C. P. On the phenomenon of sudden death in animals and man. *Psychosom. Med.* 19(3):191–198, 1957.
9. Cannon, W. B. "Voodoo" death *Psychosom. Med.* 19(3):182–190, 1957.
10. Mathis, J. L. A sophisticated version of voodoo death: Report of a case. *Psychosom. Med.* 26(2):104–107, 1964.

17

Management of Stress-Related Symptoms, Diseases and Aging

"Starve a fever and feed a cold"—or is it, "Feed a fever and starve a cold"?*

MOMMA'S MEDICAL ADVICE

1. Dress warmly, put on your boots, don't forget the umbrella, stay out of puddles, keep out of drafts, and be home by twelve!

2. Don't walk around barefoot—you'll catch yourself a death of a cold, and you'll get warts too.

3. Drink your juice—it's full of vitamins. The oatmeal is good for you—it'll coat your stomach. Chew your food slowly! Enough with the ice water!

4. Stop eating all that garbage! The problem is you eat out too much. You need more of Momma's cooking.

5. Let me give you a nice glass of warm milk with butter. It'll make you sleep better tonight.**

---

* An "old wives" saying.
** As mentioned before, this is related to the calcium and tryptophan content of the milk. Although some people recommend herbal teas, there is evidence that some types contain cancer-inducing agents (Pritikin, N. and McGrady, P. M., Jr. *The Pritikin Program for Diet & Exercise.* New York: Grosset & Dunlap, 1979).

6. Forget the alka-seltzer and the bromo-seltzer—try this chicken soup.* It's just right tonight.

7. All that running is gonna kill you. What do you want, a heart attack? You know you're not 16 anymore. Act your age! You want exercise?—take out the garbage!

8. When you go to the bathroom, remember to put paper on the seat. You don't want to catch *that* disease.

9. Stop smoking so much—you look like a chimney. And your breath stinks.

10. Brush your teeth, or you won't have any to brush. Go on, keep eating candy—your teeth will fall out.

11. Don't sit so close to the TV; you'll need glasses.

12. How can you read in the dark? Turn on some lights or you'll go blind.

13. Go out! Go out! Have a good time! Tuck in your shirt. Drive carefully. Remember, don't drink—you don't want to have a car accident. And be home by twelve!

INTRODUCTION

Probably, if we all took our mother's advice, we'd live a lot longer and be a lot healthier. There is much recent evidence that "Momma" was on the right track in many of her "do's and don't's." She believed in taking care of the whole person. The field of holistic medicine is also based on an integrated approach to symptoms and diseases. Through the use of preventive measures, psychological treatment and a "whole body" approach, many serious symptoms and diseases are either avoided, reduced in severity or successfully treated.**

These concepts are now considered. We begin with a discussion of the prevention and treatment of symptoms.

SYMPTOMS

For each of the stress-related manifestations mentioned in Chapter 4, there are specific medical treatments. The nonspecific remedies pertaining to these manifestations are discussed in this section.

---

* In a recent study it was found that chicken soup fights colds: Editorial, Hot chicken soup does fight colds, new study shows, *Med. World News* 19(14):28, July 19, 1978.

** Holistic medicine includes all three types of medical treatment. That is, allopathy (traditional medical treatment) which uses drugs and surgical procedures; homeopathy (natural healing) which uses natural methods such as herbs; and osteopathy (considered in the

Malaise

Malaise is a vague sensation of bodily discomfort that may occur with or without overt disease. Use of the relaxation response or exercise (e.g., running) can change nonserious malaise to euphoria.

Pain

Muscle-related pain is often amenable to treatment by meditation, self-hypnosis and biofeedback. Vascularly caused pain is also helped by these modalities. Exercise is an additional aid in decreasing muscle-related pain. Chronic pain from a variety of conditions has been effectively treated with hypnosis and biofeedback.[1]*

Fatigue

In Chapter 1, some terms used in physics and biology were considered (stress, strain, pressure, tension). Another term used in both these disciplines is "fatigue." The physics definition of fatigue is a weakness in metal, wood or some other material caused by prolonged stress. Biologically, there are four kinds of fatigue: (1) physical fatigue is exhaustion occurring from muscular overexertion; (2) fatigue of specific muscle units is caused by lactic acid accumulation; (3) mental fatigue is extreme mental weariness brought on by either severe mental or physical stimulation; and (4) fatigue (or exhaustion) in Selye's general adaptation syndrome (see Chapter 3) is the last stage in response to chronic unrelenting stressors.[2] The body is no longer able to adjust physiologically in the fourth type and is apt to succumb to serious or fatal disease.

The fatigue described by Selye is the most serious, and to combat it one must make every attempt to get out of the stress situation. This may not be possible. If the stressor is infection, the person is often treated with massive doses of an antibiotic and given intravenous therapy and bed rest. It is interesting that at times in order to cope with severe stress-related symptoms such as exhaustion, a

---

broader context of manipulative methods) which includes osteopathy (the professional discipline), chiropractic, acupuncture and acupressure.

* Recent findings have disclosed that natural pain-blocking substances can be produced in the brain by techniques such as electrostimulation, acupuncture and hypnosis. These substances include beta-endorphin (the "natural opiate") and l-tryptophan (the amino acid that previously had been shown to promote sleep) (Cory, C. C. Newsline: Pain: The promise of drugless pain control. *Psychol. Today* 12 (12): 26–27, 1979).

severe stressor is introduced such as shock therapy. It is almost as if the individual is shocked back into life.

For mental fatigue, the best treatment is immediately to stop the ongoing mental activity and "turn off," either listening to quiet music, watching a simple TV show or practicing the relaxation response. If mental fatigue recurs regularly, the person should work less and take more relaxation breaks.

Muscle fatigue is managed by rest of the specific muscle groups to allow for removal of the accumulated lactic acid (waste product of energy metabolism) and re-formation of muscle glycogen (a starch needed for energy). The fatigue resulting from exercise is usually a pleasant feeling, unless one is out of shape and about to collapse. With the well-trained athlete, a few hours of rest is sufficient to recharge the fatigued body. The weekend athlete may require several days of rest for complete recuperation.

Weakness

Weakness results from overexertion, being out of shape or being exposed to severe stressors such as microbial infection. It can be prevented by adequate sleep, a good diet, regular exercise and frequent relaxation breaks. Treatment of weakness includes rest, relaxation, adequate fluid and nutritional intake and moderate strength-building exercise.

Chills

One can get chills from being underclothed or from infectious diseases. Wearing warm clothing and avoiding drafts are good preventive methods (as Momma says). When one builds up his resistance, he can cope better with the infectious microbes that can cause chills. Treatment of chills includes rest, fluids and warm coverings.

Sweating

Sweating (a sympathetic nervous system response; see Chapter 3) may occur from hot weather or exercise, from taking a steam or sauna bath, from fright or as a sequel to infection.

The sweating from heat, exercise, baths or psychological stressors (e.g., fear, anxiety) can be alleviated by towel drying and relaxing in a cool place. Sweating from disease is partly relieved by cool baths, towel drying, removal of excess clothing and cool drinks.

High Fever

Body temperature rises with exercise, steam and sauna baths and infectious diseases. The nonspecific treatment is to try to cool down the body with cold baths and alcohol rubs.

Insomnia

Inability to sleep can result from mental and physical overwork, psychological stressors (e.g., worry, guilt, fear), hunger, drinking coffee and various diseases. One means of prevention is effective psychological coping during the day. (DeQuincey, said, " . . . man should forget his anger before he lies down to sleep."*)

Other preventive measures are to get regular exercise, eat balanced meals and refrain from drinking coffee at night. Treatment includes "counting sheep," meditating while lying down, self-hypnosis and drinking warm milk (as Momma says). (For a more complete discussion, refer back to Chapter 12.)**

Stomach-ache

Stomach-ache can result from psychological stressors (e.g., anxiety, worry), eating disagreeable foods, traumatic injuries and diseases. A good preventive measure is avoidance of known indigestible foods. Relaxation therapy and bed rest are helpful for treatment.

Appetite Loss

Appetite loss may be caused by psychological stressors (e.g., worry, fear, anger; "you've got me so upset I've lost my appetite"),

---

* Thomas DeQuincey (1785-1859), *Confessions of an English Opium Eater.*

** Interestingly with some rare individuals, stress causes a response opposite to insomnia, known as narcolepsy. Narcoleptics tend to fall asleep and lose bodily control (cataplexy) when confronted with stressful situations. Periodic short naps have been suggested for prevention but they tend to be ineffective. For treatment, drugs such as methylphenidate (for sleepiness) and imipramine (for cataplexy) have been used with limited success (Dement, W. C., Carskadon, M. A., GuilleMinault, C. and Zarcone, V. P., Narcolepsy. Diagnosis and treatment, *Primary Care* 3(4): 609-623, 1976).

strenuous exercise, poor body condition or diseases. With eustress mental responses, regular exercise and planned periods of relaxation, appetite generally improves. Also, the loss of appetite from strenuous exercise is usually temporary. After about an hour one can have a satisfying meal. With respect to infectious disease, once the disease is under control, the appetite generally improves.

Dizziness

Dizziness can result from psychological stressors (e.g., extreme fear, anxiety), head injuries, abruptly changing direction and diseases. When one is dizzy, he should move about slowly and cautiously, avoid sudden movements and lie down with the head lower than the legs (to increase the flow of oxygen-containing blood to the brain).

Fainting (Syncope)

Fainting (a parasympathetic nervous system response; see Chapter 3) results from lack of oxygen to the brain (cerebral anoxia). It can result from psychological stressors (e.g., apprehension at the sight of a hypodermic needle) or diseases. The person should lie down, with his legs elevated, and breathe oxygen if available. It also helps to loosen the clothes, place a cool wet compress on the head and inhale aromatic spirits of ammonia.[3]

Now that the main stress-related signs and symptoms have been covered, let us turn to a consideration of the diseases, beginning with coronary artery disease and related heart conditions.

CARDIOVASCULAR DISEASES

With cardiovascular diseases, the particular disease and the attending physician determine what specific measures should be undertaken. For prevention, the following ones seem appropriate:

1. Reduce one's intake of high-cholesterol foods such as milk, butter, eggs and beef. Some recent studies have shown increased incidence of heart attacks associated with high beef intake.[4]

2. Cut down on high sugar consumption. Studies also have shown that heart attacks are associated with increased intake of sweets.

3. Use less salt, except as a precautionary measure during activity in a hot, humid environment.

4. Stop smoking—the evidence is quite conclusive about cigarette smoking and coronary heart disease. ("Warning: The Surgeon General Has Determined That Cigarette Smoking is Dangerous to Your Health.")

5. Exercise frequently and aerobically.

6. Take regular relaxation breaks.

7. Try to avoid or evade stressors.

8. Learn to manage stressors better.

From the stress aspect, all of these things are even more important to comply with after one has had a heart attack. However, the exercise program has to be carefully monitored by a physician. Attacks of angina pectoris (pain in the chest) are often brought on by exertion. Hence, adequate periods of rest and relaxation are important for this cardiac condition.

For the prevention of hypertension, all eight of the above recommendations are applicable. For treatment of hypertension, several specific antihypertensive drugs are quite effective. One currently popular group is the beta (β)-blockers. A common β-blocker, propranolol, inhibits many of the activities of the sympathetic nervous system (which is activated during stress.)[6] Propranolol specifically blocks the endings of the noradrenaline nerve fibers. The β-blockers additionally act to inhibit palpitations. Propranolol is used in the treatment of hypertension, cardiac arrhythmias (irregular heart activity), tachycardia (rapid heart beat) and anxiety.

Herbert Benson pioneered in the use of meditation as a method to reduce blood pressure for hypertensives.[7] Since his original work, several studies have shown that various forms of meditation (TM, simple word meditation, yoga), as well as hypnosis, relaxation therapy, progressive relaxation, autogenic training and biofeedback, can lower blood pressure for hypertensives.[8] Relaxation techniques have also been shown to be of value in the treatment of cardiac arrhythmias, tachycardia and anxiety. However, the patients generally have to continue taking their medications even when these techniques are effective.

It is also known that in established cases of hypertension, the blood pressure can rise markedly in response to psychological stressors such as anger, frustration and resentment. That is why it is so important for hypertensives to learn to cope well psychologically (as discussed in Chapter 8).

MISCELLANEOUS DISEASES

For the various other stress-related diseases, there are specific medical treatments (e.g., insulin for juvenile diabetes). Nevertheless, as Hans Selye has shown, stress is the underlying cause in practically every disease.[2] Hence, all the methods of prevention and coping with stress discussed in Chapters 7–16 are appropriate to prevent the onset of a particular disease and to lessen its severity and aftereffects once the disease is present.

Certain stress-related considerations are important in particular diseases, which we shall now examine.

Asthma

Recent work has attested to the importance of psychological stressors in the development of asthma. One study showed that TM is effective in reducing severity of asthma attacks.[9] Another study showed self-hypnosis to be effective in treating asthma.[10] Thus, it would seem appropriate for an asthmatic person to have regular periods of meditation or self-hypnosis.

Diabetes

Exercise appears to be helpful in preventing the circulatory complications of diabetes.[11] However, it is essential for the diabetic person constantly to monitor his blood sugar level while exercising, to prevent serious complications.[12] Since psychological stressors can raise blood sugar, it is important for the diabetic person to cope well mentally and to have frequent relaxation breaks.

Headaches

Biofeedback and various forms of the relaxation response have been used with varying degrees of success with migraine and tension headaches. Since migraine patients tend to have attacks during periods of relaxation, meditation is not considered to be beneficial for them.[13] However, cases have been reported of successful treatment using the control methods of biofeedback and hypnosis.[14]

Ulcerative Colitis

A study of two groups of patients with colitis was reported by Adelle Davis.[15] Patients in Group A were given a controlled diet plus their usual medications. Patients in Group B were judged to have more severe colitis. They were given no specific diets and did not receive any medications. However, they received three months of regular, sympathetic psychotherapy. The results revealed more improvement, less hemorrhage, less need for surgery and fewer deaths in Group B than in Group A. Hence, this study shows that psychological consultation is beneficial in the treatment of a physical disease.

Cancer
Several uncontrolled studies and reports have shown that the mental attitude of cancer patients is very important in prognosis.[16-18] Observations showed that people who had spontaneous remissions of cancer generally could be classified as having a strong will to live; they were not depressed and had a positive outlook on life. This was contrasted to the depression and hopelessness attributed to those who succumbed to cancer.[19]

O. Carl Simonton has reported on several cases in which a mental technique was used along with conventional therapy to effect apparently complete cancer remissions.[20,21] The technique he taught included relaxation, meditation and visualization. The patients were asked to visualize their cancers as if they (the tumors) were cauliflowers or water-filled balloons. Then if the patients were undergoing radiation therapy, they were told to picture the X-rays striking and shrinking the cancerous growth. If the patients were receiving oral drugs, they were asked to visualize the medication dissolving and subsequently poisoning the cancerous cells. The patients were also asked to picture their lymphocytes (a type of white blood cell) attacking and destroying the tumor cells (see Fig. 17.1).

Simonton found that those patients who were able to visualize well and actively participated in their treatment, had successful remissions. Bright and cheerful, they had a positive outlook on life. Those

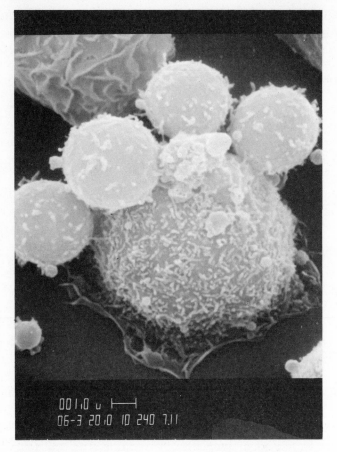

Fig. 17.1 Lymphocytes attacking a tumor cell. This scanning electron micrograph shows four T-lymphocytes attacking a malignant (cancer) cell. (Courtesy of Dr. Paul Farber, Philadelphia, Pa.).

who died tended to be uncooperative (e.g., they would not stop smoking) and had a bleak outlook on life.

Positive attitudes are important in overcoming other seemingly incurable diseases. One well-known example is that of Norman Cousins (chairman of the Editorial Board of the Saturday Review) and his conquest of the crippling disease ankylosing spondylitis.[22] Cousins self-care included massive amounts of vitamin C coupled with positive emotions such as laughter. Some 14 years after he was pronounced incurable, he is today leading a happy, active and demanding life.

Clenching, Bruxing and Myofascial Pain-Dysfunction Syndrome

These oral problems of gritting, grinding and aches of the jaw joints have been successfully treated by EMG biofeedback. These conditions are primarily caused by chronic muscle contraction of the muscles of mastication (chewing), which lend themselves to the biofeedback technique. The most important of these muscles are the masseter and the temporalis. (See Fig. 4.1.) If the patient is made aware of the contraction via a signal, he can subsequently learn to relax the muscles. Meditation and hypnosis have also been used for these conditions.[23]

Summary

Since stress is related to practically every disease, it is important that people learn to prevent and manage it. By following the suggestions given in Chapters 7–16, it is hoped that our readers will have fewer days of sickness and more days of enjoyment.

In the next section, coping with the stressors of aging is covered.

AGING*

There is a simple way to reverse aging (see end of chapter), but if that doesn't work, then heed what follows. Successfully coping with aging doesn't necessarily mean prolonging life. It does mean improving the quality of life rather than just the quantity of life (i.e., add life to years rather than only years to life).

As a person ages, he does add years, but, more important, he matures. If one really wants to worry about aging, he should start worrying as a teen-ager. It is during that time that major biological aging changes begin. But just as mental attitude is important in coping with diseases, it is of paramount importance in coping with aging. It is true that a man of 80 cannot match the physical feats of a

---

* There is one final stressful incident which is often related to aging. That is, the stress of dying. Although this book is concerned with positive ways of managing the stressors of living, we feel that we should, at least, mention that even the stress of dying can be managed positively. One helpful method, if there is time, is for the individual to place himself (or be placed) into a hypnotic trance. Then with the use of guided imagery and/or fantasy, he can take a very pleasant trip to his final resting place (Bahson, C. Guided imagery and hypnosis in the care of patients with chronic illness. Presented to the Philadelphia Society of Clinical Hypnosis, Philadelphia, May 6, 1979).

20-year-old. However, he doesn't have to—and aging changes are usually so gradual that the elderly don't even realize they are happening.

The wonderful thing is that if a person engages in certain mental and physical activities as a youth, he can continue with them thoughout his life. For example, one can enjoy running, tennis or golf as long as he lives. In fact, there are tournaments (for those who like friendly competition) for "young" 80-year-olds. Thus, you can always compete with people of your own age—so you don't have to feel inadequate.

Is it more advantageous to begin an exercise program early in life rather than in middle age or later? McCafferty and his co-workers studied the effects of physical training on the longevity of rats in an attempt to answer this question.[24] Animals that began training (running on a treadmill with an 8° incline, going at 10 m/min) before 400 days of age (i.e., younger rats) had a 74% survival rate, while nontrained sedentary rats had a 41% survival rate. Those rats that were between 450 and 600 days old when they began training (i.e., older rats) actually did worse than nontrained sedentary rats; 54% survival rate versus 83% for the controls.

Transposing these results to humans, one would be tempted to say that vigorous exercises begun in later years could be detrimental. However, in the rat experiments both young and old rats did exercises of the same severity. Most physical educators advocate decreased strenuous activities for the aged. Hence, the caution of a complete physical examination and a moderate approach for the formerly sedentary before embarking on an exercise program seems strongly indicated by these results.

If medical examination shows no abnormalities, then vigorous exercises may prove beneficial even for late starters. A recent report by investigators at San Diego State University was presented at the annual meeting of the American College of Sports Medicine.[25] Sixteen men were initially studied at the age of 45. They were put on a strenuous exercise program of one hour of exercise three times weekly at 86% of their maximum capacity. Thirteen of the men ran an average of 15 miles per week; two men combined running and swimming; and one man swam an average of six miles weekly. The men were then retested 10 years later (age 55). No deterioration in heart function was found. Their resting hearts pumped just as well as at age 45; resting blood pressure and pulse rates remained relatively constant at ages 45 and 55; an average of 18% improvement in lung function over the 10-year period was found; and all but two maintained a stable body weight.

In another study, participants at the 1975 World Masters Athletic Championships (average 50 years of age) were examined.[26] It was found that the typical Masters athlete was more fit than his contemporaries in the general population. He had less subcutaneous fat, more lean tissue, lower blood pressure, better work performance, superior aerobic power and fewer electrocardiographic abnormalities.

Life-long sedentary activities such as reading, writing, painting and collecting stamps can also prove beneficial. If one acquires a hobby early in life, it can keep him occupied and content when he retires. And sometimes hobbies such as writing and painting turn out to be financially rewarding during the retirement years.

The elderly can also maintain their interest in life by going back to school. Some have even received doctoral degrees in their eighties. "You are never too old to learn," and recent findings show you can learn well even when advanced in age.[27,28] It may take the older person a little longer, but he makes up for decreased speed by perhaps being more persistent and consistent (i.e., with experience one is more likely to maintain motivation and make fewer errors).

Geriatric scientists argue over whether the elderly should act by disengagement or activity.[28] With disengagement, the person withdraws into himself, contemplates his life, relaxes, rests and becomes a member of the "rocking-chair set." With activity, the individual actively participates in the outside world. He engages in sports, hobbies, sex, community activities and social gatherings. One study showed that active people generally had more self-esteem and a better outlook on the future.[28] The current prevailing view is that activity rather than disengagement creates the best atmosphere for older people.

In summary, we believe that the best way to cope with aging is for the individual to maintain his positive outlook and style of living. He may slow down, but he should still use those positive approaches to stress management that were discussed in Chapters 7–16. Women may find the time of retirement to be even better than earlier years, provided that they take a positive view instead of choosing depression. Many no longer have the demanding family responsibilities of home and children, and many go back to school and start new careers.*

Stress can occur to young and old alike when they have to face doctors. This is discussed in the next chapter.

REFERENCES

1. Hilgard, E. R. and Hilgard, J. R. *Hypnosis in the Relief of Pain.* Los Altos, Calif.: William Kaufmann, 1975.
2. Selye, H. *The Stress of Life,* Second Ed. New York: McGraw-Hill Book Co., 1976.
3. Morse, D. R. *Clinical Endodontology: A Comprehensive Guide to Diagnosis, Treatment and Prevention.* Springfield, Ill.: Charles C. Thomas Publ., 1974.
4. Editorial. Cutting back on meat—Probably a smart move for your heart. *Exec. Fitness Newsletter* 8(26):1–3, Dec. 17, 1977.
5. Morse, D. R. Sucrose: A common enemy. *J. Am. Soc. Prev. Dent.* 2(5):27–28, 1972.
6. Editorial. Beta-blockers in anxiety and stress. *Br. Med. J.* 2:415, 1976.
7. Benson, H. Systemic hypertension and the relaxation response. *N. Engl. J. Med.* 296:1152–1156, 1977.
8. Frumkin, K., Nathan, R. J., Prout, M. F. and Cohen, M. C. Nonpharmacologic control of essential hypertension in man: A critical review of the experimental literature. *Psychosom. Med.* 40:294–320, 1978.
9. Wilson, A. F. and Honsberger, R. The effects of Transcendental Meditation upon bronchial asthma. *Clin. Res.,* 21:278, 1973.
10. Maher-Loughnan, G. P. Hypnosis and autohypnosis for the treatment of asthma. *Int. J. Clin. Exp. Hypn.* 18:1–14, 1970.
11. Lodewick, P. A diabetic diabetologist looks at diabetes. Read before the Symposium on Diabetes, Temple University, Philadelphia, October 5, 1976.
12. Powers, P. Distance for a diabetic. *Runner's World* 11(5):10–11, 1976.
13. Dudley, D. L. and Welke, E. *How to Survive Being Alive.* Garden City: Doubleday & Co. Inc., 1977.
14. Andreychuk, T. and Skriver, C. Hypnosis and biofeedback in the treatment of migraine headache. *Int. J. Clin. Exp. Hypn.* 23:172–183, 1975.
15. Davis, A. *Let's Get Well.* New York: Harcourt, Brace and World, Inc., 1965.
16. Pelletier, K. R. *Mind as Healer Mind as Slayer: A Holistic Approach to Preventing Stress Disorders.* New York: Dell Publ. Co., Inc., 1977.
17. Arehart-Treichel, J. Can your personality kill you? *New York Magazine* 10:62–67, Nov. 28, 1977.
18. Holden, C. Cancer and the mind: How are they connected? *Science* 200:1363–1369, 1978.

*Here is that simple way to reverse aging: GNIGA. In other words, one cannot "fool Mother Nature" and the best one can do is to age gracefully.

19. LeShan, L. An emotional life-history pattern associated with neoplastic disease. *Ann. N.Y. Acad. Sci.* 125:780–793, 1966.
20. Halsell, G. Mind over cancer. *Prevention* 28(1):118–127, 1976.
21. Simonton, O. C. and Simonton, S. *Getting Well Again.* Los Angeles: J. P. Tarcher, Inc., 1978.
22. Cousins, N. What I learned from 3,000 doctors. *Prevention* 30(6):102–114, 1978.
23. Morse, D. R. and Furst, M. L. *Stress and Relaxation: Application to Dentistry.* Springfield, Ill.: Charles C. Thomas Publ., 1978.
24. McCafferty, W. B., Cosmas, A. C. and Edington, D. W. Does a "threshold age" cancel longevity hopes of exercisers? *Phys. Sportsmedicine* 3(6):70, 1975.
25. Editorial. Stopping the clock with exercise. *Phys. Sportsmedicine* 3(7):19, 1975.
26. Shephard, R. J. and Kavanagh, T. The effects of training on the aging process. *Phys. Sportsmedicine* 6(1):33–40, 1978.
27. Butler, R. N. and Lewis, M. I. *Aging and Mental Health: Positive Psychosocial Approaches.* St. Louis: C. V. Mosby Co., 1977.
28. Dibner, A. A. The psychology of normal aging. *In* Spencer, M. G. and Dorr, C. J. *Understanding Aging: A Multidisciplinary Approach.* New York: Appleton-Century-Crofts, 1975, pp. 67–90.

18

Coping with Physicians and Dentists: At the Office and in the Hospital

I'd rather have a baby than go to the dentist.*

THE SPHYGMOMANOMETER AND I**

The physical was being given on Whitehall Street in Manhattan. I started out early enough and took the IRT express at Jerome and Burnside avenues in the Bronx. But something had happened to the signal system, and the train was late in arriving downtown. I scrambled out of the station and ran for the Armed Services building.

On entering, I asked where the induction physicals were being given. The Army sergeant said it was on the third floor. I took the steps two-at-a-time and arrived panting and late. I was young and naive and a little apprehensive when the doctor put a cuff around my arm. Then he inflated it, and the pressure felt intense. I was to have this assault on my arm repeated a dozen times that day.

My psychogenic hypertension began then, 20 years ago. No one

* A fervent wish heard in dental offices every day of the week.
** By Donald R. Morse—not to be confused with Betty MacDonald's *The Egg and I*.

bothered to ask me if I had raced up the stairs. If anyone knew of the connection between exercise and elevated blood pressure readings, no one took the trouble to inform me. When the doctor gave me the bad news about my high blood pressure that first time, I sure felt anxious. And my pressure didn't go down too much for the next hour and a half.

Finally I calmed down, my pressure returned to normal, and the doctor reassured me that I didn't have heart disease. However, the die was cast, and every time for the next 20 years when I had my blood pressure taken, it was elevated. In fact, it always had to be retaken after about 15 minutes of relaxation.

Recently, I have improved. For instance, consider last year when I had my annual checkup. I arrived inside the examination room feeling "chipper." The sphygmomanometer—what a weird name for a blood pressure device—lay conspicuously displayed on a shelf. I sneaked a look at it. Then the nurse entered.

I repeated my yearly plea: "Miss Krower, let me relax for a few minutes first, or else the reading will be high." But as happens every year in that busy office, there was no time to wait, and she cheerfully replied: "It's quite all right, if it's too high, Dr. Boroden will take it again." Thirty seconds was really not enough time for me to meditate; so when I asked her the verdict, she said: "It's 158 over 80; that's all right, the bottom number's good." I thanked her and waited for the doctor.

Lately, I have devised an eyes-open meditation-hypnosis method during which I can still talk. So while the doctor was examining me for the next five minutes, I was in a trance. He then retook my blood pressure. This time it was 125 over 70. I felt better about it—but I know that for me the one stressor in a medical office that I'll always have to contend with is the blood pressure cuff. And I owe it all to my Army physical.

INTRODUCTION

Going to the dentist, physician or hospital* can create anxiety in most people. Fears are related to pain, choking, gagging, being told

* The material in this chapter applies equally to other professional offices and settings, as with osteopaths, podiatrists, optometrists, psychologists, chiropractors, clinics and nursing homes.

of having a serious disease, possible disfigurement as a result of surgery and, finally, the possibility of dying.

Whether one is going to a doctor's office or the hospital, it is of utmost importance that he have complete confidence in his doctor. If one has faith in his doctor, it is much easier to learn effective means of coping. For then, the patient doesn't have to concern himself about whether or not the procedure will be performed as well as possible.*

Finding a good physician, dentist or hospital is not easy. Unfortunately, competence or quality is not as easy to judge as the bedside or chairside manner. Most practitioners are competent, but a few are not. Those who are associated with teaching institutions and hospitals are usually well qualified. Specialists who are diplomates of their respective boards have had advanced training and have been judged by their peers to be competent.

On one's first visit to a doctor's office, he might check the walls for diplomas and see if the doctor has any additional qualifications. Is there any indication of a citation, award or special service? And one should not fail to inquire about him from friends, neighbors, other practitioners, druggists and hospitals. Finally, one should have good rapport with his doctor.

If the patient has any doubt about the suggested treatment, then he should seek another opinion. There is nothing wrong in doing this, since there is lack of consensus in medicine with respect to certain treatments. For example, it is not definitely known whether either coronary bypass surgery or the use of drugs to treat heart disease causes people to live longer.[1]

Another difference of opinion exists with respect to radical mastectomy (where breast, lymph nodes and associated tissue are removed) as opposed to simply mastectomy (breast removal only).[2] It is also believed that many tonsils and appendixes are needlessly removed.[3]

In dentistry, periodontal (gum and underlying bone) disease may be treated either surgically or conservatively depending upon the dentist and the condition.[4] The same is true for periapical disease (cysts, abscesses and areas of bone destruction at the base of the tooth root).[5]

---

* The patient is justified in his concern, since he may be the victim of iatrogenic disease—a neurotic condition (mental or physical change) induced by the diagnosis or treatment of a doctor.

Hence, it should be kept in mind that doctors are not infallible—despite the God-like image that some tend to project. In keeping with the current consumer approach to delivery of health services, it is your body, and you must take full responsibility for what is planned, how it is to be carried out and by whom.

When one is in the doctor's office, he should look around. Is the office conducive to relaxation? Is pleasant music being played? Are the magazines current? Out-of-date magazines suggest outdated practices as well as indicating lack of concern for the patient. Are the chairs comfortable? Is the equipment modern? Are office personnel friendly? All of these are important considerations if a person is to be relaxed in a doctor's office. One should never forget that he can choose whom he wants to see and whether or not he wants to enter a particular hospital. With these introductory thoughts in mind, let us now consider coping in the dental office.

AT THE DENTIST'S

Going to the dentist can create anxiety for many people. Studies have shown that blood pressure, heart rate and corticosteroid and catecholamine levels tend to become elevated in that situation.[6] Anxiety level questionnaires repeatedly show that dentistry imposes stress on a large segment of the population. The present negative image of dentistry is carried over from the frightening methods of the 1920s.

However, modern dentistry usually can be painless.[5,6] Dentists have the most effective local anesthetics available. The hypodermic needles are fine-bored and sharp, and the penetration is usually painless. In addition, the majority of dentists use topical anesthetics or pressure anesthesia to numb the gum before giving the injections.

Many dentists use other techniques to overcome fear and pain. There is nitrous oxide–oxygen relative analgesia (also known as "laughing gas"). In fact, many people look forward to going to the dentist so that they can relax with "nitrous." In other offices, intravenous sedation is used. The patient gets an injection in his arm, and soon he is in a state of tranquility and euphoria. More and more dentists are using suggestion, hypnosis, and meditation to overcome fear, induce relaxation, inhibit gagging and reduce or eliminate pain.

Other techniques employed by some dentists include audioanalgesia (i.e., the use of stereophonic music to elicit relaxation and decrease pain) and acupuncture. The author (DM) was involved in a study with acupuncture and root canal therapy.[7] Acupuncture was found to be effective for some patients, but the results were not predictable. In other studies, hypnosis and meditation were found to be reliable as well as effective.[8,9]

In addition to these techniques, many dentists prescribe sedatives (e.g., pentobarbital) and tranquilizers (e.g., Valium) to relax their patients. However, there are always side effects with drugs, therefore, they should be used sparingly and with caution.

Psychological behavior modification techniques are now being used by dentists to overcome fear.[6] Methods such as contingency management (e.g., giving a reward for good behavior) are very effective with children. However, the methods we believe are the easiest and the best to use in the dental office are the deep relaxation methods of self-hypnosis, meditation and the combined hypnosis-meditation technique discussed in Chapter 15. When one has confidence in his dentist, he merely has to close his eyes, induce the relaxation response, get his painless "Novocaine"* injection and proceed to take a pleasant, relaxing trip (see the illustration in Fig. 18.1).

The author (DM) has been involved in three clinical studies using meditation and meditation-hypnosis for patients requiring root canal therapy.[10-12] With some patients, it was possible to perform the entire root canal procedure, including removal of the "live nerve," without any anesthesia except hypnosis. The patients were completely relaxed; they didn't flinch a muscle, and they reported enjoying the procedure. Other patients only required about one-half the normal dose of "Novocaine," and they too were completely relaxed and were entirely satisfied. Therefore, regardless of whether one is a good patient or not, the method described in Chapter 15 allows a patient to have his dental work completed easily and well, while he can be on a pleasant mental trip.

This method is also of benefit to the dentist and his staff. It is much easier and more pleasant for a dentist to work on a patient when the patient's lips, tongue and cheeks are relaxed and when the patient doesn't have to get up every few minutes to rinse out his mouth (see Fig. 14.1).

---

* Although most patients and dentists refer to the local anesthetic injections as "Novocaine," this particular anesthetic is rarely used in dentistry today. Novocaine is a brand name for procaine, which was the first popular local anesthetic agent used. Within the last 15 years,

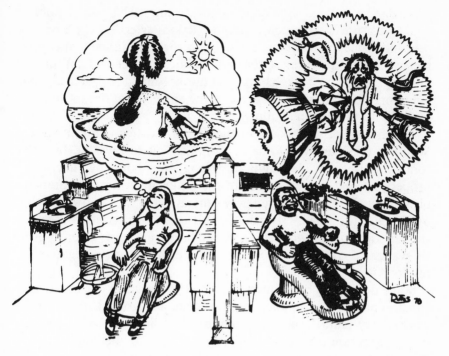

Fig. 18.1 Two views of dental treatment. Meditation is on the viewer's left; aggravation is on the viewer's right. (From Morse, D. R. and Furst, M. L., *Stress and Relaxation: Application to Dentistry,* 1978. Courtesy of Charles C Thomas, Publisher, Springfield, Illinois. Illustration by Robert "Rufus" Minor.)

Now let us go down the street to the medical doctor's office and try to cope there.

AT THE PHYSICIAN'S

Having arrived at the doctor's office, one must be ready to cope with the possible stressors present there. Throughout this book, we've emphasized the importance of preparation, which is also a key factor in the physician's office. For most people, waiting increases anxiety. And in most doctors' offices, the waiting room is just that—a place to wait.

So rather than just sit, wait and worry, one should go to the office prepared. Instead of reading an old *National Geographic* or *Life*

---

other more potent local agents have taken its place. These include Xylocaine® (a brand name for lidocaine) and Carbocaine® (a brand name for mepivicaine).

magazine, a patient should bring something of his own choice. It could be a novel, some current new fiction, science fiction or a recent magazine. Sometimes, rather than read, an individual can immerse himself in writing. Other possibilities are needlepoint, crewel, knitting, sewing or sketching. Whatever one does, actively participating in a diversion does reduce the anxiety that occurs from sitting idly in the waiting room.

Another cause of anxiety in the doctor's office is the unknown. Whether one has symptoms or not, there is always the fear that something deep inside might be wrong, might not be functioning properly. Many people adhere to the philosophy that "ignorance is bliss," but there is greater anxiety generated by "not knowing" than by "facing the facts." Hence, in this case it is better to meet the stressors by having the medical examination and tests than to avoid or evade the issue. And positive attitudes help ensure negative test results.*

Some diagnostic procedures used by the physician can create anxiety and pain. For example, rectal, vaginal and urinary tract probing can be very painful, and, as mentioned earlier, the blood pressure pumping action can create anxiety. A helpful method for these various diagnostic tests is to ask the nurse or doctor to please allow a few minutes of preparatory time. Then the person merely has to meditate or use self-hypnosis. It is amazing how much less painful is the procedure, and how much less anxious one becomes when he is deeply relaxed.

Another source of stress in all doctors' offices is financial. To reduce this stressor, the patient should ask about the fee before the examination or surgical procedure. And if possible, he should be prepared by having medical, dental or surgical insurance.

Whether surgery is performed in the doctor's office or at the hospital, it is a fear-generating procedure. As was described with respect to the word "needle" in our study at Temple University (see Chapter 1), prewarning often reduces stress.[13] Hence, if a patient is told about the anticipated surgery, the stress can usually be reduced. Even if local or spinal anesthesia is used for the surgical procedure, meditation or self-hypnosis can help relieve anxiety and allow time to "fly by."

Now let's stop off at the hospital.

* In medicine, the concern is with disease rather than with health. Hence, negative test results mean the absence of disease manifestations.

AT THE HOSPITAL

The greatest anxiety for most people occurs when they have to go to a hospital. This has been ascertained by means of stress questionnaires and studies showing that several stress-related changes occur shortly before or at the time of hospitalization.[14] These changes include higher pulse rate, increased blood pressure, more rapid platelet aggregation and elevated corticosteroid levels.

In the hospital, there are many potential stressors, including the cost of hospital care, an array of diagnostic gadgets, general anesthesia and fear of drugs, being unsure of what will be done, strange surroundings and the specter of death! The best way to avoid these stressors is to remain healthy.

If possible, alternate anesthetic methods should be considered. For instance, a woman can have natural childbirth without the risk of general anesthesia. People who require operations can learn self-hypnosis and have local or spinal anesthesia (e.g., "Novocaine") rather than general anesthesia. As a result, a shorter hospital stay and faster healing may be possible.

As mentioned with respect to the doctor, adequate medical and surgical insurance can help offset the potentially enormous financial stressors of a long hospital stay. Meditation and self-hypnosis can help reduce anxiety and lessen the pain during diagnostic tests. Just sitting or lying in a hospital bed can be deadly boring during the recovery from surgery or an illness. It can also be dangerous, since blood clots can form from inactivity.

A recent study showed that deep breathing could speed up blood flow and help prevent clots. Six hundred hospital patients recovering from surgery were instructed in deep breathing exercises.[15] Results showed that the blood flow increased by up to 33% in the patients' legs during the deep breathing sessions. Deep breathing is also an effective method of relaxation in bed.

Self-hypnosis with positive imagery can help in the recovery and also help pass the time. One could engage in useful hobbies, read or write. However, it is important not to overburden oneself. Recovery means just that, and too much mental or physical activity can interfere with the healing process.

SUMMARY

Coping with the medical and dental environment is difficult because a person is brought face to face with sickness, aging changes and death. Yet, one can learn to manage the various stressors if he practices the coping methods we have discussed. Of special importance is the use of meditation, self-hypnosis and methods of diversion such as reading and writing.

Now that the various methods of managing stress have been covered, we try to integrate them together into a unified approach, presented in Part IV.

REFERENCES

1. Editorial. Bypass: VA surgeon challenges VA study. *Med. World News* 19(7):15–16, Apr. 3, 1978.
2. Editorial. More backing for conservative treatment of breast cancer. *Med. World News* 19(14):63–64, July 10, 1978.
3. Editorial. HEW to promote second opinions on elective surgery. *Med. World News* 19(4):14, Feb. 20, 1978.
4. Schluger, S., Yuodelis, R. A. and Page, R. C. *Periodontal Disease: Basic Phenomena, Clinical Management and Occlusal and Restorative Interrelationships.* Philadelphia: Lea & Febiger, 1977.
5. Morse, D. R. *Clinical Endodontology: A Comprehensive Guide to Diagnosis, Treatment and Prevention.* Springfield, Ill.: Charles C. Thomas Publ., 1974.
6. Morse, D. R. and Furst, M. L. *Stress and Relaxation: Application to Dentistry.* Springfield, Ill.: Charles C. Thomas Publ., 1978.
7. Gross, M. A. and Morse, D. R. Acupuncture and endodontics—A review and preliminary study. *J. Endo.* 2:236–243, 1976.
8. Morse, D. R. Hypnosis in the practice of endodontics. *J. Am. Soc. Psychosom. Dent. Med.* 22(1):17–22, 1975.
9. Morse, D. R. Meditation in dentistry. *Gen. Dent.* 24(5):57–59, 1976.
10. Morse, D. R. Use of a meditative state for hypnotic induction in the practice of endodontics. *Oral Surg.* 41:664–672, 1976.
11. Morse, D. R. and Hildebrand, C. N. Case report: Use of TM in periodontal therapy. *Dent. Surv.* 52(1):36–39, 1976.
12. Morse, D. R. Nonsurgical endodontic therapy for a vital tooth with meditation-hypnosis as the sole anesthetic: A case report. *Am. J. Clin. Hypn.* (1979), in press.
13. Morse, D. R., Martin, J. M., Furst, M. L. and Dubin, L. L. A physiological and subjective evaluation of neutral and emotionally-charged words for meditation. *J. Am. Soc. Psychosom. Dent. Med.* 26(1–4): (1979), in press.
14. Volicer, B. J. Hospital stress and patient reports of pain and physical status. *J. Human Stress.* 4(2):28–37, 1978.
15. Editorial. Deep breathing: More than a sigh of relief. *Prevention* 30(6):58–62, 1978.

Part IV

Integration

Knowing about stress and how to cope with it is fine, but what is needed is a practical way to put it all together. This is covered in Part IV.

In Chapter 19, The Winning Combination, the interplay of nutritional, physical and mental factors is examined, and a concept emerges for effective management of stress.

In Chapter 20, the Personalized Assessment Stress System (PASS) is introduced. In this chapter each individual is given the opportunity to produce his own stress profile. He is also guided into ways of modifying this profile so that he can move more effectively toward the goals of health and happiness.

19

The Winning Combination

A sound mind in a sound body.*

STRESS COPING PATTERNS

A. The drive home includes a stop at the city tavern.

B. First work, then workout, then home to the wife and kids.

C. Fighting the fumes on the highway, a quick change, a run around the river, then homeward bound.

D. Leave work at five; on the bus at 5:15; the body relaxes, the eyes close, and meditation takes over till 5:40; at the house by 5:45.

E. Dinner's cooking in the oven, the table's set, and it's off to the beauty parlor for a "wash and set."

F. Today's midday break is a 50-minute session on the psychiatrist's couch.

These various stress coping patterns, which were discussed in previous chapters, can all be useful. However, many people who use

* An ancient Greek credo.

these and other coping methods tend to use only one of them and ignore the others. We've discussed stress management with many individuals and find that they often can see only their own narrow approach. Consider these examples:

1. Meditators swear by meditation for stress relief, but many of them ridicule hypnosis and especially exercise. Meditators even have vehement arguments among themselves over which method is best (e.g., TM; Yoga; Benson's relaxation response; Silva Mind Control).

2. Many runners run for relaxation and stress relief, but they often negate the benefits of meditation.

3. Weightlifters press for power, for appearance and as a stress outlet. But many of them wouldn't think of running or playing tennis.

In order to manage stress best, there must be an integrated approach. This approach is covered in the remainder of this chapter.

THE FINAL PRODUCT

Stress management begins upon awakening. The person should be aroused gradually, stretch and attend to his bathroom needs. Then a quiet spot with a comfortable chair should be chosen for an early morning meditation or self-hypnosis session. This relaxation session is important because it helps counteract any distressful reactions that may have accumulated during sleep.

A nutritional breakfast is next. Orange juice, a natural cereal with fortified skim milk and a vitamin B complex, C and E supplement is suggested (e.g., Z-BEC, StressTabs 600). If feasible, one should take public transportation to work or share the driving in a car pool.

At work, it is advantageous to have stress breaks during the day. Rather than coffee breaks, there could be meditation sessions or periods set aside in which exercises could be done. For instance, Chase Manhattan Bank has an exercise program and several businesses have "in-house" TM programs, including the GM plant in Fremont, California and Sunnydale Farms, Inc., in Brooklyn.[1] At Temple University, we are initiating daily meditation and hypnosis sessions for the students and staff. There are also well-equipped gymnasiums available during school hours, and students and staff are encouraged to use them.

Some professionals as well as blue- and white-collar workers find their jobs to be monotonous. However, the professional has certain advantages to relieve the boredom. He can alternate working hours each day, take in an associate, do part-time teaching, take continuing education courses and read the current literature during his free moments. People working in factories or offices find it more difficult to relieve the boredom.*

Some possibilities in addition to the relaxation and exercise breaks are as follows: (1) give the workers a chance to be involved in decision-making, with bonuses given for useful ideas; (2) have workers shift their activities to equivalent jobs so that they don't always do the same thing; (3) grant the workers release time to upgrade their education; and (4) let the workers have time while actively working to talk and gossip and just "let off steam," perhaps at the expense of short-term "efficiency."

These are just a few ideas. As we have said, it is important that the working day itself not be a source of continual stress. When stressors do occur, it is hoped that one can use the positive mental methods of coping that were discussed in Chapter 8 (e.g., effective action; eustress mental responses).

The housewife has stressors of her own, which very often are as bad as or worse than those of the formal working world. With dependent children, unending housework, shopping and chauffeuring, the housewife indeed has a stress-filled day. There must be stress-relief breaks built into such a day. Many means are available if there is inclination and resourcefulness. Some possibilities are as follows: meditation breaks, afternoon matinees, tennis matches, TV watching, gossip sessions, curling up with a good book, painting classes and college courses. Of course, many of these activities cost money, but if the spouse employed outside the home can have daily diversions, then the partner who must stay at home should also be provided with the means to overcome stressors. (Among the most stressed individuals of all are those who carry the double burden of homemaking and employment outside the home. Stress relief is particularly necessary for them.)

After work, either on the ride home (if someone else is driving) or

---

* A recent innovation introduced to state employees in New Jersey is called, "flexitime."[2] It permits workers to choose their own working hours within a certain framework. It has been pronounced a success and apparently will be extended.

at home, we suggest another meditation or self-hypnosis break. Kenneth Olson calls the time from arriving home until dinner begins "The Arsenic Hour."[3] It is a period when the work-stressed spouse is greeted by complaints from the wife (or husband), the children or both. At that moment, it is well nigh impossible to see the others' viewpoint, and explosions are practically inevitable. One way to avoid or evade this stressful situation is to suggest a "buffer period." During this time of relaxation, a glass of wine might be a good idea. After this interim period, the mental preparation may permit "cooler minds" to prevail.

With respect to this kind of stress situation, there was an interesting study that showed the importance of a time break before returning home. Anxiety level testing was done before and after arriving home with three groups of individuals.[4] One group stopped off at the neighborhood bar before going home. The second group went to the gym, had a work-out and shower and then went home. The third group went directly home. The results showed that those who had an interruption, either a drink or two or a work-out, had significantly lower anxiety levels than those who went right home.

This then brings us to the "why's and wherefore's" of exercise. As we see it, there are three important kinds of exercise for stress management. The first is the aerobic type. This can be either running, swimming, bicycling or engaging in an energetic game such as racketball. When one participates is an individual thing. For example, some people prefer running in the morning before work; others find later in the evening is more suitable. Still others like to ride a bike to and from work. The second important kind of exercise is the strength-building type, such as weightlifting and calisthenics. The third kind comprises those activities in which companionship is found, such as doubles tennis, golf and bowling.

Fitting a combination of these into a weekly schedule can be a problem. But if one is sufficiently motivated, it can be done despite time, work and home constraints. Although this is a personal bias, we do not like to engage in aerobic or strength-building exercises every day. We consider it better, for example, to run one day and work out with weights the next; this gives a day of rest for the different muscles involved. Also activities such as golf and tennis are ideal for the weekends. There need not be any definite pattern, but we prefer three or four days of aerobic exercise, two or three days of strength-building exercises, and possibly a complete day of rest (should replace one day set aside for strength-building). During vacations, which should be relatively frequent, there is no need to follow any strict program.

Aside from exercise, it is important for everyone to have an enjoyable hobby. Remember, a hobby is an avocation if it is done at one's leisure. Programming a hobby may transform it into just another job, and then its stress-relief purpose is lost. The same thing holds true for exercise and relaxation breaks. One should not feel so compelled or guilty that he *must* run, work out or meditate. And one should not constantly feel the need to do better; e.g., "Yesterday I ran an 8-minute mile; today I've got to beat that mark." Yes, follow a reasonable program, but if you feel in a rut, then it is all right to miss a day of exercise or a couple of meditations. In short, distress in any form should be avoided.

Eating patterns may be an important part of the "winning combination." We do not wish arbitrarily to recommend that people change their eating habits, but they should keep in mind the following points:

1. One should not eat to the point of fullness.

2. Moderation is the key. Hence, one should reduce excessive intake of animal fats (meats, milk products, eggs), sweets, salt and heavily seasoned food. On the other hand, being a fanatic about it is also not indicated—enjoy an occasional treat.

3. One should try to avoid foods with artificial additives, since some of these have been implicated as carcinogens (cancer-inducing agents). An individual should take time to read labels. Here also, one should use discretion. Actually, some additives are beneficial. For instance, natural peanuts may contain a cancer-producing agent. It is possible to add chemicals that will destroy the agent and thus permit the production of a relatively safe peanut butter.

Drinking, drug intake and smoking are addictive habits. It has been emphasized that as stress-coping methods they may be effective temporarily, but for the long term they are self-defeating. We do not have any sure-fire method of eliminating these habits, but studies have shown that when people employ meditation and self-hypnosis regularly over a period of months, they often lose their desire to drink, pop pills or smoke.[5-7]

At day's end, sleeping is the last stress-relieving method. Use of one of the various methods discussed in Chapter 12 should make for a restful night's sleep.

Beyond these various stress-coping measures to be taken at particular times, a person has to develop a stress-management philosophy to serve him as a guide. The cornerstone to this philosophy is the eustress mental approach. As Selye has emphasized, it is important to consider oneself, but not at the expense of others.[8] Earning one's neighbor's love is a major aspect of the eustress mental approach. Another key component is a positive attitude. It takes time to develop the ability to see a glass as half full rather than half empty. Such an optimistic approach to life is the key to longer life and greater happiness.

In the final chapter, the Personalized Assessment Stress System (PASS) is presented.

REFERENCES

1. Marcus, J. B. *TM* and Business: Personal and Corporate Benefits of Inner Development.* New York: McGraw-Hill Book Co., 1977.
2. Cunningham, M. It's time now for flexitime. *Philadelphia Sunday Bull.* 1B:17, Aug. 27, 1978.
3. Olson, K. *The Art of Hanging Loose in an Uptight World.* Greenwich, Conn.: Fawcett Publ. Inc., 1974.
4. Sarshik, H. Taking a stress relief break. Read before the JCC Symposium on Stress Management, Cherry Hill, N.J., Oct. 12, 1978.
5. Bloomfield, H., Cain, M. P. and Jaffe, D. T. *TM*: Discovering Inner Energy and Overcoming Stress.* New York: Delacorte Press, 1975.
6. Crasilneck, H. B. and Hall, J. A. *Clinical Hypnosis: Principles and Application.* New York: Grune & Stratton, 1975.
7. Lenox, J. R. and Bonny, H. The hypnotizability of chronic alcoholics. *Int. J. Clin. Exp. Hypn.* 24:419–425, 1976.
8. Selye, H. *Stress without Distress.* Philadelphia: J. B. Lippincott, 1974.

20

The Personalized Assessment Stress System (PASS)

As Alice walked down the path she came to a fork.
"Which road shall I take, Mr. Cheshire Cat?"
"Where are you going, Alice?," he asked.
"I don't know," she said.
"Then it doesn't make any difference," he replied.*

WHICH WAY TO GO

In Chapter 1, the reader was introduced to two possible paths: "The Stress Path of Grief, Disease and Premature Death," and "The Stress Path of Happiness, Health and Longevity." As with Alice, the fork in the road has been reached and now a decision must be made. However, unlike Alice's case, here the choice is the major concern, and how one chooses makes an important difference.

To help the reader determine "where he's at" and where he has to go to "pass," we have prepared the Personalized Assessment Stress System (PASS), which is presented in Table 20.1.

* Lewis Carrol, *Alice in Wonderland.*

Table 20.1—The Personalized Assessment Stress System (PASS)

GROUP I. Factors *Not* Within Control of Individual

1. Parents' Longevity: (See Chapter 6)

_____(0) Both parents, 75 or more at death.
_____(1) Both parents, 60–74.
_____(2) One parent, 75 or more; one before 60.
_____(3) One parent, 60–74; one before 60.
_____(4) Both parents before 60.

2. Sex: (See Chapter 2)

_____(1) Female.
_____(2) Homosexual, female.
_____(3) Male.
_____(4) Homosexual, male.

3. Age: (See Chapter 2)

_____(0) 1–12; childhood
_____(1) 21–34; getting established.
_____(2) 50–64; time of maturity.
_____(3) 13–20—the trying teens; 34–49—the midlife crisis.
_____(4) 65 and over; senior citizen.

4. Background: (See Chapter 2)

_____(0) Protestant; Caucasian.
_____(1) Catholic; Caucasian.
_____(2) Jewish, Moslem; Caucasian.
_____(3) Oriental; American Indian.
_____(4) Black American; Hispanic.

GROUP II. Factors *Partially* Within Control of Individual

5. Personality Types: (See Chapter 2)

_____(0) Internal; relaxed life style; other (no category fits): Type B.
_____(1) Negativistic; endomorph; mesomorph.
_____(2) Passive-dependent; noncompetitive; extrovert; ectomorph; masochistic.
_____(3) Introvert; external; obsessive-compulsive; asthenic; dependent-passive; narcissistic; hysterical.
_____(4) Type A; "uppers and downers"; aggressive; sociopathic; "cancer";

Table 20.1 (Cont.)

GROUP II. Factors *Partially* Within Control of Individual

5. Personality Types: (See Chapter 2)

"ulcer"; "rheumatoid arthritis"; "ulcerative colitis"; "migraine"; "depressive"; "accident-prone."

6. Principal Stress-Related Diseases: heart disease, stroke, cancer, ulcers, asthma, rheumatoid arthritis; ulcerative colitis, depression (See Chapter 4)

_____(0) Individual and parents had none of the diseases.
_____(1) Individual had none; parent(s) had one.
_____(2) Individual and parent(s) had at least one.
_____(3) Individual had at least one; parent(s) had two or more.
_____(4) Individual had at least two; parent(s) had two or more.

7. Mishaps or Accidents: (See Chapter 5)

_____(0) None in the last ten years.
_____(1) One.
_____(2) Two.
_____(3) Three to four.
_____(4) Five or more; accident-prone.

8. Negative Attitudes: (See Chapter 2)

_____(0) 0–3 negative attitudes.
_____(1) 4–8.
_____(2) 9–13.
_____(3) 14–18.
_____(4) 19–24.

9. Body Weight: (See Chapters 4 and 5)

_____(0) 1–5 lb below standard weight-height-frame values (See Table 4.4).
_____(1) (+) or (—) 5 lb from standard.
_____(2) 6–15 lb above standard.
_____(3) 16–29 lb above standard; 6–25 lb below standard.
_____(4) 30 lb or more above standard.

10. Religious Attitude: (See Chapter 2)

_____(0) Devout; belief in organized religion, personal God or fate.
_____(1) Regularly attend services.

Table 20.1 (Cont.)

GROUP II. Factors *Partially* Within Control of Individual

10. Religious Attitude: (See Chapter 2.)

_____(2) Agnostic.
_____(3) Nonbeliever (e.g., atheist).

11. Life-Change Events: (See Chapter 4)

_____(0) None within the last year.
_____(1) One "moderate" within the last year (e.g., change in residence).
_____(2) Two "moderate."
_____(3) One "severe" (e.g., death of a loved one); three or more "moderate."
_____(4) Two or more "severe."

12. Occupation: (See Chapters 2 and 4)

_____(0) "Independently wealthy"; free to engage in diversions.
_____(1) Scientist; actor; entertainer; artist; model.
_____(2) Teacher; athlete; writer; white-collar worker; salesman.
_____(3) Physician; dentist; lawyer; business executive; blue-collar worker; concert musician.
_____(4) Air traffic controller; policeman; fireman; accountant; stuntman; pilot; gambler; criminal; prisoner; unemployed.

13. Location: (See Chapters 2 and 4)

_____(0) Business and home, rural; student, rural.
_____(1) Business and home, suburbs; student, suburbs.
_____(2) Business, large city (25,000 or more); home, suburbs.
_____(3) Business and home, small city (50–250,000).
_____(4) Business and home, large city.

14. Marital Status: (See Chapter 2)

_____(0) Happily married; no questions asked; single (age 20 or less).
_____(1) Happily married; second marriage.
_____(2) Tolerable marriage.
_____(3) Single (never married); divorced; widowed.
_____(4) Twice divorced and/or widowed.

15. Chronic Stressors: e.g. guilt, anxiety, frustration, worry, noise (See Chapter 1)

Table 20.1 (Cont.)

GROUP II. Factors *Partially* Within Control of Individual

15. Chronic Stressors: e.g. guilt, anxiety, frustration, worry, noise (See Chapter 1)

_____(0) None as far as is known.
_____(1) Occasional, slight to moderate.
_____(2) Occasional, severe.
_____(3) Regular, slight to moderate.
_____(4) Regular, severe.

GROUP III. Factors Within Control of Individual

16. Alcohol: (See Chapter 5)

_____(0) None; one glass of wine per day.*
_____(1) One cocktail or two glasses of wine daily.
_____(2) Two cocktails or three glasses of wine daily.
_____(3) One-half bottle of whiskey (or other hard liquor) daily.
_____(4) Alcoholic.

17. Coffee and Other Caffeinated Products (See Chapter 5)

_____(0) None at all.
_____(1) Occasional tea or cocoa; regular decaffeinated products.
_____(2) 1-2 cups of coffee daily; 3-4 cups of tea or cocoa daily.
_____(3) 3-4 cups of coffee daily; 5-6 cups of tea or cocoa daily.
_____(4) 5 or more cups of coffee daily; 7 or more of tea or cocoa daily.

18. Drugs: (See Chapter 5)

_____(0) None of any type.
_____(1) An occasional pill.
_____(2) Take pills a couple of times a week.
_____(3) Take pills several times a week.
_____(4) Take pills daily ("hooked").

19. Smoking: (See Chapter 5)

_____(0) None at all.
_____(1) On rare occasions.
_____(2) Less than a pack a day; regular pipe or cigar user.

* A glass of beer is an acceptable substitute but it contains more calories than wine.

Table 20.1 (Cont.)

GROUP III. Factors Within Control of Individual

19. Smoking: (See Chapter 5)

_____(3) Up to two packs daily.
_____(4) Over two packs per day.

20. Eating: (See Chapters 5 and 10)

_____(0) Low fat, low sugar, low salt, no snacks, balanced diet.
_____(1) Little fat, low sugar, low salt, no snacks, balanced diet.
_____(2) Moderate fat, moderate sugar and salt, some snacks, balanced diet.
_____(3) Moderate fat, moderate sugar and salt, high snacks, unbalanced diet.
_____(4) High fat, high sugar and salt, high snacks, unbalanced diet.

21. Companionship: (See Chapter 2)

_____(0) Many friends and acquaintances.
_____(1) Many acquaintances, few friends.
_____(2) One friend, a few acquaintances.
_____(3) No friends, a few acquaintances.
_____(4) A "loner," no friends or acquantances.

22. Consultations: (See Chapter 8)

_____(0) Regularly with family, friends, professionals.
_____(1) A few times a week.
_____(2) On occasion; perhaps with a crisis.
_____(3) Rarely.
_____(4) Never.

23. Sleep: (See Chapter 12)

_____(0) 8 hours per night; no problems.
_____(1) 7–7½ or 8–8½ including daytime naps.
_____(2) 6–6½ or 8½–9 including naps.
_____(3) Over 9 including naps.
_____(4) Less than 6 total.

24. Relaxation Response: (See Chapters 13–16)

_____(0) Twice daily; meditation, self-hypnosis or biofeedback.
_____(1) Once a day.

Table 20.1 (Cont.)

GROUP III. Factors Within Control of Individual

24. Relaxation Response: (See Chapters 13–16)

_____(2) Once every other day.
_____(3) Once a week.
_____(4) Never; or more than 3 hours each day.

25. Diversions: (See Chapter 9)

_____(0) Daily, regular diversions; periodic vacations (e.g., bimonthly).
_____(1) Daily, regular diversions; occasional vacations.
_____(2) Occasional diversions; vacations, rare.
_____(3) Diversions, rare; no vacations.
_____(4) No diversions or vacations.

26. Exercise: (See Chapter 11)

_____(0) Regularly; combination of aerobics, weightlifting and collaborative (e.g., golf or doubles tennis).
_____(1) Regular aerobics; irregular others.
_____(2) Occasional all three types of exercise.
_____(3) Rarely all three types.
_____(4) Never.

27. Positive Psychological Coping: e.g., reasonable goals; eustress mental response; effective action; mental preparation; positive attitudes (See Chapter 8)

_____(0) Regularly act constructively and effectively.
_____(1) Usually cope well.
_____(2) Occasionally cope well.
_____(3) Rarely cope well.
_____(4) Never seem to be able to cope well.

TAKE THE TEST: "PASS OR FAIL"

As in the case of the risk factors for coronary heart disease (Table 4.3), the weight given to the various factors in the assessment system was not obtained by a scientifically proven method. Rather, it was an arbitrary determination, based on the best available information. At any rate, it will give the reader a guide to his stress coping ability and show him directions to take in order to improve his score.

INSTRUCTIONS FOR SCORING

There are 27 factors in the system, and the 5-point scales run from values of "0" (the best) to "4" (the worst) for each factor. The reader should take a sheet of paper and number it from 1 through 27. Then he should read the description of each factor and judge where he best fits, being as judicious as possible. The assigned value should be based on the reader's best evaluation of where he belongs on a particular factor. With some factors (e.g., occupation), the reader may find that nothing fits exactly. In those cases, he should make an educated guess about which point on the scale is personally appropriate. The point score determined from each factor should be placed next to the appropriate factor number (1–27). When all 27 factors are rated, the values are summed, and a total is obtained.

The reader should see where his total score falls according to the following ranges and thus get a rating of his coping abilities.

Excellent	Very good	Good	Average	Poor	Bad
1–18	19–36	37–54	55–72	73–90	91–107

COMPUTATION AND CONSIDERATIONS

Now that you have computed your score, if you fall in the range of good or better, you should be pleased. Not only do you seem to be dealing well with stress, but you should feel well inside, and really be enjoying life.

If your score indicates that you fall in the bad to average range, then you should seriously consider changing your life style. You're probably not feeling well and you know that changes are needed. The factors under Group I are not really within your control, but those listed under Groups II and III are things that you can do something about.

It would be helpful to those who have achieved poor scores or those who want to improve their good scores to reread those sections of the book in which the controllable factors are found. Then each of those individuals should attempt to follow the given advice. In six month's time, the test should be retaken. Not only should an improved score be made, but each person will undoubtedly feel better physically and mentally. Good luck and good health!

APPENDIX

How The Authors Cope

Those who can *do,* those who can't *teach!*

Why don't you practice what you preach?

Do as I say, not as I do!*

BREAKING THE "MORSE"CODE**

Let's look at an average day. After awakening and taking care of pressing needs, I head toward my special chair for the morning meditation. Next, I spend a few minutes in stretching exercises. After washing and brushing, it's breakfast time. A typical breakfast consists of orange juice downed with a multiple vitamin-mineral supplement, followed by cold cereal (e.g., Product 19® , bran, wheat

---

* Some oft-repeated utterances that impugn the integrity of those who tell others how to
  behave. While we do not hold ourselves up as paragons, we try to follow our own advice.
** By Donald R. Morse.

germ and raisins) drowned in fortified skim milk. Then it's off to work.

Although it's preferable to go by train, I drive because I have to stop off on the way home. The drive to work is a mix of "distress and eustress." The heavy traffic is the depressing part; listening to classical music on the car stereo adds the enjoyable component.

My primary position is as teacher in the specialized field of endodontology (root canal therapy). I help train dentists to become specialists. It is a rewarding field as I have the opportunity to counsel, lecture, do research, prepare exams, write and give and take courses. I also have a secondary occupation; that is, as an endodontist I engage in clinical practice. It works out to four days of teaching and two days per week of clinical practice.

Before arriving at my current occupational blend, I had a few other careers. After college and before entering dental school I worked as a taxicab driver in New York. That was a nerve-racking six months. I remember once crossing the intersection of 135th Street and Amsterdam Avenue as another car went through the red light. I put on my brakes, and the cab came to a screeching halt. My passenger lunged forward—in those days, we didn't know about seat belts—and as she and the car stopped, these famous words echoed from her mouth, "Oh! My back."

I pacified my passenger and got out of the cab. Fortunately, I didn't hit anyone or anything. Along with my adrenaline racing, I saw something else racing—the cab's right front wheel was heading full-speed down Amsterdam Avenue. That's right, not a flat or a blowout—but an escaped wheel! So, I calmly (?) found a phone booth and called the cab company. And for the next three hours, my passenger, I and the many curious onlookers were stuck in that busy intersection. Oh! By the way, the wheel made up for my good fortune in not hitting anything; it smacked into the window of a food store and did a nice bit of damage. That incident was my formal introduction to severe stressors.

During the summers of the five years at college and dental school I worked as a waiter. Nothing really stressful then, except I saw three customers "stuff" themselves and have heart attacks in the dining room. During other odd times, I've been employed as a soda jerk, druggist's assistant, factory worker, newspaper carrier, bellhop, chauffeur, day camp counselor, athletics teacher, frozen food salesman and day laborer.

In college, I was "into" wrestling and was captain of a national championship weightlifting team; I also played a little semipro baseball. Academically, I majored in microbiology and minored in English.

Upon completing dental school, I served in the Army at Fort Campbell, Kentucky. In those years, I was a golf and squash fanatic. I also built some office furniture, which I used in my first office. (The furniture did outlive the first office.)

That first office was a general practice in a neighborhood community in Long Island. Later I went back to school and became an endodontist. Then I disbanded my first practice and opened a new office as a specialist. After two years, I started a second specialty practice in another Long Island community, which seemed more to my liking. A short time later I got the "itch" again and went back to school for three years at night for a master's degree in microbiology (my original college major). I subsequently sold my second specialty practice and used the available time to teach microbiology part-time in New York. Two years later, I sold my first endodontic practice and, against W. C. Field's advice,* headed for Philadelphia.

While teaching and practicing in Philadelphia, I found the time to take graduate courses in such widely divergent fields as immunology, physiological psychology, figure drawing, judo, acrylic painting, creative writing, hypnosis and meditation. Fortunately my college minor in English helped in my writing endeavors.

With respect to career, I've definitely become conservative in my middle years as I've been teaching at Temple University for nine years. Athletically, for the last twelve years my main interest has been tennis, although I still lift weights. In the last three years, I've taken up running, and I swim at irregular intervals in my own peculiar style.

I consider that my various jobs, careers and interests are the result of my being a Gemini. Dr. Furst calls that pure rationalization. Although I've had great variety in my life, most of the changes have been enjoyable. Changes can induce stress—but for me, it has definitely been eustress.

This whole discussion of career changes is in itself a diversion from the narrative of my daily stress-coping strategy; so let us return to that subject. After work (either teaching or practice) I stop off at

---

* It is purported that on W. C. Fields's tombstone there is inscribed the following, "I'd rather be here than in Philadelphia."

the gym on my way home. One day I run (usually about six miles), and the next day I work out with weights (light weights, high "reps"). Generally I take a sauna and shower, and I have a once-weekly massage. Sandwiched in this schedule somewhere (usually the weekends), I find time for a couple of tennis matches.

When I arrive home, after greetings, I find that chair again and remain secluded for the second meditation. My wife and I then have a glass of wine and a leisurely dinner. We generally "eat out" once a week, go to shows frequently and take about three family vacations a year.

Although it sounds like I have very little free time, that is really not the case. The reason is that I rarely watch TV (except for an occasional sports presentation or a special). Evenings are for relaxation, conversation, reading and writing (lately it's been more of the last two). I generally sleep about seven and one-half hours per night.

I've been called a Type A and a workaholic, but I really enjoy my many pursuits. Aside from an occasional outburst, I try to "keep my cool" and see the sunny side of life. The central theme I live by is: "Seek and savor life."

IN THE "FURST" PERSON*

All my life, I've been *Furst*. There's more to name magic than one would suppose. It may be that I did well at school because of both the joking and the expectation that I would be *first*. How then could it be otherwise?

Throughout this book, the "fight-or-flight" response has been mentioned repeatedly. While it may be more heroic to fight, it might be more prudent to flee. As far I'm concerned, getting out of a stress situation is preferable to "going down with the ship." Part of my coping philosophy is in keeping with this attitude; I literally practice physical withdrawal and evasion. Generally, I let the type A's carry the flag and the burden—but I counsel them to bring their compulsive behavior under control.

To counter stressors, I also do more positive things now. For instance—since 1970, when I discovered running (influenced by Cooper's book on aerobics)—I run and run and run, and as I run I

* By Larry Furst.

meditate. I try to run six miles every other day, generally starting at 6:30 A.M. Actually, I don't like exercise in itself, and running can be boring. (At the moment, I'm trying to find out what the secret is of those who report feelings of euphoria.) But with the conditioning of running I'm ready to engage in competitive sports, during which I'm so busy trying to win that I'm getting the benefits of physical exercise. My favorite sport is tennis—I'm a weekend hacker—and I play four-wall handball or three-man basketball on occasion (at the present time I find them a bit strenuous).

Regular periods of meditation are not for me, but I do manage to close out the outside world when a stressful situation threatens. Actually, I operate well under "pressure." I have my own brand of hypnosis-meditation, which I find extremely helpful (an eclectic culling from my experiences with "touching and feeling" encounter groups). In fact, I've had most of my dental procedures done (since 1970) with a minimum of "Novocaine," and some major surgery was performed with only a local anesthetic.

I have many interests and diversions. Currently, I'm promoting a very large tennis racquet of my own invention, which is designed for a two-handed forehand as well as backhand (see Fig. A.1). Apart from the obvious advantage of greater reach, beginners or mediocre players—those of us who are aging need some advantage—find it is *fun* and physically beneficial to keep the ball in play (thus avoiding the frustration that is ordinarily experienced in missing the tennis ball).

I also make attempts at stained glass windows, picture framing, calligraphy, drawing and writing. Working with my hands seems to provide the proper balance to my intellectual pursuits. Finally, my diet is moving toward a low-fat, high-carbohydrate, little sugar and salt, little meat and high-fish, vegetable and salad approach. My staples are granola, yogurt and fruit.

My parting thought is that I have found being a tortoise isn't all that bad—being Furst—if you keep the fate of the hare in mind.

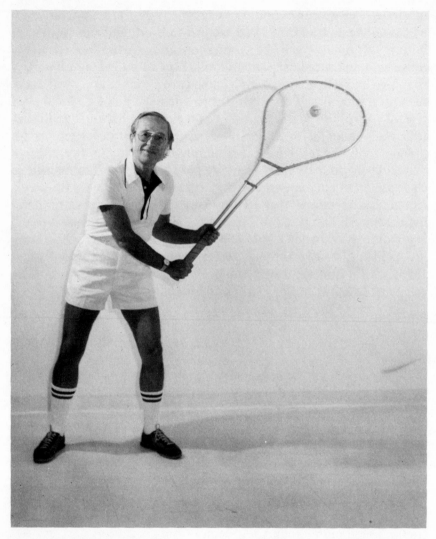

Fig. A.1 The author (MF) is seen holding a very large tennis racquet of his own invention. Yes, it's "for real"—and it's legal! More important, tennis is a diversion—combining humor, craftsmanship and exercise—which can be enjoyed for a lifetime.

Afterword

James Carney was in a depressed mood. He had just received the results of his lab tests: blood pressure was 220/140; cholesterol level was 540 mg%; the EKG indicated some heart abnormalities; and the urine test showed the presence of sugar.

When James reached home, he knew he was about to do something drastic. He took off his clothes, went into the bathroom, looked at himself in the full-length mirror—and could hardly bear the sight. James Carney had been a college football star, but like many former athletes had let himself "go to pot"—the mirror reflected what could only be described as a "fat slob."

He looked in the medicine cabinet for the sleeping pills. James knew about overdosing on barbiturates. As he was about to grab the bottle, he caught a glimpse of a moving figure from the bathroom window. James put his hand down and moved to the window. The fleeting image was that of a runner: A middle-aged man was "running for his life." James took it as a sign. Maybe this would be his last chance. And if it didn't work, he could still "fall back" on the pills.

James Carney became a runner. The first day he could barely last a quarter of a mile. But each day it got easier. Not only did the pounds begin to melt away, but James felt better mentally. Miraculously, when he went for another physical six months later, the lab tests showed marked improvement.

James was elated. He went to the sporting goods store and bought the place out: two pairs of the best running shoes, fancy sweat suits, socks, T-shirts, jocks and shorts. And everything was color-coordinated. James even bought himself an expensive chronograph so he would be able to time his daily runs.

When James got home that afternoon and undressed, he smiled at the vision in the mirror. He then donned one of his classy running outfits and headed for the park.

The next day's newspaper had a small item of little general interest: "Middle-aged runner killed by car while crossing 5th and Charles at the entrance to Woodmere Park."

The moral of this story is not that, "When your number's up, that's it," or, "It's all in the stars." Our final message is that if a person can learn to manage stress by using some of the methods outlined in this book, it all goes for naught if he doesn't look where he's going. Stress is only one of the potential hazards of life. It's great to learn how to cope—but please keep your eyes open and your ears attuned to the rest of the world.

Suggested Readings

EXERCISE

1. Anderson, J. L. and Cohen, M. *The West Point Fitness and Diet Book*. New York: Rawson Associates, 1977.
2. Cooper, K. H. *The Aerobics Way*. New York: M. Evans and Co. Inc., 1977.
3. Cureton, T. K., Jr. *Physical Fitness and Dynamic Health,* Second Ed. New York: Dial Press, 1973.
4. Fixx, J. F., *The Complete Book of Running*. New York: Random House, 1977.
5. Gallwey, T. *The Inner Game of Tennis*. New York: Random House, 1974.
6. Runner's World Editors. *The Complete Runner,* Second Ed. Mountain View Calif.: World Pubns., 1975.
7. Sheehan, G. *Running and Being*. New York: Simon & Schuster, 1978.

NUTRITION

1. Cheraskin, E., Ringsdorf, W. M. and Clark, J. W. *Diet and Disease.* Emmaus, Pa.: Rodale Books, 1968.
2. Howard, R. B. and Herbold, N. H. *Nutrition in Clinical Care.* New York: McGraw-Hill Book Co., 1978.
3. Pauling, L. *Vitamin C, the Common Cold and the Flu.* San Francisco: W. H. Freeman and Co., 1976.
4. Rosenberg, H. and Feldzamen, A. N. *The Doctor's Book of Vitamin Therapy: Megavitamins for Health.* New York: Putnam's Sons, 1974.
5. Williams, R. *Nutrition Against Disease: Environmental Prevention.* New York: Pitman, 1971.
6. Pritikin, N. and McGrady, P. M., Jr. *The Pritikin Program for Diet & Exercise.* New York: Grosset & Dunlap, 1979.

RELAXATION

1. Benson, H. *The Relaxation Response.* New York: William Morrow, 1975.
2. Bloomfield, H. H., Cain, M. P. and Jaffe, D. T. *TM*: Discovering Inner Energy and Overcoming Stress.* New York: Delacorte Press, 1975.
3. Bowers, K. S. *Hypnosis for the Seriously Curious.* Monterey, Calif.: Brooks/Cole, 1976.
4. Carrington, P. *Freedom in Meditation.* Garden City: Doubleday & Co., Inc., 1977.
5. Green, E. and Green, A. *Beyond Biofeedback.* New York: Delacorte Press/Seymour Lawrence, 1977.
6. Hilgard, E. R. and Hilgard, J. R. *Hypnosis in the Relief of Pain.* Los Altos, Calif.: William Kaufmann, 1975.
7. Luthe, W. *Autogenic Training.* New York: Grune & Stratton, 1969.
8. Marcus, J. B. *TM* and Business: Personal and Corporate Benefits of Inner Development.* New York: MacGraw-Hill Book Co., 1977.
9. White, J. *Everything You Want to Know About TM Including How to Do It.* New York: Pocket Books, 1976.

SELF-HELP

1. Dychtwald, K. *Body-Mind.* New York: Jove Publ., Inc., 1978.
2. Dyer, W. W. *Your Erroneous Zones.* New York: Funk and Wagnalls, 1976.
3. Dyer, W. W. *Pulling Your Own Strings.* New York: Thomas Y. Crowell Co., 1978.
4. Gould, R. *Transformations.* New York: Simon & Schuster, 1978.
5. Kiley, J. C. *Self-Rescue.* New York: McGraw-Hill Book Co., 1977.
6. Olson, K. *The Art of Hanging-Loose in an Uptight World.* Greenwich, Conn.: Fawcett Publ., Inc., 1974.
7. Ringer, R. J. *Looking Out for #1.* New York: Fawcett Crest Books, 1977.
8. Sheehy, G. *Passages: Predictable Crises of Adult Life.* New York: Dutton, 1976.

STRESS

1. Brown, B. *Stress and the Art of Biofeedback.* New York: Harper & Row, 1977.
2. Dudley, D. L. and Welke, E. *How to Survive Being Alive.* Garden City: Doubleday & Co., 1977.
3. Friedman, M. and Rosenman, R. H. *Type A Behavior and Your Heart.* New York: Knopf, 1974.
4. Lewis, H. R. and Lewis, M. E. *Psychosomatics: How Your Emotions Can Damage Your Health.* New York: Viking Press, 1972.
5. McCamy, J. C. and Presley, J. *Human Life Styling: Keeping Whole in the 20th Century.* New York: Harper & Row, 1975.
6. McQuade, W. and Aikman, A. *Stress: What It Is: What it Can Do to Your Health: How to Fight Back.* New York: E. P. Dutton Co., 1974.
7. Pelletier, K. R. *Mind as Healer Mind as Slayer: A Holistic Approach to Preventing Stress Disorders.* New York: Dell Publ. Co. Inc., 1977.
8. Selye, H. *The Stress of Life,* Second Ed. New York: McGraw-Hill Book Co., 1976.

9. Selye, H. *Stress Without Distress.* New York: J. B. Lippincott Co., 1974.
10. Sharpe, R. and Lewis, D. *Thrive on Stress: How to Make It Work to Your Advantage.* New York: Warner Books Inc., 1977.
11. Wolf, S. and Goodell, H. *Harold G. Wolff's Stress and Disease,* Second Ed. Springfield, Ill.: Charles C. Thomas Publ., 1968.
12. Woolfolk, R. L. and Richardson, F. C. *Stress, Sanity and Survival.* New York: Simon & Schuster, 1978.

Name Index

Abbey, M. L., 122
Adam, 3
Adams, A. K., 15, 153
Adler, A., 18, 20
Aikman, A., 121, 135, 360
Akers, T. K., 15, 153
Akutsu, K., 278, 300
Alexander, F., 79
Allen, F., 7, 8
Almog, C. H., 47, 80, 121
American Heart Association, 89, 121, 202
American Medical Joggers Association, 207
American Society for Clinical Hypnosis, 254
American Society of Psychosomatic Dentistry and Medicine, 254
Anand, B. K., 278, 300
Anderson, D. W., 198
Anderson, J. L., 217, 359
Anderson, L., 197
Anderson, T. W., 183, 197
Anderson, W. A. D., 57
Andreychuk, T., 324
Antelman, S. M., 79
Anthropometrics Heart Clinic, 211

Arehart-Treichel, J., 47, 122, 324
Arthur, R. J., 120
Aumüller, G., 34, 47

Bagchi, B. K., 278
Bahson, C., 321
Banquet, 278, 300
Barber, T. X., 261
Barmash, I., 43, 48
Barney, V. S., 216
Barzilay, J., 47, 80, 121
Bassler, T. J., 217
Beary, J. F., 279, 300, 301
Beaton, G. H., 197
Bedouins, 67
Beck, F. M., 135
Beeker, B. J., 19
Beecher, H. K., 79
Bell, B., 148
Belloc, N. B., 126, 128, 130, 134, 146, 149, 202, 216, 220, 225
Benjamin, L. S., 47
Bennett, J. E., 280, 301
Benson, H., 69, 80, 228, 237, 239, 241, 269, 270, 273, 278, 279, 288, 290, 296, 298, 300, 301, 302, 317, 324, 338, 360

Berkman, L., 44
Bernheim, 253
Biersner, R. J., 79, 123
Blackwelder, W. C., 198
Bloomfield, H. H., 241, 299, 342, 360
Bonny, H., 342
Borg, B., 228
Borland, L. R., 26
Boswell, 200
Bowers, K. S., 260, 360
Brady, J. V., 41, 48, 108, 122
Braid, J., 253
Brandt, M., 78
Brazier, M. A. B., 300
Breuer, J. 253
Brewer, H. B., Jr., 198
Bricklin, M., 180, 216, 302
Broad, W. J., 187
Brock, A. J., 49
Brosse, 277
Brown, B. B., 79, 122, 300, 310, 361
Brown, W. A., 78
Brush, E. S., 46
Budyznski, T., 310
Buonassis, V., 47
Burch, J. G., 122
Butler, R. N., 149, 325

363

Subject Index